PREGNANCY AND INFANTS: MEDICAL, PSYCHOLOGICAL AND SOCIAL ISSUES SERIES

DRUGS DURING PREGNANCY

PREGNANCY AND INFANTS: MEDICAL, PSYCHOLOGICAL AND SOCIAL ISSUES SERIES

Focus on Milk and Infants
Viroj Wiwanitkit
2009. ISBN: 978-1-60741-106-2

Infectious Pregnancy Complications
Richard N. Canfield (Editor)
2009. ISBN: 978-1-60471-038-6

Drugs During Pregnancy
Bengt Källén
2009. ISBN: 978-1-60876-154-8

PREGNANCY AND INFANTS: MEDICAL, PSYCHOLOGICAL AND SOCIAL ISSUES SERIES

DRUGS DURING PREGNANCY

BENGT KÄLLÉN

Nova Biomedical Books
New York

For permission to use material from this book please contact us:
Telephone 631-231-7269; Fax 631-231-8175
Web Site: http://www.novapublishers.com

NOTICE TO THE READER

LIBRARY OF CONGRESS CATALOGING-IN-PUBLICATION DATA

Källén, Bengt.
Drugs during pregnancy / Bengt Källén.
p. ; cm.
Includes bibliographical references and index.
ISBN 978-1-60876-154-8 (hardcover)
1. Fetus--Effect of drugs on. 2. Pregnant women--Drug use. I. Title.
[DNLM: 1. Pregnancy--drug effects. 2. Abnormalities, Drug-Induced--etiology. 3. Drug Therapy--contraindications. 4. Pharmaceutical Preparations--adverse effects. WQ 200 K14d 2009]
RG627.6.D79K35 2009
618.3'2--dc22

2009029265

Published by Nova Science Publishers, Inc. ✦ New York

CONTENTS

PREFACE

There are many scientific articles on the possible association between maternal drug use during pregnancy and risks for the unborn child and also many books which summarize this literature in a more or less critical way. My interest in the subject was raised in the early 1960s when the thalidomide catastrophe happened and caused the birth of about 130 severely malformed infants in Sweden. The scientific society and the administrative agencies were mainly unprepared for this event and the Swedish National Board of Health (at that time called Medicinalstyrelsen) was no exception. I was called to a meeting to discuss possible actions to be taken in order to protect the public from a similar disaster. At this discussion, I suggested that a surveillance register should be set up so if a new similar event occurred it should be detected rapidly and actions could be taken. This was done and together with a colleague, Jan Winberg, we got the task to arrange and run such a register with a beginning in 1964, not the first in the world but one of the early ones. We realized, however, that such a surveillance register could only detect a situation similar to that with thalidomide – a marked increase in the risk of a previously rare malformation or combination of malformations. There was a need for epidemiological analyses in order to detect less obvious statistical associations between maternal drug use and infant malformations. One way to get such material was to run a prospective recording of drug use during pregnancy and together with another colleague, Stig Kullander, we tried this in the early 1960s in one Swedish medium-sized city, Malmö, close to the university where I worked as a professor in embryology. It was a tough undertaking, notably considering the primitive computer possibilities which existed at that time. The number of pregnancies we could follow was limited, only a little more than 5000, a couple of papers were produced, some of which are still quoted in the literature. Such a small study had of course a low statistical power and I started to dream about a nation-wide recording of maternal drug use. In the meantime, the classical book from the Collaborative Perinatal Project in US was published, describing drug use and malformations in more than 55 000 pregnancies, a ten times larger material than ours. This book is still valuable but of course out-dated considering the arrival of many new drugs since that study was made. Perhaps the present book can supplement it.

In 1973, the Swedish Medical Birth Register was started but initially was concentrated on perinatal problems. In 1982, data content was increased to deal also with maternal characteristics but my efforts to include also information on drug use were not successful until in 1994 when it became possible to do so, partly because of the advancement of computer technology. With this, a possibility to get a nation-wide recording of maternal drug use opened up and my old dream came true. After a couple of years, enough data were collected to permit analysis of at least rather common drugs and a long series of scientific articles have been published, based on data from the register.

Now, data for more than a dozen years are available and every year data on another 100 000 deliveries are added. For a couple of years I have been thinking of writing this book which will summarize all available data (nearly) up to and including 2006 and when I got an offer from the publisher, I decided to try. My thought is that the data presented (and the conclusions I have dared to draw) can be of help for people interested in the scientific issue of drugs during pregnancy, but also for administrative agencies and for interested clinicians.

There is no ideal way to attack these problems and I have tried to underline methodological problems and uncertainties in conclusions drawn from such data. Furthermore, the data are of course limited to drugs used in Sweden and for many such drugs usage during pregnancy is low and therefore data are scanty. A typical example is illegal drug use which is certainly heavily underreported.

The analyses I have made have followed a basic pattern with some modifications. Data are there, however, and refined or different analyses can be made *ad hoc*.

The studies could not have been made without the co-operation of the Swedish National Board of Health and Welfare and the Swedish Medical Drug Agency for which I am thankful. Also thanks to my eldest son, Anders Källén, and my old friend Elisabeth Robert-Gnansia for valuable comments. The studies were made possible by grants from Evy and Gunnar Sandberg Foundation, Sweden.

Lund, April 2009

Bengt Källén
Professor Emeritus in Embryology, University of Lund, Sweden

ABBREVIATIONS USED

ACE	acetylcholine esterase
ASD	atrium septum defect
ATC	Anatomical, Therapeutic,Chemical classification of drugs
BMI	body mass index
CNS	central nervous system
CoA	coarctatio of aorta
END	early neonatal death (<7 days)
FV1	document from delivery
FV2	document from paediatric examination of newborn
IBD	immunological bowel disease
ICD	International Classification of Diseases and Injuries
HBRA	hypnotic bensodiazepine receptor agonists
HDC	high density cholesterol
HELLP	haemolytic anemia, elevated liver ensymes, low platelet count
LDC	low density cholesterol
LGA	large for gestational age
LMP	last menstrual period
MHV1	first document from antenatal care clinic
MHV2	second document from antenatal care clinic
NSAID	non-steroid antiinflammatory drug
NTD	neural tube defect
OR	odds ratio
OTC	over the counter drugs
PDA	patent ductus arteriosus
PPHN	persistent pulmonary hypertension of the newborn
RR	risk ratio
SB	stillbirth
SD	standard deviation
SGA	small for gestational age
SNRI	serotonin and noradrenalin reuptake inhibitor
SSRI	selective serotonin reuptake inhibitor
SUA	single umbilical artery
TGV	transposition of great vessels
TIS	teratology information system
VATER	"syndrome" of congenital malformations with vertebral, anal, tracheo-oesophageal, and limb reduction defects.
VSD	ventricular septum defect

Chapter 1

A Short History of the Study of Maternal Drug use and Delivery Outcome

Up to the end of the 1950s, little attention was paid to the possibility that maternal use of drugs could harm the developing embryo or foetus. In a review by Joseph Warkany [1] two types of drugs were discussed: antimetabolites and the masculinising effect of some gestagens. It was generally thought that, with these exceptions, drugs could without risk be used during pregnancy. It was well known that in animal experiments, teratogenic effects could be found but usually only in dosages which far exceeded those used in clinical practice.

Everything was changed with the appearance of thalidomide, an apparently non-toxic sleeping drug which was put on the market in Germany in 1957 as an over-the-counter drug. In 1961, a cluster of cases was described consisting of severe limb reduction defects [2] and in December the same year two publications [3,4] identified the cause: that the mothers of the children had used thalidomide during early pregnancy. Many thousands of children were damaged by this drug worldwide until it was withdrawn from the market (even though it has been used and is still used under very special circumstances).

After the thalidomide catastrophe, many efforts were made to reduce the risk for the introduction of a drug with a strong teratogenic effect by compulsory laboratory testing on pregnant animals. The efficacy of animal experiments to identify a possible human teratogenicity is not very high and teratogenic drugs may still come into clinical use in spite of extensive animal tests. Furthermore, many drugs which have been used for a long time have never been thoroughly tested. It has therefore always been thought necessary to follow-up the possible results of drug use by pregnant women.

Various methodologies have been used. A relatively recent methodological discussion is available [5]. Only a short summary will be given here:

The Alert Clinician

Clinical observation and case descriptions have seldom resulted in the identification of drugs with teratogenic properties in the human. Except thalidomide just mentioned, some examples can be given: the association between anticonvulsants and infant orofacial clefts [6] and between valproic acid and spina bifida [7]. In order to detect an association this way it is usually necessary that the drug has a strong teratogenic effect and that the outcome is unusual. Formal epidemiological studies are more effective in investigations of effects of moderate strength and on relatively common outcomes.

Epidemiological Studies

Such studies can be made in different ways. Basically, one wants to compare the occurrence of specific outcomes after specific exposures. One therefore counts the number of exposed outcomes (cases) and, one way or another, compares it with the expected number of cases under the null hypothesis that no association between outcome and exposure exists. The expected number can be estimated from the total population under the assumption that all individuals have been characterized both according to outcome and exposure. If such data are not available, one can make similar estimates from a sample of the population. If the outcome rate and the exposure rate in the population are not known, they can be estimated from representative samples drawn from the total population. In *case-control* studies (case-referent studies) one compares exposure rate among cases with exposure rate in a sample from the population (controls or referents). With this design, one can use the same material of cases and study many different exposures, for example, look for an excess of exposure for a number of different drugs among cases consisting of infants with a certain malformation. In *cohort* studies instead, the outcome in exposed infants is compared with the expected outcome calculated from non-exposed infants. In this design, many different outcomes (e.g., different types of congenital malformations) can be studied after a defined exposure.

If data are available for all individuals in a population, both types of analyses can of course be made on the same material. If one is only interested in one specific outcome and one exposure, the expected number of exposed outcomes will be the same if you calculate it from the exposure rate among controls or from the outcome rate among non-exposed individuals.

Data for a whole population is sometimes available by record linkage between registers of delivery outcome and of prescriptions when the two data sets can be linked, for instance by the use of individual identification numbers [8-10]. In other studies, such data were obtained by interviews of all pregnant women. The first large such study [11] was performed as part of the Collaborative Perinatal Project which collected information from 12 American hospitals in 1958-1965 on about 55 000 pregnancies, a still useful information source, notably for older drugs. Other small similar studies exist but their number of interviewed individuals is usually small and they therefore have a low statistical power to detect anything but very strong effects. The data presented in this book were collected from a medical birth register which covers practically all births in Sweden and which is supplemented with data from other health registers.

All analyses of data necessitate as unbiased information as possible, both on outcome and on exposure. Case-control studies are usually made retrospectively, after the birth of the damaged infant, and therefore carry a risk for recall or interviewer bias and often also a significant non-response rate. In the Hungarian case-control study, a mixture of prospective and retrospective information is used and the studies are based on all identified malformed infants in Hungary during 1980-1996 [12] and selected controls. Cohort studies are usually based on prospective recording of drug use while outcome data often are obtained by interviews or in other ways some time after the birth of the infant.

In both designs, a bias can easily be obtained from non-responders, notably when the rate of non-responders is high.

In the final analysis of data, it is important to consider the possibility that women using a specific drug have characteristics which by themselves influence the outcome. If a factor co-varies with both exposure and outcome it is called a *confounder* and if adjustment is not made for it, false results can be obtained. Maternal use of sedatives increases with age and so does the risk for having an infant with Down syndrome. Without adjustment for maternal age in the analysis, an association between the use of sedatives and the birth of infants with Down syndrome appears but it is only secondary to the age factor and disappears if adjustment for age is made.

In later chapters I will describe in more detail the background to the studies reviewed in this book and list the pros and cons of the approach.

REFERENCES

[1] Warkany J. Environmental teratogenic factors. In: Fishbein M (ed): *First International Conference on Congenital Malformations.* Lippincott, Philadelphia and Montreal, pp 99-105.

[2] Wiedemann H-R. Hinwise auf eine derzeitige Haufung hypo- und aplastischer Fehlbildungen der Gliedmassen. *Med Welt* 1961; 37: 1863-1866.

[3] Lenz W. Kindliche Misbildungen nach Medikament-Einnahme während der Gravidität? *Dtsch Med Wochenschr* 1961; 86:2555-2556.

[4] McBride WG. Thalidomide and congenital abnormalities. *Lancet* 1961; 2: 1358.

[5] Källén B. Methodological issues in the epidemiological study of teratogenicity of drugs. *Congen Anomal* 2005; 45: 44-51.

[6] Meadow SR. Congenital abnormalities and anticonvulsant drugs. *Proc Roy Soc Med* 1968; 63: 12-49.

[7] Robert E, Guibaud P. Maternal valproic acid and congenital neural tube defects. *Lancet* 1982; 2: 937.

[8] Sørensen HT, Steffensen FH, Olesen C, Nielsen GL, Pedersen L. Pregnancy outcome in women exposed to calcium channel blockers. *Reprod Toxicol* 1998; 12: 383-384.

[9] Rosa F. Databases in the assessment of the effects of drugs during pregnancy. *J Allergy Clin Immunol* 1999; 103: S360-361.

[10] Oberlander TF, Warburton W, Misri S, Ahgajanian J, Hertzman C. Neonatal oucomes after prenatal exposure to selective serotonin reuptake inhibitor antidepressants and maternal depression using population-based linked health data. *Arch Gen Psychiatry* 2006; 63: 898-906.

[11] Heinonen OP, Slone D, Monson RR, Hook EB, Shapiro S. *Birth Defects and Drugs in Pregnancy.* Publishing Sciences Group, Inc., Littleton, Mass.

[12] Bártfai Z, Kocsis J, Puhó EH, Czeizel AE. A population-based case-control teratologic study of promethazine use during pregnancy. *Reprod Toxicol* 2008; 25: 276-285.

Chapter 2

THE PRACTICAL CONSEQUENCES OF DRUG EFFECTS ON DELIVERY OUTCOME

Epidemiological or other studies may be able to identify risks associated with drug exposure during pregnancy. The significance and meaning of such risk estimates varies with the situation when an evaluation of the risk is needed. One then has to distinguish between the *individual risk* and the *attributive risk*, associated with a specific exposure. The *individual risk* tells how large the risk is that the infant is damaged if the mother has used the drug during pregnancy. The *attributive risk* tells to what extent use of the drug would contribute to the total number of damaged infants in the population.

A drug may have a rather strong teratogenicity and a high individual risk (e.g., Accutane) but only few exposures will occur in the population if the drug is handled with great care, and therefore only few infants will be damaged by the drug. If, on the other hand, the pregnant woman has used the drug, the individual risk is so large that it may be wise to consider a termination of the pregnancy.

Another drug or other agent may have a relatively low risk to cause damage but is widely used, a good example is maternal smoking which carries a moderate risk for effects on foetal growth and survival and a weak effect on the risk for a congenital malformation. The latter may be so low that for the individual it plays no role, but if the exposure is common it will cause many damaged infants in the population.

1. INTRODUCTION OF A NEW DRUG INTO A MARKET

When a new drug is introduced on the market, preclinical tests have nowadays been made in order to identify possibly risks connected with its use during pregnancy. Even if tests have shown no ill effects in animals, there may still be a risk when humans are using it – species variations in response are well known. If the drug has not been used on another market, little or no experience of its use during pregnancy usually exists. At the clinical work up of the drug, exposures of pregnant women are avoided if the drug is not to be specifically used in pregnant women. As in this situation both the individual and attributive risks are of interest, even moderate ill effects must be weighted against the significance of the new drug in comparison with what is already available on the market. If, for instance, the alleged association between paroxetine and infant cardiac defects is true and paroxetine is to be launched on a new market, it would seem prudent to avoid introducing paroxetine when there are a number of other SSRI drugs which probably lack an effect on cardiac development.

2. A Woman has used the Drug in Early Pregnancy

A common situation is that a woman becomes pregnant and knows she has used some drug during the organogenetic period. She is often concerned over this and may consider terminating her pregnancy because of the possible risk to have damaged her embryo. In this situation, only the individual risk is of interest: how large is the probability that the embryo will be damaged and what results are expected? Every pregnant woman runs the risk that her child gets malformed, the question is if the use of the drug has increased this probability in a noticeable way and if the damage is of clinical significance for the child when born. If we suppose that the general risk for a child to be born with a relatively severe malformation is around 3-4%, even a 50% risk increase means that the absolute risk is only 4.5-6%. If the risk for a spina bifida is increased 10 times after a specific drug use, it is still low and would not motivate a termination of the pregnancy – but well an intense search for a neural tube defect using prenatal diagnosis. The greatest problems arise when one is dealing with a drug when no or very little epidemiological data are available. If pregnancy outcome among, say, 100 women who had used the drug appeared normal, it is still possible that the drug is teratogenic but the individual risk must be rather low and it seems unnecessary to discuss the possibility of pregnancy termination. For this type of data, the materials from teratology information organizations (TIS) have proved rather effective. – My rule of thumb is that if I cannot tell the patient roughly how high the risk for a malformation is and what type of malformation is caused by the drug, there is no reason to discuss a termination of pregnancy. If moderate risks exist, their significance for the individual patient must be taken into consideration.

3. To Prescribe a Drug to a Pregnant Woman

In this situation both the individual and attributive risk is of importance. If a certain drug is often prescribed to pregnant women and carries a risk for the embryo or foetus, even a small risk increase will be of importance, even though perhaps of little practical interest for the individual woman. This situation is relatively rare in early pregnancy, when malformations can arise. First, the prescribing doctor – and perhaps even the woman – may be unaware of the pregnancy. Second, in many instances it is possible to postpone drug use until the organogenetic period is over. When the situation necessitates drug treatment in early pregnancy, drugs where data on teratogenicity exist and the risk seems to be low should be chosen among alternative drugs, if such are available. An example: even though the possible association between the use of paroxetine and the origin of mild cardiac defects is still under debate, it may be wise to avoid paroxetine and replace it with another SSRI if a woman, still in the first trimester, needs an antidepressant. During the later part of the pregnancy, the use of drugs with harmful effects should when possible be avoided. If we take the example with SSRI, it is known that use of such drugs in late pregnancy may affect the newborn infant in a negative way – this short-term effect must be weighted against the woman's need for treatment of a depression or anxiety, conditions which may, if untreated, threaten the life and well-being of the woman and perhaps in themselves may be harmful for the foetus.

4. A Malformed Infant was Born and the Mother Remembers having taken a Specific Drug. A Causal Effect?

Many women have used some drugs in early pregnancy, many infants are born with congenital malformations. The random association of these two phenomena will be quite common and often causes concern. The parents who have had a damaged child seek an explanation to their misfortune. A rather small proportion of such parents can get a simple and straight-forward explanation, e.g., heredity, the other parents and their doctors try to find an explanation and the use of drugs in early pregnancy is a common alternative. If the drug-malformation association is known from the scientific literature, the situation is simple and the parents can get an adequate explanation. It should be remembered, however, that if the risk increase of malformation A after maternal use of drug B is less than 2, in the individual case there is still a larger probability that no causality exists in the individual case than that it exists. If the risk increase is 5 times, for instance, there is a high probability that the drug actually caused the malformation in the individual case. If no association is known between the drug use and the origin of the malformation in question, causality may still exist but it is also possible that it is just a case of a random association as mentioned above. Such an individual case cannot be interpreted but may be of significance for the identification of a previously unknown relationship. Especially when one is dealing with a relatively rare drug and a relatively rare malformation, the association may seem impressive – but it could still be random. Such associations should, however, be reported as adverse drug reactions. If a number of such associations between the same drug and the same anomaly appear, this may be a sensitive way to detect a rare teratogenic effect of a drug. It is important to realize, that one cannot evaluate the probability for a causal association just from the frequency of the malformation and the frequency of the drug use. When an association has occurred, it is not possible to calculated how likely it is random. There are many unusual drugs and many unusual outcomes which can coincide and some will occur by chance. The analysis of the rate of exposure and the rate of outcome can estimate how likely one exposed infant is to have this outcome before the outcome has occurred – not after it has occurred.

According to my experience, one has to be very careful when discussing these matters with the parents. If they get the impression that a causality may exist when it is uncertain, this may give problems. One possibility is that they engage in legal activities which have small chances to result in anything. Another is that the woman may blame herself for having taken those tablets and thereby damaging her baby, a trauma which may be devastating for her and her relationship with the child.

Chapter 3

THE SWEDISH HEALTH REGISTERS USED AND VARIABLES STUDIED

The main register used is the Swedish Medical Birth Register. This register was started in 1973 and contains data on the pregnant women, the deliveries, and the neonatal conditions in all Sweden. Since 1982, the register is based on copies of standardized medical records, identical in all parts of Sweden. When the medical records are completed, copies are produced which after delivery are collected and sent to the National Board of Health and Welfare for computerization. During the last few years data are also transferred as computer files.

THE FOLLOWING RECORDS ARE INCLUDED:

MHV1

A form used at the first visit to the antenatal care system, which is free of charge and is used by practically all women who will give birth. The first visit usually occurs between weeks 8 and 12 and 90% of all attendance will occur during the first trimester This form summarizes data obtained from a midwife interview with the pregnant woman, which usually takes half an hour or more. All such data are not computerized, thus, for instance, information on alcohol use is regarded as so unreliable that it is not included. Information of drug use during pregnancy, based on the midwife interviews, was collected from July 1, 1994 onwards.

MHV2

One or more forms used during the following antenatal care. Information on prescribed drugs during pregnancy is recorded with a beginning in 1994.

FV1

A form for data on delivery – in case of multiple births, each infant will have its own form.

FV2

A form for the examination of the newborn. All liveborn infants and many stillbirths are examined by a paediatrician. If the infant is transferred to a neonatal unit, the discharge diagnoses should be given in this form.

Each year, 90-110 000 births occur in Sweden. All copies are not forwarded to the National Board of Health and Welfare. In order to be included in the Medical Birth Register, at least the delivery form has to be present. A few per cent of all deliveries are completely missing in the register. The forms from the antenatal care centres are missing in around 4.7%. As information on drug use was obtained from the antenatal care forms, all records with totally missing antenatal care information were excluded from the analyses shown in this book.

THE FOLLOWING DATA WERE USED

Year of Delivery

The study is restricted to the eleven year period 1996-2006.

Maternal Age

Calculated from the date of birth of the woman and the date of delivery. Woman's date of birth enters her personal identification number, a number which every person living in Sweden gets. Participation in the Medical Birth Register is compulsory but a few women refuse to have their id. numbers recorded and maternal age will then be unknown. Such deliveries will be included in the study but in all analyses where adjustments for maternal age are performed, women with unknown age will be excluded. Maternal age will be grouped in 5-year groups: <20, 20-24, etc. with ≥45 as one group.

Parity

With parity will be meant the parity after delivery – thus, a woman who has her first child will be said to be of parity 1. Information on parity is linked from the official birth register of Statistic Sweden. When the woman's id.number is missing or incomplete, the parity information is instead taken from the MHV1 form as the sum of previously born infants +1. Parity is grouped as 1, 2, 3, ≥4.

Smoking in Early Pregnancy

This information is obtained from MHV1 and is based on midwife interview. Data are grouped as unknown, none, <10 cigarettes/day, and ≥10 cigarettes per day.

Number of Previous Miscarriages

Data from MHV1 and based on midwife interviews. Grouped as none, 1, 2, ≥3.

Body Mass Index (BMI)

Information of woman's weight is obtained from MHV1 and is either based on stated pre-pregnancy weight or actual weighing at the first antenatal visit. As this occurs very early in pregnancy, little difference is seen. Woman's height is also obtained from MHV1 and the BMI is calculated as weight/(height^2) where weight is expressed in kg and height in m. As a normal BMI is regarded 19.8-25.9. In most instances BMI is grouped as unknown, <19.8, 19.8-25.9, and ≥26.

Country of Birth

Race or ethnicity must not be registered in Sweden. Country of birth for the woman is, however, available and obtained by linkage with the birth register of Statistics Sweden. If the woman's id. number is missing or incomplete, such linkage cannot be made. In the analyses, three groups are used: born in Sweden, in another Nordic country, and born in a Non-Nordic country. Most of the latter women were born outside Europe.

Family Situation

As marriage is nowadays a poor description of family situation, four groups are used instead: unknown, co-habiting, living alone, and living in other circumstances. Information is obtained from MHV1, based on midwife interviews in early pregnancy.

Work Outside Home

Also this information is based on MHV1 and midwife interview. Grouped as unknown, full-time work, part-time work, and no work outside home.

Maternal Education

Maternal level of education is linked from a national education register (Statistics Sweden). Such linkage was made in 2002 and gave education level for women who gave birth up to and including 2001. Since then no further linkage has been made. The education information concerns the situation in 2002, thus the woman's "final" education, not necessarily the education when she was pregnant. These data can thus only give an idea of the education level for women who gave birth during the period 1996-2001 and cannot be used for adjustments for the total material. Grouped as unknown, <12 years, 12 years, 13-14 years, and ≥14 years.

Maternal Drug Use

Drugs reported at the first antenatal visit, based on midwife interviews, and drugs prescribed by the antenatal care during pregnancy are included and stored separately. Drugs are coded as ATC codes when possible – if not possible, the drug name is given in clear text. Information on dosage and exact timing of drug use in early pregnancy is often incomplete or missing or stated in such an unspecific way that it cannot be used, e.g., "when needed". For drugs prescribed during pregnancy, usually both dosage and pregnancy weeks when used are available.

Multiple Births

Number of infants in birth.

Maternal Delivery Diagnoses

Up to 12 delivery diagnoses can be given and are coded as ICD codes. Up to 1997, ICD-9 was used, after that ICD-10. The transition between ICDs used occurred gradually during 1997. Among the diagnoses, the following ones were routinely analysed (Table 3:1):

Table 3.1. List of pregnancy diagnoses which are routinely analysed and the ICD codes used to identify the conditions

Diagnosis	ICD-9 codes	ICD-10 codes
Pre-existing diabetes	250, 648.0	E10, O24.0-24.3
Gestational diabetes	648.8	O24.4
Chronic hypertension	642.0-642.2	O11 or O12
Pre-eclampsia	642.4-642.7	O13-O15
Hyperemesis	643	O21
Placenta previa:	641.0 or 641.1	O44.
Abruptio placentae	641.2	O15
Antepartum bleeding	640, 641	O46
Intrapartum bleeding	not available	O67
Postpartum bleeding:	666	O77

Delivery Mode

Induction of the delivery with exception of deliveries starting with a caesarean section, and caesarean section (irrespective of previous induction of delivery).

Pregnancy Duration in Completed Weeks

In most cases determined from second trimester sonography. When such is missing, based on last menstrual period. Values below 23 or above 44 weeks are regarded as missing data. Grouped (when known) into preterm (<37 completed weeks) and term. Only analysed in singleton pregnancies.

Infant Sex

Male, female, indeterminate or missing.

Birth Weight in Gram

Values below 300 or above 6700 are regarded as missing data. Grouped into low birth weight (<2500 g) and other birth weight (≥2500g), and into high birth weight (≥4500g) and other birth weight (<4500g). Only analysed in singletons.

Intrauterine Growth

Determined from standard graphs constructed from data in the Medical Birth Register[1]. Small for gestational age (SGA) is <-2 standard deviations from expected weight for that pregnancy week according to sex and parity (1st and.higher parity), large for gestational age is >2 standard deviations from expected weight. Since these graphs were constructed, women have reduced their smoking during pregnancy and increased their average BMI why infants now show fewer SGA and more LGA than expected from 2 SD limits.

Infant Neonatal Diagnoses

Up to 12 diagnoses can be given and are coded according to ICD-9 or ICD-10 (see above under Maternal diagnoses). Among the diagnoses, the following ones were routinely analysed (Table 3:2):

Table 3.2. List of neonatal diagnoses which are routinely analysed and the ICD codes used to identify the conditions

Diagnosis	ICD-9 codes	ICD-10 codes
Hypoglycaemia	777.1	P70
Respiratory diagnoses	768-770	P20-P28.
CNS diagnoses	779.0-779.3	P90, P91.3-P91.9, P92
Neonatal jaundice	773 or 774	P57-P59

Table 3.3. List of congenital malformations which are excluded at the definition of relatively severe malformations

Diagnosis	ICD-9 codes	ICD-10 codes
Preauricular tag	744.1	Q17.0
Patent ductus arteriosus in preterm infant	747.0	Q25.0
Single umbilical artery	747.5	Q27.0
Tongue tie	750.0	Q38.1
Undescended testicle	752.5	Q53
Hip (sub)luxation, unstable hip	754.3	Q65
Nevus	757	Q82.5

Table 3.4. List of malformations which were routinely analysed when numbers were large enough (usually more than three)

Diagnosis	ICD-9 codes	ICD-10 codes
Any CNS malformation	740-742	Q00-Q05
Neural tube defects	740, 741, 742.0	Q00-Q01, Q05
Eye malformations	743	Q11
Ear malformations	744	Q16-Q19
Any cardiac defect except PDA in preterm infants and SUA	745-747 except 747.5 and 747.0 (preterm)	Q20-Q28 except Q25.0 (preterm) and Q27.0
VSD and/or ASD	754.4, 745.5	Q210, Q211
Unspecified cardiac defects	746.9	Q249
Orofacial cleft	749	Q35-Q37
Oesophageal atresia/stenosis	750.3	Q39.0-Q39.3
Small gut atresia/stenosis	751.1	Q41
Anal atresia/stenosis	751.2	Q42
Abdominal wall defects	756.7	Q79.2-Q79.4
Diaphramatic hernia	756.6	Q79.0
Hypospadias	752.6	Q54
Kidney agenesis/dysgenesis	753.0	Q60
Cystic kidney	753.1	Q61
Pes equinovarus	754.5	Q66.0
Polydactyly or syndactyly	755.0-1	Q69-Q70
Limb reduction defect	755.2-755.4	Q71-Q73
Hip (sub)luxation or unstable hip	754.3	Q65
Craniostenosis	754.0	Q750
Chromosome anomalies	758	Q9

Low Apgar Score

Apgar score at 1 and 5 minutes are usually registered, sometimes also Apgar at 10 minutes. If Apgar 1 is over 8 and Apgar 5 is missing, the latter is assumed to be 9. Apgar scores may be completely missing.

Congenital Malformations in Infants

Included are conditions coded in ICD-9 as 740.0-759.9 and in ICD-10 coded beginning with a Q.

In the Medical Birth Register, codes for congenital malformations may be missing. The data were therefore supplemented with data from the Swedish Register of Birth Defects (previously called Register of Congenital Malformations) and with data from the Hospital Discharge Register. Linkage was made with the use of maternal or infant personal identification numbers. In this way the total rate of infants with diagnoses of congenital malformations increased from 3.5 to 4.6% for the whole period. The following types of congenital malformations were routinely tabulated:

Any congenital malformation

Relatively severe congenital malformations. A number of not so important conditions were then excluded (Table 3:3), also because they are variably registered. Excluded were thus infants with only one or more of these malformations.

Specific malformation diagnoses were analysed *ad hoc*, either because they had been specifically associated with an exposure in the literature or because a major group which appeared to occur in excess should be broken up in its components, e.g., cleft lip/palate and median cleft palate among orofacial clefts and gastroschisis and omphalocele among abdominal wall defects.

Chapter 4

ADVANTAGES AND DISADVANTAGES OF THE STUDY MATERIAL

The material used for analysis has advantages and disadvantages.

ADVANTAGES

Data on exposures are collected during pregnancy without knowledge of the delivery outcome. From this point of view it can thus be characterized as prospective. It is possible, however, that events before or in early pregnancy like IVF or early pregnancy bleeding may affect the completeness and correctness of the recording of drug use.

The size of the study material is large and is continually growing.

The data contain information on characteristics of the women which may act as confounders in the analysis. These characteristics are also collected in a prospective way or obtained by linkage with independent administrative registers.

Outcome data are collected separately from the collection of exposure data and are in principle independent of information on exposure. In special circumstances like maternal epilepsy or diabetes, the knowledge of the maternal disease may affect the completeness and correctness of the registration of, for instance, congenital malformations. This risk will reasonably more strongly affect the registration of mild and variable conditions than that of serious malformations. It is at least to some extent balanced by the fact that information on congenital malformations is also collected from other sources than the Medical Birth Register.

DISADVANTAGES

Exposure Information

Information on drug use is certainly not complete. At the midwife interview in early pregnancy, the woman may not tell about drugs used or the midwife may not record it. Some drugs may be especially sensitive to this source of error. To this category belong street drugs which are probably heavily underreported. It may also be true for other drugs, e.g., drugs used for psychiatric diseases. The recording of drug use later in pregnancy is based on notes in the records of the antenatal care. They to a large extent consist of prescriptions or recommendations made by the attending staff and it is not certain that the advice given has been followed. Furthermore, the patient may have had prescriptions from other sources which are not recorded in the MHV2 records.

The effect of incomplete recording of drug use will be a loss of power in the study but will affect risk estimates rather little if the exposure rate in the population is low. It will mean that some women who have used the drug are regarded as non-exposed but in most instances they will make up only a small part of the material used for comparison. This is graphically illustrated in Figure 4.1 which shows the effect of various degrees of incomplete recording on the risk ratio estimate of 2.0 at different rates of exposure.

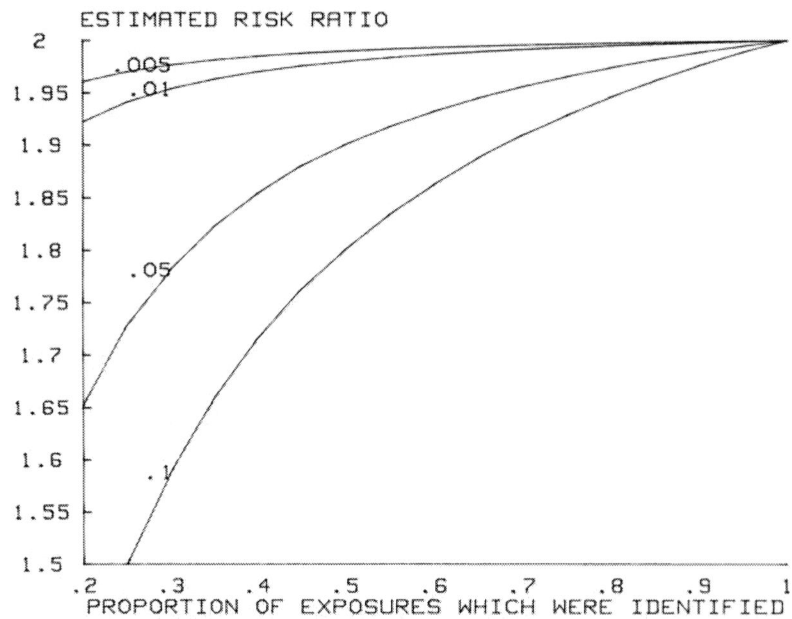

Figure 4.1. Estimated risk at a true risk of 2 depending on the proportion of identified exposures for different true rates of exposure in the population (marked in association with the graphs).

The next problem is that the exact time of drug exposure will usually not be known. As the early pregnancy use of drugs is ascertained at the first antenatal care visit which usually takes place during weeks 10-12, most of these exposures will have occurred during the first trimester. Some, however, may have occurred before organogenesis – or even before pregnancy like some drugs used for ovarian stimulation – or after organogenesis. So, for instance, neural tube defects are formed during weeks 4-5 after LMP and if the woman reports the use of a drug in week 7, it can not have caused a neural tube defect. This error will falsely increase the number of infants which are regarded as exposed and therefore bias risk estimates towards 1. It will be most important for drugs which are used temporarily like hypnotics, analgesics or antibiotics, and will play a minor role for drugs which are used chronically. In some circumstances, drug use is related to a pregnancy complaint which does not occur until after the formative period of, for instance, neural tube defects. A typical example is antiemetics used for nausea and vomiting in pregnancy which seldom starts before week 6. Even a very large material of a drug used for this condition, e.g., meclozine, cannot exclude the possibility that the drug increases the risk for a neural tube defect if used during weeks 4-5, for instance because of motion sickness.

There is little information on the amount of drug taken. Drugs may have teratogenic effects which depend on drug amounts taken. An example is benzodiazepines which seem to have little teratogenic effect at normal use [1] but which, at very high usage, may have an ill effect on the foetus [2].

Outcome Information

Also an incomplete recording of the outcome will occur, leading to a reduction in power but giving little effect on risk estimates (see above). This is a rather small problem concerning congenital malformations because these are ascertained from multiple sources but some late apparent effects will be incompletely ascertained and depend on the follow-up time of the children. This is true, for instance, for mild cardiac defects.

Information on pregnancy duration, birth weight, infant sex and mortality are of high quality with little data loss. Neonatal diagnoses, however, may be incompletely recorded but loss of diagnoses is hardly affected by maternal drug use. The same is true for maternal diagnoses of complications during pregnancy. Such loss will again reduce power but only little affect risk estimates.

One important deficiency in the outcome data is the lack of information on foetuses, aborted after prenatal detection of a congenital malformation. Such cases are reported to the Register of Birth Defects, but Swedish law prohibits their registration with identification number and it has therefore not been possible to get information on drug use in early pregnancy. This will mean that there will be no possibility to identify an association between drug use and foetuses with a congenital malformation (e.g., anencephaly) which is practically always aborted. If foetuses with a malformation are sometimes but not always aborted (e.g., spina bifida), the power of the study will decrease but it will still be possible to identify associations with drug use (e.g., valproic acid).

Information on Confounding Factors

Some confounders used will be of high quality like year of birth, maternal age, and parity. The quality of smoking information is more dubious for two reasons. One is that it is based on reports from the woman and some under-recording of smoking probably occurs. The other problem is the rather crude grouping of smoking into less than 10 and 10 or more cigarettes per day. If drug use is strongly associated with smoking, it can be expected that within both groups and notably within the ≥10 cigarettes per day group, the amount smoked will be higher among drug users than among other women and the adjustment will be incomplete. Also for BMI, rather crude groups are routinely used but when needed, more subgroups can be applied.

There is rather detailed information on maternal education but only for births up to and including 2001. Therefore, this variable cannot be used for analysis of the whole period.

The following maternal characteristics are routinely tabulated or shown as diagrams: maternal age, parity, smoking, previous miscarriages, BMI, subfertility, country of birth, education, family situation, and working conditions. These data are given not only in order to identify possible confounders but also in order to characterise the women. Some features, e.g., working situation, may be secondary to the underlying disease; other, e.g., smoking, may be actually contributing to the underlying disease and therefore to drug use.

References

[1] Norstedt Wikner B, Stiller C-O, Bergman U, Asker C, Källén B. Use of benzodiazepines and benzodiazepine receptor agonists during pregnancy: neonatal outcome and congenital malformations. *Pharmacoepidemiol Drug Safety* 2007; 16: 1203-1210.

[2] Laegreid L, Olegård R, Walström J, Conradi N. Teratogenic effects of benzodiazepine use during pregnancy. *J Pediatr* 1989; 114: 126-131.

Chapter 5

STRATEGY OF ANALYSIS

Each drug chapter will be introduced with a very short literature review. This is in no way comprehensive but may give the reader some introduction into the literature and can bring out some pertinent article of importance for the rest of the chapter.

The first step in the analysis is to describe the actual drugs within each drug group which were recorded and the number of women who had reported each drug. Also the simultaneous use of two or more drugs of different categories but within the drug group is described. As most of the following analysis is made on all drugs in the drug group and perhaps on subgroups, it is regarded as important to show which drugs represented the major part of the group.

The next step in the analysis of a group of drugs is to compare women who reported such drugs in early pregnancy with all women who gave birth. The odds ratios according to maternal age, parity, smoking in early pregnancy, BMI, previous miscarriages, subfertility, country of birth of the woman, family situation, and work outside home are determined. There are two reasons: to describe her situation in the beginning of the pregnancy and to identify variables which could be important confounders in the analysis of delivery outcome. Maternal education could not be used as a confounder, as data were available only up to and including 2001. The odds ratios are determined after adjustment for other women characteristics and also the year of delivery.

The reporting of the use of other drugs in early pregnancy is then analysed. For a number of drug groups, the number of women using them together with the target drugs is compared with the number of women using that drug group among all women. In the analysis, adjustment is made for year of delivery, woman's age, parity, and smoking habits. In this way, co-medication with other drugs can be identified. There may be different explanations to an association between the uses of two drugs. They may be used for treatment of the same condition, e.g., antiasthmatic drugs and antibiotics, or they may be associated because of co-morbidity between the indications of the drugs, e.g., diabetes and hypothyreosis.

Such co-medication can have an impact on the estimated risks for various outcomes. This problem is usually solved by a repeated analysis after exclusion of women with the selected associated drugs.

In the next step, maternal diseases during pregnancy are studied. These could be the reason for drug use (e.g., pre-existing diabetes, chronic hypertension) or could be the result of the drug or underlying disease (e.g., gestational diabetes, preeclampsia, and placenta previa). Finally, also some information on mode of delivery and delivery complications are analyzed: bleeding around delivery, caesarean section, and induction of vaginal delivery. When associations during late pregnancy are studied, the drugs can also have been used to treat the complication.

The outcome of the pregnancy is studied from various points of view:

Infant sex ratio is relevant because at some conditions (e.g., nausea and vomiting in pregnancy) it is skewed against a female excess.

Multiple births can also be an indicator of some conditions (e.g., nausea and vomiting in pregnancy) but is especially the result of infertility treatment (ovarian stimulation and in vitro fertilization). If an association between drug use and multiple births is not seen after exposure in early pregnancy but after later exposure, the explanation is reasonably that the drug has been used because of complications arising from the multiple gestation.

The risk for preterm birth (<37 weeks) and low birth weight (<2500g) are studied in singletons because of the increased occurrence in multiple births. Also high birth weight (≥4500g) can be an effect of underlying pathology (e.g., pre-existing diabetes or gestational diabetes) and can also be a direct drug effect (suggested after tricyclic antidepressants). Small-for-gestational age and large-for-gestational age is studied as indicators for effects on intrauterine growth. An association with drug use can be due to treatments in order to delay a threatened preterm birth.

Some selected neonatal diagnoses are analyzed as they may indicate neonatal effects of maternal drug use. When enough data are available on drug use after the first antenatal care visit, effects from drugs are usually expected to be more prominent than after first trimester exposure, but usually more cases are available of early exposure than after later exposure.

Finally, the analysis concentrates on congenital malformations, usually only in association with early exposures as most malformations originate during the first trimester. There are some exceptions (e.g., pylorostenosis, microcephaly, hydrocephaly) which may originate late during pregnancy.

The malformation analysis begins with the risk for the infants to have any malformation diagnosis. In the next step a number of common minor conditions are removed from the analysis, among other things because their registration may vary considerably between hospitals. After this, specific conditions are tabulated, either specific malformations (e.g., hypospadias) or groups of malformations (e.g., neural tube defects). Specific malformations are usually only tabulated if at least three cases have occurred.

When a group of drugs are analysed, each specific drug is tabulated with risk estimates for any relatively severe malformation and sometimes for specific malformation groups. When an increased risk is noticed, the actual malformations present are scrutinized.

Statistical Notes

In order to adjust for putative confounders, the Mantel-Haenszel [1] technique is used which gives a weighted average odds ratio for a number of different strata. The approximate 95% confidence interval was regularly estimated using Miettinen's method [2]. The Mantel-Haenszel method was preferred to modelling methods because the latter are often complex and not straight line regressions, as exemplified in Chapter 6. Another advantage was that the same method of analysis could easily be used throughout the book. The main draw-back with the Mantel-Haenszel method is the loss of data, if controls are not available in a stratum. As controls in the present analysis are made up of all births in the population (with the exception of the rather few exposed ones) this is a very unlikely event.

The Mantel-Haenszel method is based on a $\chi 2$ analysis and therefore necessitates a normal approximation. When the expected number of outcome was low (<10), therefore the expected number was calculated (with due consideration to the selected confounders) and the observed number of outcome was compared with the expected number as a risk ratio. Its exact 95% confidence interval was then determined from Poisson distributions (SABER software).

In the majority of cases, no prior hypothesis exists and therefore associations with apparent formal statistical significance may arise by chance. Sometimes there are already some associations identified in the literature which can be tested in the present material which reduces – but does not eliminate – the risk for false statistical significances. If many such tests based on prior data are made, still some may reach statistical significance by chance. This must always be kept in mind in the interpretation of the results. In the book by Heinonen et al. [3] which described a similarly collected material, it was nicely put (p. 7): "None of the associations presented in this book should be regarded as anything more than hypotheses requiring independent confirmation."

Another fact which should be remembered in the interpretation of data is that after splitting a material into subgroups, one subgroup may show "statistical significance" and the other may not. This does not mean that the first group necessarily shows a stronger effect than the second group: in order to demonstrate that, it must be shown that the two risks cannot be estimates from the same average risk. Such comparisons will be made using two-tailed z tests based on variances estimated from the Mantel-Haenszel tests.

REFERENCES

[1] Mantel N, Haenszel W. Statistical aspects of the analysis of data from retrospective studies of disease. *J Natl Cancer Inst* 1959; 22: 719-748.

[2] Miettinen OS. Simple interval estimation of risk ratio. *Am J Epidemiol* 1974; 100: 515-516.

[3] Heinonen OP, Slone D, Monson RR, Hook EB, Shapiro S. *Birth Defects and Drugs in Pregnancy*. Publishing Sciences Group, Inc., Littleton, Mass.

Chapter 6

DATA ON WOMEN AND INFANTS RECORDED IN THE MEDICAL BIRTH REGISTER DURING 1996-2005

During this period, 1 015 537 women with deliveries were recorded in the register. Among them, 968 307 (95.3%) contained data from the antenatal care clinics and these were used for the further analysis because drug information was obtained from the antenatal care records. The average percentage of records without information from the antenatal care was thus 4.7% but this varied with year of delivery: from 2.2% in 1996 to 7.8% in 2005 with values between 6.8 and 7.3 % also in 1998, 2000 and 2004.

In adjusted analyses, women without a known age were excluded. There were 551 women without information of age (1.8 per 1000).

Data on some maternal characteristics are given in Table 6.1

Among these women, 361 316 reported the use of some drug in early pregnancy (37%) and 658 666 had some drug prescribed during antenatal care (68%).

Table 6.1. Characteristics of women in the register

Variable	Number	Per cent
Maternal age		
<20	17945	1.9
20-24	134363	13.9
25-29	318771	32.9
30-34	328625	34.0
35-39	141699	14.6
40-44	25349	2.6
≥45	988	0.1
Parity		
1	422807	43.7
2	350098	36.2
3	134207	13.9
≥4	60628	6.3

Table 6.1. Characteristics of women in the register (Continued)

Variable	Number	Per cent
Smoking in early pregnancy		
Unknown	28075	2.9
None	833650	86.1
<10 cigarettes/day	73430	7.6
≥10 cigarettes/day	33585	3.5
Number of previous miscarriages		
None	770745	79.6
1	151363	15.6
2	32991	3.4
≥3	12641	1.3
Body Mass Index		
Unknown	105034	10.9
<19.8	75301	7.8
19.8-25.9	554791	57.3
≥26	232641	24.0
Years of unwanted childlessness		
0	897903	92.8
1	19256	2.0
2	20572	2.1
3	11310	1.2
4	6442	0.7
≥5	12259	1.3
Maternal country of birth		
Unknown	8756	0.9
Sweden	787842	81.4
Other Nordic country	22035	2.3
Non-Nordic country	149107	15.4
Family situation		
Unknown	20566	2.1
Cohabiting	897610	92.8
Living alone	24702	2.6
Other	24782	2.6
Work outside home		
Unknown	136784	14.1
Full time	444726	46.0
Part time	223449	23.1
No	162781	16.8
Maternal education level (1996-2005, n=506238)		
Unknown	15815	3.1
<9 years	9344	0.2
9 years	49829	9.8
"Gymnasium"*, 12 years	260807	51.5
2 years post-gymnasium	27460	5.4
≥3 years post-gymnasium	140320	27.7
Research studies	2663	0.5

*Swedish gymnasium corresponds roughly with upper secondary high school in UK and senior high school in US.

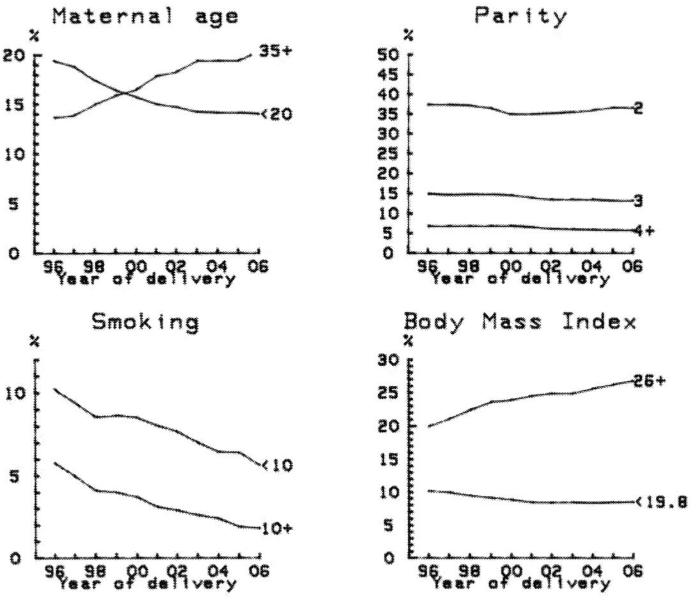

Figure 6.1. The yearly distribution of the first four characteristics. It can be seen that the group of women aged 35 or more increases and the group with an age below 25 decreases during the studied period, parity distribution is relatively constant, smoking in early pregnancy decreases and over-weight increases.

Data on Pregnancy Outcome in all Deliveries in the Medical Birth Register During 1996-2005

1. Preterm birth, low birth weight, large birth weight, intrauterine growth

Gestational duration was mainly estimated from second trimester sonography. Among all singleton births, 4.9% were preterm, that is, born before week 37. There was little variation between delivery years. Low birth weight (<2500g) among singleton births was found in 3.1% which did not vary between years and large birth weight (≥4500g) in 4.1%, small for gestational age (<-2 standard deviations, SGA) in 2.2% and large for gestational age (>2 standard deviations, LGA) in 6.1%. The slightly low rate of SGA and the high rate of LGA depends on the fact that the reference graph was determined for the years 1985-1989, and since then smoking has decreased among pregnant women and BMI has increased (se above), both factors which increase birth weight. The impact of various maternal characteristics on the crude percentages of the various outcomes is given in Table 6.2.

Information on SGA and LGA according to parity is not given because intrauterine growth is adjusted for parity (1st vs. ≥1).

Some of these variables co-vary strongly, e.g., maternal age and parity. Figure 6.2 shows that the effect on preterm birth, low birth weight, and high birth weight varies for each maternal age group according to parity. Furthermore, the graphs are basically U-shaped.

Table 6.2. Preterm birth (<37 weeks), low birth weight (<2500g), high birth weight (≥4500g), small for gestational age (SGA), and large for gestational age (LGA) according to some maternal characteristics. Only singleton births Percentages of all with known gestational duration or birth weight, respectively

Variable	Low Preterm birth	High birth weight	Birth weight	SGA	LGA
Maternal age					
<20	6.7	5.0	2.0	4.2	6.1
20-24	5.6	3.6	2.9	2.7	6.4
25-29	4.9	3.0	3.9	2.1	7.5
30-34	4.7	3.0	4.6	1.9	8.9
35-39	5.4	3.6	4.9	2.1	10.2
40-44	6.5	4.8	4.8	2.7	11.1
≥45	7.0	6.0	5.0	3.5	11.9
Parity					
1	6.3	4.3	2.67	-	-
2	3.8	2.2	4.9	-	-
3	4.1	2.5	6.0	-	-
≥4	5.9	3.54	6.0	-	-
Smoking					
Unknown	8.3	5.4	3.9	2.4	6.4
None	4.6	2.8	4.4	1.9	6.4
<10 cigarettes/day	6.1	4.9	2.6	3.8	3.8
≥10 cigarettes/day	7.2	6.3	1.9	4.5	3.4
Body Mass Index					
Unknown	6.6	4.3	4.0	2.4	6.2
<19.8	5.4	4.5	1.3	3.4	1.9
19.8-25.9	4.5	2.9	3.4	2.0	5.0
≥26	5.4	3.1	6.8	1.9	10.2
Years of unwanted childlessness					
0	5.0	3.2	4.1	2.1	6.2
1	5.9	3.9	3.9	2.5	5.2
2	6.0	4.1	3.8	3.0	5.1
3	6.5	5.0	3.6	3.5	4.4
4	7.0	5.5	4.2	3.6	5.1
≥5	8.4	6.2	3.2	4.6	4.2
Country of birth					
Unknown	9.3	7.0	2.1	4.7	3.8
Sweden	5.0	3.6	3.3	2.6	5.1
Other Nordic	5.6	3.6	4.3	2.2	6.6
Non-Nordic	5.0	3.0	4.5	1.9	6.6
Family situation					
Unknown	8.5	5.6	3.7	2.6	6.1
Co-habiting	4.8	3.0	4.2	2.1	6.2
Living alone	6.1	4.7	3.0	3.7	4.5
Other	6.1	4.6	2.9	3.6	3.7
Work outside home					
Unknown	6.3	4.1	4.0	2.4	6.3
Whole time	5.0	3.1	3.9	2.3	5.2
Part time	4.4	2.6	4.8	1.6	7.7
No	5.0	3.5	3.9	2.5	6.3

It can be noted that for first parity, the percentage of preterm birth or low birth weight is high at high maternal age while for parity 3 the percentage is high at young age.

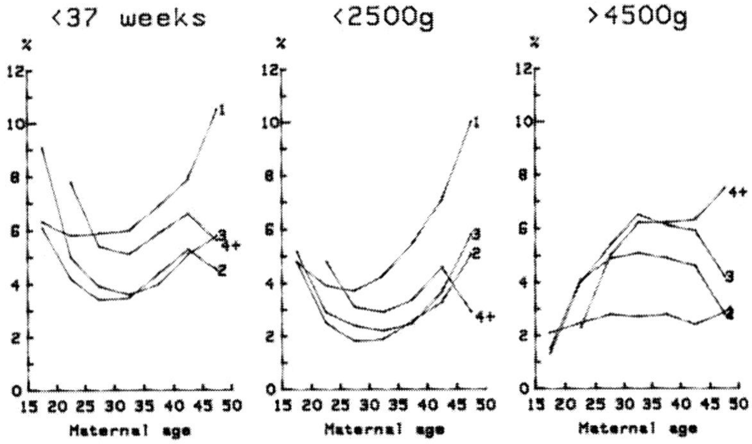

Figure 6.2. Percentage of singleton infants with gestational duration <37 weeks or with birth weight <2500g or ≥4500g at different maternal age and different parities (1, 2, 3, and 4+).

Table 6.3. Diagnoses and other outcomes among all deliveries with information on maternal age

Outcome/diagnosis	Number	Denominator	Rate per 100
Maternal diagnoses			
Pre-existing diabetes	12112	967 742	1.3
Pre-existing hypertension	10811	967 742	1.1
Preeclampsia	43429	967 742	4.5
Gestational diabetes	8590	967 742	0.9
Placenta previa	10426	967 742	1.1
Abruptio placentae	11377	967 742	1.2
Antepartum bleeding	12947	967 742	1.3
Intrapertum bleeding	19162	967 742	2.0
Postpartum bleeding	54970	967 742	5.7
Delivery induction	102853	898 063	11.5
Caesarean section	150702	967 742	15.7
Outcomes			
Preterm birth (<37 weeks)[a]	46310	952 848	4.9
Low birth weight (<2500g)[a]	29471	949 489	3.1
High birth weight (≥4500g)[a]	39274	949 489	4.1
SGA[a]	20368	949 111	2.2
LG[a]	58068	949 111	6.1
Stillbirth	3245	982 456	0.3
Early neonatal death	2006	982 456	0.2
Neonatal diagnoses			
Hypoglycaemia	35102	982 456	3.6
Respiratory diagnoses	49451	982 456	5.1
Low Apgar score	19636	973 456	2.0
CNS diagnoses	6032	982 456	0.6
Jaundice	39589	982 456	4.0
Adrenal insufficiency	7756	982 456	0.8

[a]Only singletons.

2. Infant Sex and Multiple Births

Among all infants born, sex was unknown or indeterminate in 330, 504 267 were male and 477 857 female which gives a sex ratio (males/females) of 1.06. There were 14 453 twin deliveries (1.5%), 187 triplet deliveries and two quadruplet deliveries.

3. Maternal and Infant Diagnoses and Infant Outcome

Table 6.3 gives number of diagnoses/outcomes, the denominators, and the rates. Sometimes information was missing, sometimes rates were calculated on subgroups (delivery induction only on women whose deliveries did not began with a caesarean section).

Table 6.4. Number of different categories of congenital malformations and rates among all 982 454 infants

Congenital malformation	Number	Rate per 1000 birth
Chromosome anomalies	1911	1.9
In absence of a chromosome anomaly:		
Any CNS malformations	1197	1.2
Neural tube defects	381	0.4
Eye malformations	959	1.0
Ear malformations	2306	2.3
Or facial cleft	1788	1.8
All cardiovascular defects	10408	10.6
Some severe cardiovascular defects	833	0.8
VSD and/or ASD	5475	5.6
Unspecified	1062	1.1
Oesophageal atresia	289	0.3
Small gut atresia	244	0.2
Anal atresia	379	0.4
Pylorostenosis	704	0.7
Abdominal wall defect	252	0.3
Diaphragmatic hernia	231	0.2
Hypospadias	2803	2.9
Kidney agenesis or dysgenesis	277	0.3
Cystic kidney	381	0.4
Pes equinovarus	1400	1.4
Poly/syndactyly	1990	2.0
Limb reduction defect	570	0.6
Hip (sub)luxation, unstable hip	6130	6.2
Caniostenosis	589	0.6

4. Congenital Malformations

The total rate of congenital malformations detected during the observation period was 4.7% (n=46 289). There was a clear-cut decline in rate with year of birth from 5.4% in

1996 to 4.2% in 2006. This is the result of a shorter follow-up and therefore less effective identification from the Hospital Discharge Register.

Among the infants with a diagnosis of a congenital malformation, some had only one or more of some common, mild and variably registered conditions, namely preauricular appendix, PDA at preterm birth, undescended testicle, unstable hip, tongue tie, single umbilical artery or nevus. If such infants were not counted (n=31 737) the rate decreases to 3.2%, again with a time trend from 4.0% in 1996 to 2.8% in 2005.

The number and rate of some selected groups of malformations are seen in Table 6.4.

The maternal characteristics will vary for each type of malformation. For example there is a strongly increasing rate of some chromosome anomalies with maternal age while for gastroschisis the opposite is seen.

Chapter 7

ANTACIDS

The use of antacids during pregnancy is not associated with any certain observable risk.

Antacids are commonly used drugs which most probably are incompletely identified in the register. During early pregnancy nausea and vomiting is common and may result in the use of antacids, and during late pregnancy the expanding uterus may cause gastric acidity and gastro-oesophageal reflux. Little is published on the use of antacids in early pregnancy, usually regarded as harmless [1]. In an early study, an increased risk for abnormality after 1st trimester use of antacids was noted [2].

Table 7.1. Number of women identified with use of antacids

Total:	9294
Reported use in early pregnancy	4569
Got prescription later in pregnancy	5218
Both early and late use	493

CHARACTERISTICS OF WOMEN USING ANTACIDS

Based on women reporting the drug in early pregnancy (n=4569) Each variable is adjusted for all other variables and year of delivery. Comparison with all women who gave birth during the period and with information from the first antenatal care (n=967 742). The odds ratios for maternal age, parity, smoking in early pregnancy, number of previous miscarriages, BMI, subfertility, and country of birth are adjusted for all other variables and are shown in Figure 7.1.

Some further characteristics were analyzed, adjusting for year of delivery, maternal age, parity, smoking and BMI (Table 7.2)

The women are thus slightly older and more often than expected of first parity, they smoke less and have a higher BMI than expected. They work outside home less often than expected.

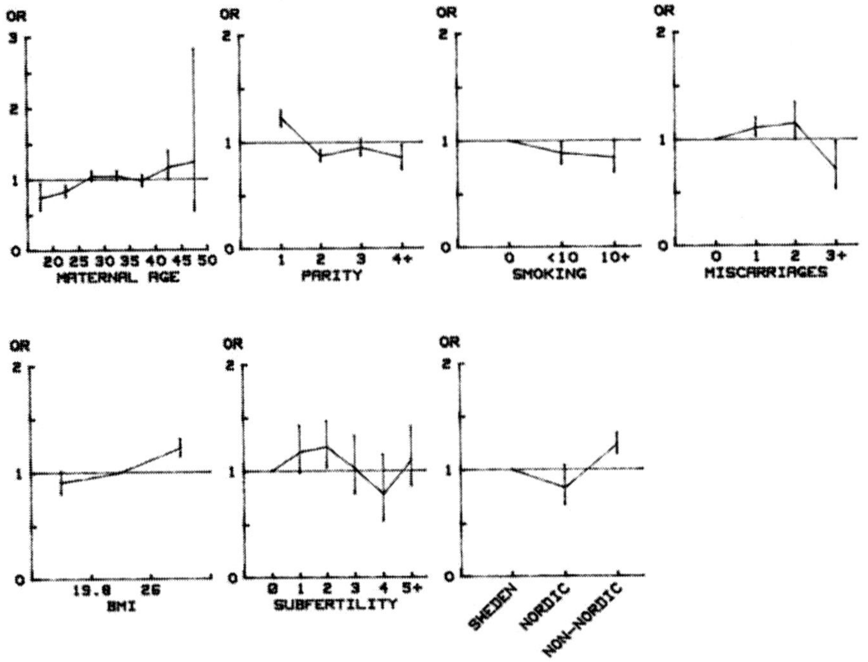

Figure 7.1. Odds ratios for seven maternal characteristics. The odds ratios (OR) for each variable are adjusted for the other variables and year of delivery. Vertical lines mark 95% confidence intervals. For maternal age and parity, each class is compared with all other classes.

Table 7.2. Some further characteristics of women using antacids in early pregnancy

Variable studied	Number	OR	95% CI
Education (1996-2001, 2 059 women with drugs, 526 695 in population)			
Unknown	54	-	
<12 years	213	0.98	0.84-1.15
12 years	1079	1.00	reference
13-14 years	93	0.77	0.62-0.96
≥14 years	620	0.94	0.85-1.04
Family situation			
Unknown	69	-	
Co-habiting	4235	1.00	reference
Living alone	90	0.88	0.71-1.09
Other family situation	117	1.01	0-82-1.24
Work outside home			
Unknown	562	-	
Full time	2086	1.00	reference
Part time	1066	1.06	0.98-1.15
None	797	1.17	1.03-1.23

Table 7.3. Concomitant drug use (early pregnancy)

Drug group	Number	OR	95% CI
Drugs for stomach ulcer and reflux	394	10.8	9.90-11.7
Drugs for inflammatory bowel disease	5	0.38	0.16-0.87
Multivitamins	421	1.07	0.98-1.17
Folic acid	297	1.02	0.41-1.23
Drugs for hypertension	13	0.71	0.41-1.23
Oral contraceptive	15	1.19	0.71-1.98
Progestogens	16	0.80	0.49-1.31
Gonadotrophins	9	0.83	0.43-1.60
Systemic corticosteroids	15	0.88	0.53-1.47
Thyroid drugs	34	0.51	0.37-0.92
Antibiotics	163	1.07	0.91-1.25
NSAID	137	1.79	1.51-2.12
Opioids	40	1.63	1.19-2.23
Minor analgesics	1033	3.81	3.56-4.07
Drugs for migraine	7	0.54	0.26-1.12
Anticonvulsants	5	0.36	0.16-0.82
Neuroleptics	57	3.42	2.67-4.38
Sedatives, hypnotics	26	1.29	0.88-1.89.
Antidepressants	39	0.69	0.50-0.94
Drugs for rhinitis	147	2.19	1.86-2.58
Antiasthmatics	132	0.91	0.76-1.08
Cough medicines	49	1.95	1.48-2.58
Antihistamines	799	3.45	3.21-3.71
For NVP	703	3.96	3.67-4.27
For allergy	126	1.95	1.48-2.58

Table 7.4. Maternal delivery diagnoses associated with the use antacids

Diagnosis	Drug in early pregnancy			Drug later in pregnancy		
	Number	OR	95%CI	Number	OR	95% CI
Pre-existing diabetes	66	1.05	0.82-1.35	87	1.09	0.87-1.35
Chronic hypertension	69	1.23	0.97-1.56	85	1.13	0.91-1.41
Gestational diabetes	57	1.33	1.02-1.73	53	0.93	0.71-1.23
Preeclampsia	275	1.25	1.11-1.42	303	1.29	1.14-1.45
Hyperemesis gravidarum	66	1.39	1.09-1.78	97	1.56	1.28-1.92
Placenta previa	63	1.11	0.92-1.53	70	1.00	0.78-1.27
Abruptio placentae	68	1.17	0.92-1.50	75	0.96	0.76-1.22
Antepartum bleeding	73	1.16	0.92-1.46	75	0.96	0.76-1.21
Intrapartum bleeding	111	1.09	0.90-1.32	141	1.12	0.94-1.33
Postpartum bleeding	256	0.98	0.87-1.12	274	1.02	0.95-1.16
Delivery induction	577	1.14	1.05-1.25	726	1.39	1.28-1.51
Caesarean section	797	1.06	0.98-1.14	1019	1.28	1.19-1.38

The association with drugs for stomach ulcer and gastro-oesophageal reflux is obvious. Some drugs like some analgesics may increase symptoms which motivate the use of antacids. There is an association with antihistamines used for NVP, a condition when also antacids are used. This may also explain the association with neuroleptics, often used at NVP, and drugs for rhinitis, used among other things for pregnancy rhinitis which can be associated with NVP. Some other drug associations may be caused by the fact that women who report antacids may be more careful than other women in their reporting of some other drugs like cough medicines but one would then expect a similar phenomenon for vitamins which is not seen.

There are a number of conditions which are associated with the use of antacids, including hyperemesis gravidarum and the rates of delivery inductions and caesarean sections are increased, notably after late exposure.

Outcome after Maternal use of Antacids

Infant Sex

When the mother had used antacids in early pregnancy, 2337 infants were male and 2305 female (1 unknown sex) which gives a sex ratio of 1.01 (95% CI 0.96-1.07), a slightly low sex ratio even if the normal sex ratio of 1.06 is contained within the confidence interval. This indicates an excess of pregnancies with strong nausea and vomiting which is associated with an excess of female infant sex. When drug use has occurred later in pregnancy, the sex ratio was normal: 2754 males, 2570 females (four unknown) which give a sex ratio of 1.08 (95% CI 1.02-1.14).

Multiple Births

There were 74 twin pairs after maternal use of antacids in early pregnancy. The odds ratio for twin delivery was 1.07 (95% CI of 0.85-1.35). After antacid use later in pregnancy, there were 86 twin deliveries, OR = 1.11 (95% CI 0.90-1.38).

Table 7.5. Pregnancy duration and infant birth weight at maternal use of antacids. Only singleton births

Variable studied	Drug use in early pregnancy			Drug use later in pregnancy		
	Number	OR	95% CI	Number	OR	95% CI
<37 weeks	205	0.92	0.80-1.06	279	0.88	0.77-1.01
<2500g	131	0.94	0.79-1.12	137	0.85	0.72-1.01
≥4500g	184	0.97	0.84-1.13	230	1.04	0.91-1.19
SGA	109	1.12	0.93-1.36	96	0.87	0.75-1.07
LGA	279	1.02	0.90-1.15	299	0.90	0.80-1.01

No certain effect on these variables is seen when the mother had used antacids.

There is thus no increased perinatal death risk but actually a decrease after exposure in late pregnancy.

Table 7.6. Infant mortality after maternal use of antacids

Variable studied	Drug use in early pregnancy			Drug use later in pregnancy		
	Number	OR	95% CI	Number	OR/RR	95% CI
Stillbirth	15	0.96	0.58-1.59	11	0.58	0.32-1.06
Early neonatal death	4	0.60	0.16-1.15	3	0.38	0.08-1.12#

#observed over expected number with exact Poisson confidence interval.

Table 7.7. Neonatal diagnoses after maternal use of antacids

Diagnosis	Drug use in early pregnancy			Drug use later in pregnancy		
	Number	OR	95% CI	Number	OR	95% CI
Hypoglycaemia	165	0.95	0.81-1.11	173	0.90	0.78-1.05
Respiratory diagnoses	191	0.81	0.70-0.94	215	0.84	0.73-0.96
Low Apgar score	44	0.48	0.36-0.65	69	0.71	0.56-0.90
CNS diagnoses	18	0.59	0.37-0.93	39	1.12	0.81-1.54
Jaundice	215	1.11	0.97-1.28	230	1.05	0.92-1.20

There were thus no signs of an increased risk for neonatal symptoms after maternal use of antacids. Some estimates were actually low – this may be due to an association with nausea and vomiting in pregnancy which has been shown to be associated with a better than expected outcome.

Table 7.8. Congenital malformations in infants whose mothers used antacids

Congenital malformations	Number	OR/RR	95% CI
All drugs			
All malformations	193	0.88	0.76-1.02
Relative severe malformations	134	0.90	0.75-1.05
Chromosome anomalies	6	0.65	0.24-1.42
Without chromosome anomalies:			
Neural tube defects	4	2.26	0.62-5.79#
Eye malformations	4	0.93	0.25-2.39#
Ear malformations	6	0.58	0.26-1.28#
Any cardiovascular defect	56	1.13	0.87-1.49
VSD and/or ASD	30	1.11	0.77-1.60
Unspecified cardiac defects	7	1.55	0.62-3.18#
Orofacial cleft	4	0.48	0.13-1.22
Esophageal atresia	3	2.27	0.47-6.64#
Anal atresia	3	1.75	0.36-5.13#
Pylorostenosis	4	1.15	0.31-2.94#
Hypospadias	8	0.55	0.28-1.08
Severe kidney malformations	4	1.42	0.39-3.63#
Pes equinovarus	3	0.44	0.09-1.30
Polydactyly/syndactyly	9	0.97	0.44-1.84#
Limb reduction defect	4	1.44	0.39-3.68#
Hip (sub)luxation, unstable hip	30	1.01	0.71-1.45

#observed over expected number with exact Poisson confidence interval.

There are thus no signs of teratogenicity.

Summary

Use of antacids during pregnancy is apparently not associated with any noticeable harm.It should be remembered that even though drug ascertainment in early pregnancy is prospective with regard to pregnancy outcome, it is likely that the registration of antacids is rather incomplete as such drugs are OTC drugs and generally regarded as harmless.

References

[1] Mahadevan U, Kane S. American Gastroenterological Association Institute technical review on the use of gastrointestinal medications in pregnancy. *Gastroenterology* 2006; 131: 283-311.

[2] Nelson MM, Forfar JO. Associations bewen drugs administered during pregnancy and congenital abnormalities in the foetus. *BMJ* 1971; i: 523-527.

Chapter 8

DRUGS USED FOR GASTRIC ULCER AND GASTRO-OESOPHAGEAL REFLUX

Use of drugs for gastric ulcer and gastro-oesophageal reflux seem to be without own ill effects on pregnancy outcome. Only little information is available on the use of misoprostol for this indication. If possible, exposure should be avoided but if such exposure has occurred in early pregnancy it is hardly a reason to discuss an interruption of pregnancy.

Table 8.1. Number of women identified with use of drugs for gastric ulcer and gastrointestinal reflux

Total:	11360
Reported use in early pregnancy	7914
Got prescription later in pregnancy	4658
Both early and late use	1212

Type of drug	ATC code	Early use	Later use
Histamine-2 antagonists	A02BA	2128	797
Cimetidine	A02BA01	95	28
Ranitidine	A02BA02	1619	676
Famotidine	A02BA03	426	94
Nizatidine	A02BA04	7	0
Prostaglandines	A02BB	15	1
Misoprostol	A02BB01	15	1
Proton pump inhibitors	A02BC	4793	2853
Omeprazole	A02BC01	3686	2264
Pantoprazole	A02BC02	106	53
Lansoprazole	A02BC03	800	446
Rabeprazole	A02BC04	12	3
Esomeprazole	A02BC05	261	127
Other drugs	A02BX	1283	1200
Sucralfate	A02BX02	1267	1135
Alginic acid	A02BX13	18	67
Unspecified	A02B	15	1

These drugs are used for the prevention and treatment of gastritis and gastric ulcer but also for gastro-oesophageal reflux. A number of drugs increase the risk for such complaints and may therefore co-vary with the use of the anti-ulcer drugs. Furthermore, during early pregnancy nausea and vomiting is common and may result in the use of such drugs, and during late pregnancy the expanding uterus may cause gastric acidity and gastro-oesophageal reflux.

A number of publications exist in the literature on pregnancy outcome after maternal use of these drugs without any risks being identified [1-5].

Some women thus used two or more drugs of this category

	Prosta-glandin	Proton pump inhibitor	Other
Early pregnancy use			
H2-antagonist	1	145	48
Prostaglandin		1	
Proton pump inhibitor			101
Late pregnancy use			
H2-antagonist		60	34
Proton pump inhibitor			94

Five women reported the use of H2-antagonist, proton pump inhibitor, and other in early pregnancy and three got such prescriptions later in pregnancy.

Characteristics of Women using Drugs for Gastric Ulcer or Gastro-Oesophageal Reflux

Based on women reporting the drug in early pregnancy (n=7913, one missing maternal age). Each variable is adjusted for all other variables and year of delivery. Comparison with all women who gave birth during the period and with information from the first antenatal care (n=967 742). The odds ratios for maternal age, parity, smoking in early pregnancy, number of previous miscarriages, BMI, subfertility, and country of birth are adjusted for all other variables and shown in Figure 8.1.

Some further maternal characteristics were analysed, adjusting for year of delivery, maternal age, parity, smoking, and BMI (Table 8.2).

Characteristics of women using drugs for stomach ulcer and gastro-oesophageal reflux is thus a higher use with increasing age, a low use at parity two, an association with smoking and low education, an increased use among non-cohabiting women and women who did not work outside home.

Thus women using drugs for stomach ulcer or gastro-oesophageal reflux use many other types of drugs in excess. There may be different explanations to this. One is methodological, that women who reported this drug category may be extra careful in reporting other drugs as well but that should have been apparent for multivitamins and folic acid. Some drugs like some analgesics may increase symptoms which motivate the use of drugs for gastric ulcer or gastro-oesophageal reflux. Some drugs like psychoactive drugs may indicate co-morbidity between stomach ulcer symptoms and psychiatric problems.

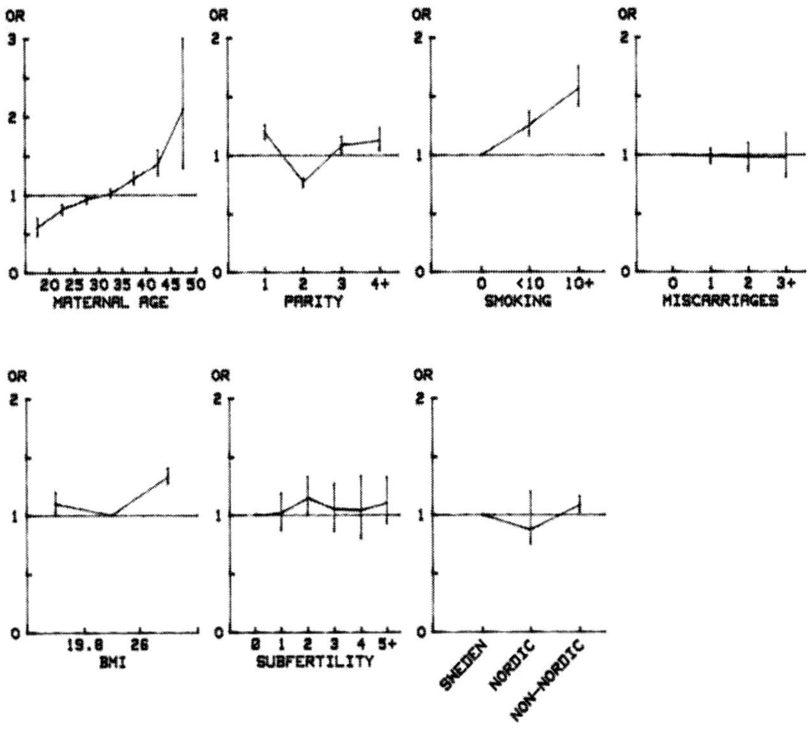

Figure 8.1. Odds ratios for seven maternal characteristics. The odds ratios (OR) for each variable are adjusted for the other variables and year of delivery. Vertical lines mark 95% confidence intervals. For maternal age and parity, each class is compared with all other classes.

Table 8.2. Some further characteristics of women using drugs for gastric ulcer or gastro-oesophageal reflux in early pregnancy.

Education (1996-2001, 3696 women with drugs, 526 695 in population)			
Unknown	87	-	
<12 years	545	1.20	1.08-1.33
12 years	1974	1.00	reference
13-14 years	157	0.74	0.63-0.88
≥14 years	933	0.81	0.75-0.88
Family situation			
Unknown	132	-	-
Co-habiting	7161	1.00	reference
Living alone	263	1.25	1.10-1.43
Other family situation	236	1.14	0.99-1.32
Work outside home			
Unknown	1069	-	-
Full time	3527	1.00	reference
Part time	1784	1.05	0.98-1.12
None	1412	1.10	1.03-1.18

Table 8.3. Concomitant drug use (early pregnancy)

Drug group	Number	OR	95% CI
Antacids	394	10.8	9.98-11.7
Drugs for inflammatory bowel disease	72	3.42	2.79-4.27
Insulin	27	0.92	0.63-1.35
Multivitamins	446	0.87	0.79-0.92
Folic acid	394	0.95	0.85-1.05
Drugs for hypertension	66	1.95	1.53-2.48
Oral contraceptive	49	1.97	1.49-2.60
Progestogens	26	0.70	0.47-1.02
Gonadotrophins	19	1.01	0.64-1.59
Systemic corticosteroids	84	2.82	2.29-3.47
Thyroid drugs	128	1.12	0.94-1.34
Antibiotics	377	1.48	1.34-1.65
NSAID	316	2.08	1.86-2.33
Opioids	202	4.46	3.90-5.09
Minor analgesics	903	1.44	1.34-1.54
Drugs for migraine	78	3.34	2.69-4.15
Anticonvulsants	36	1.53	1.10-2.13
Neuroleptics	153	5.40	4.66-6.25
Sedatives, hypnotics	158	3.87	3.33-4.50
Antidepressants	316	2.92	2.61-3.26
Drugs for rhinitis	173	1.50	1.29-1.75
Antiasthmatics	407	1.59	1.44-1.76
Antitussives	65	1.51	1.18-2.88
Antihistamines	1131	2.71	2.60-2.98

Table 8.4. Maternal delivery diagnoses associated with the use of drugs for stomach ulcer or gastro-oesophageal reflux

Diagnosis	Drug in early pregnancy			Drug later in pregnancy		
	Number	OR	95%CI	Number	OR	95% CI
Pre-existing diabetes	124	1.05	0.87-1.26	87	1.09	0.87-1.35
Chronic hypertension	125	1.14	0.95-1.36	85	1.13	0.91-1.41
Gestational diabetes	102	1.21	0.99-1.47	53	0.93	0.71-1.23
Preeclampsia	474	1.21	1.10-1.33	303	1.29	1.14-1.45
Hyperemesis gravidarum	134	1.47	1.23-1.74	97	1.56	1.28-1.92
Placenta previa	125	1.21	1.01-1.45	70	1.00	0.78-1.27
Abruptio placentae	134	1.19	1.00-1.41	75	0.96	0.76-1.22
Antepartum bleeding	145	1.19	1.01-1.41	75	0.96	0.76-1.22
Intrapartum bleeding	208	1.12	0.97-1.28	141	1.12	0.94-1.33
Postpartum bleeding	462	1.01	0.92-1.11	274	1.02	0.91-1.16
Delivery induction	1055	1.21	1.13-1.30	726	1.39	1.28-1.51
Caesarean section	1628	1.26	1.19-1.36	1019	1.28	1.19-1.38

There is thus an increased rate of pre-existing diseases but also of conditions associated with the pregnancy, resulting in an increased risk of caesarean section and delivery induction in deliveries that did not start with a caesarean. There are no major differences between early and later exposure.

Outcome after Maternal use of Drugs for Stomach Ulcer or Gastro-Oesophageal Reflux

Infant Sex

When the mother had used drugs for stomach ulcer or gastro-oesophageal reflux in early pregnancy, 4036 infants were male and 4009 female (two with unknown sex) which gives a sex ratio of 1.01 (95% CI 0.96-1.05), a slightly low sex ratio. This indicates an excess of pregnancies with strong NVP which is associated with an excess of female infants. When drug use has occurred later in pregnancy, the sex ratio was slightly low: 2398 males, 2335 females (one unknown sex) which gives a sex ratio of 1.03 (95% CI 0.97-1.09) but the normal sex ratio (1.06) lies within the confidence interval.

Table 8.5. Pregnancy duration and infant birth weight at maternal use of drugs for stomach ulcer or gastro-oesophageal reflux. Only singleton births

Variable studied	Drugs	Drug use in early pregnancy			Drug use later in pregnancy		
		Number	OR	95% CI	Number	OR	95% CI
<37 weeks	All	499	1.27	1.16-1.40	269	1.17	1.03-1.32
	A02BA	116	1.06	0.88-1.28	37	0.92	0.66-1.29
	A02BC	332	1.40	1.25-1.56	179	1.27	1.09-1.48
	A02BX	62	1.05	0.81-1.36	66	1.12	0.87-1.44
<2500g	All	307	1.20	1.06-1.34	165	1.12	0.95-1.31
	A02BA	73	1.07	0.81-1.30	24	0.97	0.64-1.47
	A02BC	202	1.28	1.11-1.48	109	1.19	0.98-1.45
	A02BX	40	1.08	0.79-1.49	37	0.98	0.70-1.37
≥4500g	All	352	1.07	0.96-1.19	194	0.95	0.82-1.10
	A02BA	82	0.94	0.76-1.18	26	0.69	0.46-1.02
	A02BC	220	1.11	0.97-1.28	110	0.95	0.70-1.18
	A02BX	64	1.12	0.87-1.45	57	1.09	0.83-1.43
SGA	All	201	1.12	0.97-1.29	114	1.15	0.95-1.39
	A02BA	50	0.97	0.73-1.29	18	1.07	0.66-1.72
	A02BC	122	1.11	0.82-1.33	76	1.23	0.97-1.55
	A02BX	33	1.35	0.95-1.92	23	0.94	0.62-1.43
LGA	All	508	1.05	0.96-1.15	328	1.08	0.96-1.21
	A02BA	130	1.05	0.87-1.26	57	1.01	0.79-1.34
	A02BC	304	1.05	0.93-1.18	192	1.05	0.90-1.22
	A02BX	94	1.07	0.86-1.34	92	1.18	0.95-1.47

A02BA = histamine-2 antagonists, A02BC = proton pump inhibitors, A02BX = other, mainly sucralfate.

Multiple Births

There were 128 twin pairs and two triplet sets after maternal use of drugs for stomach ulcer or gastro-oesophageal reflux in early pregnancy. The OR for twin delivery was 1.04

with a 95% CI of 0.87-1.24. After such drug use later in pregnancy, there were 74 twin and one triplet delivery. The OR for twin delivery was 1.04, 95% CI 0.83-1.32.

The total group ("All") shows an excess of preterm births which is of the same order of magnitude after exposure in early or late pregnancy and which apparently is restricted to exposure to proton pump inhibitors.

Table 8.6. Infant mortality (Including multiple births)

Variable studied	Drug use in early pregnancy			Drug use later in pregnancy		
	Number	OR	95% CI	Number	OR	95% CI
Stillbirth	35	1.16	0.83-1.62	12	0.68	0.39-1.21
Early neonatal death	7	0.55	0.22-1.13	1	0.13	0.01-0.75#

#observed over expected number with exact Poisson confidence interval.

Infant mortality is thus if anything low.

Table 8.7. Neonatal diagnoses after maternal use of drugs for stomach ulcer and gastro-oesophageal reflux

Diagnosis	Drug use in early pregnancy			Drug use later in pregnancy		
	Number	OR	95% CI	Number	OR	95% CI
Hypoglycaemia	271	0.88	0.78-0.99	162	0.90	0.77-1.05
Respiratory diagnoses	374	0.90	0.81-1.00	209	0.91	0.79-1.04
Low Apgar score	104	0.65	0.53-0.78	70	0.79	0.62-1.01
CNS diagnoses	65	1.23	0.96-1.58	43	1.25	0.91-1.70
Jaundice	411	1.23	1.11-1.36	250	1.27	1.12-1.44

The only increased risk was for jaundice and possibly for CNS diagnoses (although not statistically significant) while for other diagnoses even low risks were indicated.

Sucralfate

The only significantly increased risk estimate concerns sucralfate, a prescription drug in Sweden, which acts locally with only little systemic absorption. Among five infants with chromosome anomalies, three had Down syndrome (maternal age 33, 33, and 37 years), one had trisomy 18 (maternal age 32) and one had Wolf-Hirchhorn syndrome (maternal age 28).

Among the 55 infants with other relatively severe malformations, 21 had cardiovascular defects, five had hypospadias, four had limb reduction defects, and three had orofacial clefts. .

Only two of these infants had been exposed to a drug with known or suspected teratogenicity. One infant had bile duct atresia and subaortic valve stenosis. The mother had also reported the use of carbamazepine. The second infant had craniostenosis and VSD and the mother had also used propylthiouracil. Among other maternal concomitant drug use in this group of infants were mainly found antihistamines.

Table 8.8. Congenital malformations in infants whose mothers used drugs for stomach ulcer or gastro-oesophageal reflux

Congenital malformations	Number	OR/RR	95% CI
All drugs			
All malformations	400	1.05	0.95-1.16
Relative severe malformations	288	1.10	0.98-1.24
Chromosome anomalies	17	0.97	0.60-1.57
Without chromosome anomalies:			
Any CNS malformation	10	1.08	0.52-1.98#
Neural tube defects	3	1.03	0.21-3.02#
Eye malformations	9	1.18	0.54-2.24#
Ear malformations	13	0.70	0.40-1.20
Orofacial clefts	8	0.55	0.28-1.09
Cardiovascular defect	110	1.28	1.06-1.55
VSD and/or ASD	52	1.14	0.86-1.50
Unspecified cardiac defects	13	1.70	0.99-2.94
Oesophageal atresia/stenosis	3	1.31	0.27-3.83#
Small gut atresia/stenosis	6	2.92	1.07-6.37#
Anal atresia/stenosis	4	1.19	0.32-3.04#
Pylorostenosis	5	0.94	0.30-2.19#
Hypospadias	23	0.97	0.64-1.48
Severe kidney malformations	4	0.82	0.22-2.10#
Pes equinovarus	10	0.83	0.45-1.56
Poly/syndactyly	14	0.84	0.49-1.44
Limb reduction defect	10	2.15	1.03-3.96#
Hip (sub)luxation, unstable hip	49	1.00	0.75-1.32
Craniostenosis	6	1.23	0.45-2.67#
Histamine-2 antagonists (n=2159)			
All malformations	114	1.10	0.91-1.33
Relatively severe malformations	73	1.01	0.81-1.29
Cardiovascular defects	25	1.09	0.73-1.63
Hypospadias	5	0.81	0.26-1.88#
Proton punp inhibitors (n=4872)			
All malformations	219	0.95	0.83-1.09
Relatively severe malformations	161	1.02	0.87-1.20
Cardiovascular defects	64	1.21	0.94-1.56
Hypospadias	15	1.02	0.60-1.73
Other drugs (n=1312)			
All malformations	81	1.31	1.05-1.65
Relatively severe malformations	62	1.47	1.13-1.70
Cardiovascular defects	22	1.62	1.06-2.48
Hypospadias	5	1.45	0.47-3.38#

#observed over expected number with exact Poisson confidence interval.

Effects of Concomitant Drug Use

In order to see to what extent these effects are due to concomitant drug use in excess of what could be expected, the analyses of outcome after 1st trimester exposure were repeated after exclusion of cases where exposure was reported for one or more of the following drugs: drugs for immunological bowel disease, hypertension, oral contraceptives, systemic corticoids, thyroid drugs, antibiotics, NSAID, analgesics, neuroleptics, sedatives, hypnotics, anticonvulsants, drugs used for rhinitis or asthma, or cough medicines. A total of 4 789 infants remained born of 4 616 women (Table 8.10).

Table 8.9. Relatively severe malformations and individual drugs (at least 50 exposures)

Drug	Number of infants				
	Malformed	Total	Per cent	OR/RR	95%CI
Cimetidine	4	96	6.4	1.21	0.33-3.09#
Ranitidine	53	1640	3.4	0.98	0.74-1.29
Famotidine	16	436	4.1	1.08	0.66-1.79
Omeprazole	129	3746	2.3	1.02	0.89-1.27
Pantoprazole	1	110	1.1	0.29	0.01-1.63#
Lansoprazole	27	811	3.7	1.04	0.70-1.55
Esomeprazole	7	268	3.0	0.85	0.34-1.74#
Sucralfate	60	1295	4.6	1.44	1.15-1.86

#observed over expected number with exact Poisson confidence interval.

Table 8.10. Maternal and infant characteristics after maternal use of drugs for stomach ulcer and gastro-oesophageal reflux after removal from the analysis of women who used some other specified drugs

Outcome	Number with outcome	OR	95% CI
Maternal diagnoses			
Pre-existing diabetes	73	1.19	0.88-1.42
Chronic hypertension	68	1.12	0.88-1.43
Gestational diabetes	63	1.35	1.05-1.74
Preeclampsia	263	1.17	1.03-1.33
Placenta previa	74	1.29	1.02-1.62
Abruptio placenta	76	1.21	0.96-1.53
Antepartum bleeding	86	1.21	0.98-1.50
Intrapartum bleeding	118	1.13	0.94-1.35
Postpartum bleeding	296	1.12	0.99-1.26
Delivery induction	571	1.11	1.01-1.21
Caesarean section	870	1.15	1.07-1.24
Infant characteristics			
<37 weeks	253	1.08	0.95-1.23
<2500 g	164	1.08	0.90-1.27
≥4500g	204	1.06	0.92-1.22
SGA	104	1.00	0.79-1.17
LGA	282	1.00	0.89-1,14
Hypoglycaemia	158	0.87	0.74-1.02
Respiratory diagnoses	211	0.86	0.75-0.99
Low Apgar score	53	0.55	0.81-1.21
CNS diagnoses	36	1.15	0.83-1.60
Jaundice	235	1.11	1.03-1.35
Any congenital malformation	227	0.98	0.86-1.12

Thus, the only statistically significant effect on the infants which remained was jaundice. It is probable that the effects seen were due to confounding by associated conditions, apparent as the use of other drugs. On the other hand, the odds ratios for maternal complications remained basically unchanged, indicating a direct association between conditions which caused use of drugs for gastric ulcer or gastro-oesophageal reflux in early pregnancy and certain maternal complications.

SUMMARY

The use of drugs for gastric ulcer or gastro-oesophageal reflux seems to have no certain ill effects on the infants born. In the crude analysis, an increased risk for preterm birth, low birth weight, and neonatal pathology was seen but these effects appear to be secondary to conditions which co-vary with the use of such drugs. No general teratogenic effect was seen but an increased risk was noted after the use of sucralfate which is unlikely to be causal because there is little systemic absorption. An association between the use of this type of drugs in early pregnancy and some maternal pregnancy complications was seen, probably due to a confounding by indication.

REFERENCES

[1] Diav-Citrin O, Arnon J, Shechtman S, Schaefer C, van Tonningen MR, Celmenti M, de Santis M, Robert-Gnansia E, Valti E, Malm H, Ornoy A. The safety of proton pump inhibitors in pregnancy: a multicentre prospective controlled study. *Aliment Pharmacol Ther* 2005; 21: 269-75.

[2] Källén B. Delivery outcome after the use of acid-suppressing drugs in early pregnancy with special reference to omeprazole. *Br J Obstet Gynaecol* 1998; 105:877-81.

[3] Källén BA. Use of omeprazole during pregnancy no hazard demonstrated in 955 infants exposed during pregnancy. *Eur J Obstet Gynecol Reprod Biol* 2001; 96:63-8.

[4] Mahadevan U, Kane S. American Gastroenterological Association Institute technical review on the use of gastrointestinal medications in pregnancy. *Gastroenterology 2006; 131: 283-311.*

[5] Ruigómez A, García Rodríguez LA, Cattaruzzi C, Troncon MG, Agostinis L, Wallander MA, Johansson S. Use of cimetidine, omeprazole, and ranitidine in pregnant women and pregnancy outcomes. *Am J Epidemiol* 1999; 150: 476-81.

Chapter 9

DRUGS USED FOR FUNCTIONAL INTESTINAL SYMPTOMS

Use of spasmolytics during pregnancy is relatively rare and even if a tendency to an increased rate of pregnancy complications could be seen, the confidence intervals were large. There were no signs of a teratogenic effect of these drugs. Propulsives consisted mainly of metoclopramiDe which has a major indication at nausea and vomiting in pregnancy. It is therefore understandable that a strong association with this drug and hyperemesis gravidarum existed. No evidence exists for a teratogenic effect of metoclopramide which is in agreement with the data in the literature. In many countries, this drug is the drug of choice in the treatment of nausea and vomiting in pregnancy. Both for spasmolytics and propulsives, an increased risk for caesarean section or delivery induction was seen. These effects may be the result of underlying pathology, e.g., hyperemesis gravidarum.

This group of drugs contains anticholinergic drugs (spasmolytics) and propulsives. An association between use of anticholinergic drugs and minor malformations in the offspring was indicated in an early study with a 30% over-risk [1]. More recent data are available on the use of the propulsive drug metochlorpramide without any signs of ill effects on the delivery outcome [2-4], but most of these studies are of limited size.

CHARACTERISTICS OF WOMEN USING DRUGS FOR FUNCTIONAL INTESTINAL SYMPTOMS

Based on women reporting the drug in early pregnancy (n=2412, 1815 of them with propulsives, 597 with spasmolytics). Each variable is adjusted for all other variables and year of delivery. Comparison with all women who gave birth during the period and with information from the first antenatal care (n=967 742) (Table 9.2)

Table 9.1. Number of women identified with use of drugs for functional intestinal symptoms

Total:	3250
Reported use in early pregnancy	2412
Got prescription later in pregnancy	1249
Both early and late use	406

Type of drug	ATC code	Early use	Later use
Anticholinergics	A03AB, A03BA, A03BB	207	91
Propantheline	A03AB05	4	0
Mepenzolate	A03AB12	113	58
Hyoscyamine	A03BA03	58	28
Butylscopolamine	A03BB01	34	6
Spasmolytics of papaverine type	A03AD	374	276
Papaverine	A03AD01	373	276
Moxaverine	A03AD30	1	0
Spasmolytics with psycholeptics		20	5
Clinidium	A03CA02	18	3
Oxyphencyclimine	A03CA03	2	2
Propulsives	A03FA	1815	884
Metoclopramide	A03FA01	1713	858
Cisapride	A03FA02	103	26
Unspecified	A03	6	6

Some women used two drugs of different categories

	Papaverine-like	Spasmolytic + psyhcoleptic	Propulsives
Early pregnancy use			
Anticholinergics	5	1	1
Papaverine-like		3	
Late pregnancy use			
Anticholinergics	7		2
Papaverine-like			4

The two groups of drugs thus show some markedly different associations with use of other drugs. Thus, for instance, there is a positive association with vitamin/folic acid use and spasmolytics but an opposite association with propulsives. Had the association been caused by reporting bias (women reporting one drug may be more apt to report vitamins), one would expect similar associations for both drug uses. Antibiotics are associated with spasmolytics but not with propulsives. Antihistamines are strongly associated with propulsives but less markedly with spasmolytics. The latter phenomenon is due to the use of metoclopramide at NVP: the association is specifically strong with antihistamines mainly used for NVP like meclozine and much weaker for antihistamines mainly used for allergy.

Table 9.2. Characteristics of women using drugs for functional intestinal symptoms in early pregnancy

Variable	Spasmolytics			Propulsives		
	Number of women with drug	OR	95% CI	Number of women with drug	OR	95%CI
Maternal age						
<25	98	0.99	0.79-1.25	271	1.13	0.98-1.29
25-34	392	1.00	reference	1227	1.00	reference
≥35	107	1.04	0.89-1.32	317	0.89	0.79-1.02
Parity						
1	277	1.20	1.01-1.43	654	0.68	0.62-0.76
≥2	320	1.00	reference	1161	1.00	reference
Smoking						
Unknown	24	-		38	-	
None	480	1.00	reference	1673	1.00	reference
Yes	93	1.75	1.23-2.48	104	0.46	0.32-0.68
Earlier miscarriages						
None	468	1.00	reference	1356	1.00	reference
Yes	129	1.04	0.85-1.27	459	1.31	1.18-1.46
BMI						
Unknown	66	-		158	-	
<19.8	51	1.39	1.03-1.88	209	1.57	1.35-1.82
19.8-25.9	275	1.00	reference	1022	1.00	reference
≥26	205	1.72	1.42-2.08	408	0.91	0.81-1.02
Subfertility (years of unwanted childlessness)						
0	545	1.00	reference	1687	1.00	reference
Any subfertility	52	1.20	0.89-1.61	128	1.10	0.91-1.32
Education (1996-2001 , 297 women with spasmolytics, 879 with propulsives, 526 695 in population						
Unknown	8	-		33	-	
<12 years	40	1.12	0.77-1.62	111	1.12	0.77-1.62
12 years	167	1.00	reference	443	1.00	reference
13-14 years	9	0.47	0.24-0.92	36	0.47	0.24-0.92
≥14 years	73	0.74	0.56-0.99	256	0.74	0.56-0.99
Country of birth						
Unknown	4	-		22	-	
Sweden	507	1.00	reference	1324	1.00	reference
Other Nordic country	13	0.90	0.52-1.56	32	0.89	0.62-1.27
Non-Nordic country	73	0.75	0.59-0.95	437	1.65	1.48-1.84
Family situation						
Unknown	12	-		25	-	
Co-habiting	563	1.00	references	1706	1.00	referens
Living alone	20	1.03	0.64-1.65	41	1.02	0.74-1.39
Other family situation	2	0.11	-	43	0.95	0.70-1.28
Work outside home						
Unknown	93	-		246	-	
Full time	233	1.00	reference	736	1.00	reference
Part time	158	1.37	1.10-1.69	462	1.08	0.96-1.21
None	113	1.33	1.05-1.67	371	1.27	1.12-1.45

It can be noted that very different effects are seen of some variables between the drug groups, e.g., parity, smoking, high BMI, woman being born in a non-Nordic country.

Table 9.3. Concomitant drug use (early pregnancy)

Drug group	Spasmolytics			Propulsives		
	Number	OR/RR	95% CI	Number	OR/RR	95%CI
Drugs for stomach ulcer and reflux	47	8.29	6.09-11.0	133	9.99	8.63-11.6
Drugs for inflammatory bowel disease	7	5.00	2.01-10.3#	2	0.79	0.01-2.87#
Insulin	1	0.50	0.01-2.77#	8	1.36	0.59-2.67#
Multivitamins	37	1.37	0.95-1.99	56	0.57	0.43-0.76
Folic acid	38	1.62	1.15-2.28	68	0.84	0.65-1.07
Drugs for hypertension	4	1.59	0.43-4.06#	12	1.77	0.91-3.09#
Oral contraceptive	6	2.87	1.05-6.25#	4	0.65	0.18-1.67#
Progestogens	4	1.50	0.41-3.85#	16	2.40	1.37-3.90#
Gonadotrophins	2	1.45	0.18-5.24#	6	1.53	0.56-3.32#
Systemic corticosteroids	2	0.96	0.12-3.46#	14	2.17	1.18-3.64#
Thyroid drugs	5	0.67	0.22-1.56#	26	1.15	0.78-1.69
Antibiotics	37	2.03	1.46-2.81	60	1.09	0.84-1.41
NSAID	33	3.14	2.22-4.44	41	1.34	0.98-1.82
Opioids	36	10.8	7.23-14.9	41	4.81	3.45-6.53#
Minor analgesics	67	1.49	1.15-1.92	203	1.53	1.32-1.77
Drugs for migraine	2	1.02	0.12-3.68#	19	3.91	2.35-6.10#
Anticonvulsants	0	0.00	0.00-2.10#	5	1.05	0.34-2.46#
Sedatives, hypnotics	15	1.95	1.09-3.22#	25	3.44	2.23-5.08#
Antidepressants	12	1.57	0.81-2.74#	50	2.54	1.92-3.34
Drugs for rhinitis	14	1.68	0.92-2.82#	16	0.65	0.40-1.07
Antiasthmatics	35	1.79	1.27-2.51	64	1.22	0.95-1.56
Antitussives	2	0.66	0.08-2.37#	9	0.98	0.45-1.87
Antihistamines	60	1.87	1.44-2.44	881	15.9	14.5-16.5
For NVP	43	1.74	1.28-2.36	800	16.6	15.5-17.8
For allergy	21	2.31	1.51-3.53	165	6.58	5.71-7.57

#observed over expected number with exact Poisson confidence interval.

Table 9.4. Some maternal delivery diagnoses associated with the use of spasmolytics

Diagnosis	Drug in early pregnancy			Drug later in pregnancy		
	Number	OR	95%CI	Number	OR	95% CI
Pre-existing diabetes	11	1.25	0.62-2.23#	3	0.50	0.10-1.45#
Gestational diabetes	12	1.79	0.92-3.12#	3	0.68	0.14-1.99#
Preeclampsia	37	1.26	0.90-1.77	16	0.84	0.51-1.40
Hyperemesis	12	1.70	0.88-2.98#	4	0.82	0.22-2.09#
Chronic hypertension	10	1.15	0.55-2.12#	6	1.05	0.38-2.28#
Placenta previa	11	1.42	0.71-2.54#	4	0.74	0.20-1.90#
Abruptio placentae	13	1.49	0.79-2.55#	6	1.01	0.37-2.20#
Antepartum bleeding	14	1.49	0.81-2.49#	5	0.83	0.27-1.94#
Intrapartum bleeding	20	1.52	0.97-2.38	88	0.83	0.36-1.64
Postpartum bleeding	48	1.39	1.03-1.86	22	1.04	0.68-1.60
Delivery induction	90	1.45	1.15-1.82	53	1.32	0.99-1.27
Caesarean section	121	1.27	1.03-1.56	65	1.02	0.78-1.34

For spasmolytics, many conditions show ORs around 1.5 but due to small numbers, few are statistically significant and all refer to first trimester exposures. Both delivery inductions and caesarean sections occur in excess. For propulsives, most ORs lie around 1.0 after first trimester exposures with an exception for hyperemesis, placenta abruption and antepartum bleeding and after later exposure the majority lie below 1.0 with the exception of hyperemesis. Also after these drugs, delivery induction and caesarean section occur in excess.

Table 9.5. Some maternal delivery diagnoses associated with the use of propulsives

Diagnosis	Drug in early pregnancy			Drug later in pregnancy		
	Number	OR	95%CI	Number	OR	95% CI
Pre-existing diabetes	30	1.30	0.91-1.98	9	0.71	0.37-1.38
Gestational diabetes	23	1.41	0.95-2.28	6	0.71	0.26-1.74#
Preeclampsia	85	1.13	0.80-1.31	39	0.96	0.70-1.34
Hyperemesis	73	4.17	3.35-5.19	32	3.34	2.38-4.69
Chronic hypertension	23	1.11	0.70-1.83	8	0.72	0.36-1.45
Placenta previa	24	1.18	0.33-1.79	6	0.55	0.25-1.22
Abruptio placentae	29	1.32	0.84-1.89	10	0.86	0.46-1.62
Antepartum bleeding	33	1.36	1.02-2.09	9	0.75	0.39-1.45
Intrapartum bleeding	41	1.12	0.79-1.57	21	1.05	0.68-1.63
Postpartum bleeding	94	0.94	0.75-1.18	27	0.55	0.38-0.70
Delivery induction	226	1.26	1.07-1.46	127	1.37	1.14-1.65
Caesarean section	325	1.24	1.07-1.40	165	1.24	1.05-1.48

#observed over expected number with exact Poisson confidence interval.

OUTCOME AFTER MATERNAL USE OF DRUGS FOR FUNCTIONAL INTESTINAL SYMPTOMS

Infant Sex

When the mothers had used spasmolytics in early pregnancy, 325 of the children were male and 280 female, a sex ratio of 1.16 (95% CI 0.99-1.36) and when they had used it in late pregnancy there was a male excess: 217 males and 154 females, sex ratio 1.41 (95% CI 1.15-1.74). The normal sex ratio is 1.06. When the mothers had used propulsives in early pregnancy there were 860 males and 998 females, sex ratio 0.86 (95% CI 0.79-0.94) and when they had used it in late pregnancy, there were 429 males and 478 females, a sex ratio 0.90 (95% CI 0.79-1.02). The low sex ratio is expected after the use of metoclopramide which is often given at NVP.

Multiple Births

After maternal use of spasmolytics in early pregnancy, there were nine twin deliveries and no higher order multiples. The OR for twinning was 1.00 (95%CI 0.52-1.93). After maternal use of propulsives, there were 43 twin pairs. The OR for twinning was 1.60 (95% CI 1.18-2.17). The high twinning risk after propulsives is expected after the use of metoclopramine for NVP (42 of the 43 twin pairs), a condition which is more common in twin pregnancies than in singleton pregnancies.

After maternal use of spasmolytics, an increased risk for low birth weight is seen both in early and later pregnancy. After use of propulsives, an increased rate of SGA was seen (significant only after later exposure). No other outcome showed a statistically significant effect.

Table 9.6. Pregnancy duration and infant birth weight at maternal use of drugs for functional intestinal symptoms. Only singleton births

Variable studied	Drugs	Drug use in early pregnancy			Drug use later in pregnancy		
		Number	OR	95% CI	Number	OR	95% CI
<37 weeks	Spasmolytics	35	1.19	0.85-1.68	25	1.42	0.94-2.13
	Propulsives	88	1.09	0.88-1.35	48	1.22	0.91-1.64
<2500g	Spasmolytics	28	1.47	1.01-2.16	19	1.71	1.08-2.91
	Propulsives	49	0.96	0.73-1.28	30	1.26	0.88-1.82
≥4500g	Spasmolytics	18	0.70	0.44-1.12	17	1.07	0.66-1.73
	Propulsives	82	1.09	0.87-1.36	37	0.97	0.70-1.35
SGA	Spasmolytics	19	1.38	0.97-2.18	9	1.18	0.54-2.25#
	Propulsives	39	1.20	0.87-1.65	25	1.61	1.08-2.39
LGA	Spasmolytics	36	0.97	0.64-1.36	19	0.78	0.49-1.24
	Propulsives	127	1.09	0.91-1.31	56	0.94	0.72-1.24

#observed over expected number with exact Poisson confidence interval.

Table 9.7. Infant mortality after maternal use of drugs for functional intestinal symptoms

Variable studied	Drug	Drug use in early pregnancy			Drug use later in pregnancy		
		Number	OR	95% CI	Number	OR	95% CI
Stillbirth	Spasmolytics	3	1.39	0.29-4.05 #	4	1.28	0.85-7.99#
	Propulsives	6	1.09	0.40-2.38#	3	1.20	0.25-3.51#
Early neonatal death	Spasmolytics	0	-	-	1	0.56	0.04-9.98#
	Propulsives	3	1.17	0.24-3.41#	0	-	-

#observed over expected number with exact Poisson confidence interval.

There are no firm evidence of an increased perinatal mortality but due to low number of deaths, confidence intervals are wide.

Table 9.8. Neonatal diagnoses after maternal use of drugs for functional intestinal symptoms

Diagnosis	Drugs	Drug use in early pregnancy			Drug use later in pregnancy		
		Number	OR	95% CI	Number	OR	95% CI
Hypoglycaemia	Spasmolytics	29	1.30	0.89-1.88	20	1.49	0.95-2.33
	Propulsives	62	1.01	0.79-1.31	31	1.00	0.70-1.44
Respiratory diagnoses	Spasmolytics	35	1.10	0.78-1.55	13	0.72	0.41-1.25
	Propulsives	112	1.32	1.09-1.60	48	1.20	0.89-1.60
Low Apgar score	Spasmolytics	11	0.89	0.49-1.62	9	1.33	0.61-2.53#
	Propulsives	47	1.43	1.07-1.91	13	0.85	0.49-1.46
CNS diagnoses	Spasmolytics	9	1.52	0.69-2.88#	3	1.17	0.24-3.41#
	Propulsives	21	1.39	0.90-2.14	9	1.44	0.66-2.72#
Jaundice	Spasmolytics	31	1.15	0.80-1.64	19	1.12	0.71-1.79
	Propulsives	97	1.29	1.05-1.58	61	1.59	1.23-2.06

#observed over expected number with exact Poisson confidence interval.

After maternal use of propulsives (mainly metoclopramide), an increased risk is seen for respiratory diagnoses and low Apgar score and for jaundice. No other deviations reach statistical significance.

There is no statistically significant increase in the rate of any congenital malformation, neither after the use of spasmolytics, nor propulsives (Table 9.9). There were two infants with limb reduction defects after maternal use of spasmolytics. Both had absent hands, one of them also epidermolysis bullosa letalis. Both mothers had used papaverine. Two children had abdominal wall defects (one of them also had diaphragmatic hernia and double outlet right ventricle, the other also had ventricular septum defect). Both mothers had used metoclopramide.

Table 9.9. Congenital malformations in infants whose mothers used drugs for functional intestinal symptoms

Congenital malformations	Number	OR/RR	95% CI
Spasmolytics			
All malformations	33	1.11	0.75-1.66
Relative severe malformations	24	1.09	0.68-1.75
Chromosome anomalies	2	2.05	0.25-7.39#
Without chromosome anomalies:			
Cardiovascular defect	8	1.34	0.63-2.84#
Hypospadias	4	2.04	0.56-5.23#
Limb reduction defect	2	5.74	0.69-20.7#
Propulsives			
All malformations	80	0.92	0.72-1.16
Relative severe malformations	55	0.87	0.65-1.15
Chromosome anomalies	3	0.84	0.17-2.46#
Without chromosome anomalies:			
Cardiovascular defect	20	1.18	0.76-1.84
Orofacial cleft	2	0.56	0.07-2.03#
Oesophageal atresia/stenosis	2	3.90	0.47-14.1#
Abdominal wall defect	2	4.16	0.50-15.0#
Hypospadias	3	0.62	0.12-1.65#
Pes equinovarus	2	0.83	0.10-3.00#

SUMMARY

Very few abnormalities were noticed after the use of drugs for functional intestinal symptoms. After maternal use of spasmolytics, a tendency to high odds ratios for many pregnancy and delivery complications was seen. Use of propulsives was significantly associated with hyperemesis gravidarum which is obviously due to the use of metoclopramide for NVP. For both groups, delivery induction and caesarean sections occurred in excess. An increased risk for low birth weight was seen after spasmolytics both early and later in pregnancy. After late use of propulsives, an increased risk for small-for-gestational age was seen. It is unclear to what extent these possible effects are related to the drugs or to underlying conditions.

REFERENCES

[1] Heinonen OP, Slone D, Shapiro S. *Birth Defects and Drugs in pregnancy*. Publishing Sciences Group, Inc. Littleton, Mass. 1977.

[2] Asker C, Norstedt Wikner B, Källén B. Use of antiemetic drugs during pregnancy in Sweden. *Eur J Clin Pharmacol* 2005; 61:899-906.

[3] Berkovitch M, Mazzota P, Greenberg, Elbirt D, Addis A, Schuler-Faccini L, Merlob P, Arnon J, Stahl B, Magee L, Moretti M, Ornoy A. Metoclopramide for nausea and vomiting of pregnancy: a prospective multicenter international study. *Am J Perinatol* 2002; 19: 311-316.

[4] Sørensen HT, Nielsen GL, Christensen K, Tage-Jensen U, Ekbom A, Baron J & the Euromap study group. Birth outcome following maternal use of metoclopramide. *Br J Clin Pharmacol* 2000; 49: 264-268.

Chapter 10

ANTI-EMETIC DRUGS

Relatively little knowledge exists on the possible risks associated with the use of the anti-emetic drug ondansetron and still less for granisetron. It is therefore not possible to exclude a teratogenic effect and the drugs should be avoided, notably in early pregnancy. If exposure has already occurred during the first trimester, there is no evidence that it is harmful and therefore a discussion of a termination of pregnancy is not motivated. The same is true for the use of scopolamine.

This chapter deals with drugs listed under the ATC code heading of A04A which excludes some common drugs used as antiemetics, especially antihistamines, metoclopromide, dixyrazine, prochloperazine. These are dealt with in other chapters of this book.

There are two main reasons for the use of antiemetic drugs during pregnancy: postoperaive vomiting or vomiting related to chemotherapy or irradiation and vomiting associated with pregnancy: NVP. The first indications are relatively uncommon in pregnancy and at NVP usually other drugs are preferred. Therefore, the number of women using these drugs will be low. Relatively little information is available in the literature on the use of this drug category during pregnancy [1,2] with the exception of scopolamine for which an early study found no teratogenic effect based on 309 first trimester exposures [3]. In Sweden, scopolamine is used as an anti-emetic administered as a plaster and is used for moving sickness but also for NVP.

Table 10.1. Number of women identified with use of anti-emetics

Total	171
Reported use in early pregnancy	124
Got prescription later in rpegnancy	87
Both early and late use	40

Type of drug:	ATC code	Early use	Later use
Serotonin (5-HT3) receptor			
antagonists	A0AA	102	82
Ondansetron	A04AA01	101	81
Granisetron	A04AA02	1	1
Parasympathicometic	A04AD	17	5
Scopolamine	A04AD01	17	5
Unspecified	A04A	5	0

Because of the low number of women using these drugs (124), only some characteristics could be analyzed (Table 10.2).

Table 10.2. Characteristics of women using antiemetics

Variable	Number of women with drug	OR	95% CI
Maternal age			
<25	25	2.41	1.50-3.87
25-34	99	1.00	reference
≥35	30	1.28	0.83-1.96
Parity			
1	38	0.51	0.35-0.75
≥2	86	1.00	reference
Smoking			
Unknown	5	-	
None	117	1.00	reference
Any smoking	2	0.23	-
Earlier miscarriage			
None	96	1.00	reference
Yes	28	1.05	0.68-1.61
BMI			
Unknown	14	-	
<19.8	12	1.46	0.79-2.69
19.8-25.9	68	1.00	reference
≥26	30	0.93	0.61-1.41
Subfertility			
None	117	1.00	reference
Yes	7	0.85	0.40-1.84
Country of birth			
Unknown	2		
Sweden	80	1.00	reference
Other Nordic country	2	-	
Non-Nordic country	26	1.33	0.86-2.07
Variable	Number of women with drug	OR	95% CI
Family situation			
Unkown	1	-	
Co-habiting	119	1.00	reference
Living alone	4	1.55	-
Work outside home			
Unknown	15	-	
Full time	40	1.00	reference
Part time	22	0.73	0.43-1.23
None	39	1.60	1.04-2.46

There is thus an excess of low maternal age and multiparity. Other characteristics are based on so low numbers that no statistical significance is reached. A low smoking rate and a trend for decreasing use with increasing BMI is suggested but can thus be random. Women not working outside home had an increased risk of using these antiemetics.

Table 10.3. Concomitant drug use (early pregnancy)

Drug group	Number	RR	95% CI
Antacids	4	7.84	2.14-20.1#
Drugs for stomach ulcer and reflux	20	18.5	11.3-28.6#
Multivitamins	7	0.60	0.27-1.35
Folic acid	5	0.61	0.20-1.41#
Antibiotics	9	1.04	0.48-1.98#
NSAID	3	1.62	0.33-4.34#
Minor analgesics	9	1.04	0.48-1.98#
Antideprssants	8	1.05	0.45-2.06#
Other antiemetic drugs*	51	18.6	14.1-24.6

*Included drugs: metoclopramide, dixyrazine, prochlorperazine, dimenhydrinate, prometazine, cyclicine, meclizine.
#observed over expected number with exact Poisson 95% confidence interval.

The strong association with other antiemetic drugs suggests that the majority of exposures were actually due to NVP. Ondansetron may have been used as a mode stabilizer together with antidepressants.

One woman had also used azathioprine together with drugs for immunological bowel disease. None had used any other cytotoxic drug.

Table 10.4. Some maternal diagnoses associated with the use of anti-emetics

Diagnosis	Drugs in early pregnancy			Drug later in pregnancy		
	Number	OR/RR	95% CI	Number	OR/RR	95% CI
Preeclampsia	6	1.31	0.43-3.06#	4	1.02	0.28-2.61#
Chronic hypertension	0	0.00	0.00-2.60#	2	1.77	0.21-6.39#
Hyperemesis gravidrum	4	3.20	0.87-8.19#	5	5.32	1.73-12.4#
Placenta previa	1	0.70	0.02-3.92#	0	-	-
Intrapartum bleeding	3	1.05	0.12-3.82#	1	0.49	0.01-2.72#
Postpartum bleeding	7	0.63	0.13-1.85	3	0.86	0.23-2.21#
Delivery induction	18	1.40	0.84-2.34	18	2.18	1.28-3.71#
Caesarean section	23	1.21	0.78-1.88	19	1.41	0.87-2.29

#observed over expected number with exact Poisson 95% confidence interval.

There were no cases of pre-existing diabetes, gestational diabetes, abruption of placenta, or antepartum bleeding. The only statistically significant effect is thus for an increased risk of delivery induction after the use of antiemetics in late pregnancy and for hyperemesis after such drug use in late pregancy.

Outcome after Maternal use of Antiemetic Drugs

Infant Sex

After use of antiemetics in early pregnancy, 63 infants were male and 63 female, a sex ratio of 1.00 which is low but the 95% confidence interval (0.70-1.42) includes the normal sex ratio (1.06). A low sex ratio is typical at NVP. After exposure later in pregnancy, there were 51 male and 39 female infants, a sex ratio of 1.31 (95% CI 0.87-2.02).

Multiple Births

After the use of antiemetics in early pregnancy there was only two twin births among the 126 deliveries, after late exposure there were three among 90.

Table 10.5. Pregnancy duration and infant birth weight at maternal use of antiemetics

Variable studied	Drug use in early pregnancy			Drug use later in pregnancy		
	Number	RR	95% CI	Number	RR	95% CI
<37 weeks	8	1.47	0.64-2.90	7	1.79	0.72-3.70
<2500g	6	1.88	0.69-4.08	0	-	-
≥4500g	8	1.51	0.65-2.97	6	1.74	0.43-4.08
SGA	4	1.93	0.53-4.95	1	0.65	0.02-2.59
LGA	15	1.73	0.97-2.85	11	2.06	1.03-3.69

All outcome risks are based on small numbers. The most suggestive finding is an increased probability for LGA infants, suggested after early and significant after late exposure.

Table 10.6. Infant mortality after maternal use of antiemetics

Variable studied	Drug use in early pregnancy			Drug use later in pregnancy		
	Number	RR	95% CI	Number	RR	95% CI
Stillbirth	1	3.29	0.08-18.3	2	9.11	1.10-32.9
Early neonatal death	0	-	-	0	-	-

Only few deaths occurred and risk estimates are uncertain.

Table 10.7. Neonatal diagnoses after maternal use of antiemetics

Diagnosis	Drugs use in early prgnancy			Drug use later in pregnancy		
	Number	RR	95% CI	Number	RR	95% CI
Hypoglycaemia	8	1.93	0.83-3.81	4	1.33	0.36-3.41
Respiratory diagnoses	8	1.45	0.63-2.86	5	1.24	0.40-2.90
Low Apgar score	4	2.11	0.57-5.39	2	1.34	0.16-4.85
CNS diagnoses	5	5.81	1.89-13.6	1	1.49	0.04-8.32
Jaundice	8	1.48	0.64-2.91	6	1.51	0.55-3.79

Numbers are low and confidence intervals wide. The only outcome which reaches statistical significance is CNS diagnoses after early pregnancy exposure but this is based on only five cases. Two of these were twins. Four infants had feeding problems, one convulsions.

Only six infants whose mothers used antiemetic drugs in early pregnancy had a diagnosis of congenital malformations which gives a risk ratio of 1.11 (95% CI 0.41-2.41). The malformations of six infants and the drugs used in early pregnancy were:

1) Pylorostenosis. Scopolamine plaster.
2) Hip dysplasia. Ondansetron.
3) Ventricular and atrium septum defect. Ondansetron, metoclopramide, lansoprazole.
4) Undescended testicle. Ondansetron, prochlorperazine.

5) Anal and ileum stenosis/atresia. Ondansetron.
6) Ventricular septum defect. Ondansetron

Thus five of the malformed infants were exposed to ondansetron (RR = 1.18, 95% CI 0.38-2.75).

SUMMARY

No certain ill effects on delivery outcome was found. Two outcomes showed statistically significant risk increases. One was delivery induction after late use of the drugs, another was an increased risk for CNS diagnoses in the infant after early exposure. The latter observation was based on only five cases and may well be a random event in spite of the formal statistical significance. Furthermore, four of the five cases only had feeding problems. There is still only little information on the malformation risk after early use of ondansetron, and some care should be taken in order to avoid such exposure. The estimated odds ratio has a wide confidence inteval with an upper limit of nearly 3.

REFERENCES

[1] Einarson A, Maltepe C, Navioz Y, Kennedy D, Tan MP, Koren G. The safety of ondansetron for nausea and vomiting of pregnancy: a prospective comparative study. *BJOG* 2004; 111: 940-943.
[2] Asker C, Norstedt Wikner B, Källén B. Use of antiemetic drugs during pregnancy in Sweden. *Europ J Clin Pharmacol* 2005; 61: 899-906.
[3] Heinonen OP, Slone D, Shapiro S. *Birth Defects and Drugs in Pregnancy*. Publishing Sciences Group, Inc. Littleton, Mass. 1977.

Chapter 11

BILE ACID PREPARATIONS

No certain teratogenic effect has been demonstrated of bile acid preparations but enough data are not available to discard such an effect. Therefore, the use of bile acid preparations in early pregnancy should be avoided. If exposure has occurred, there is no reason to discuss a termination of pregnancy. Due to signs of ill effects both on mother an infant after use in late pregnancy, the drugs should be avoided if not necessary for the treatment of the woman.

The primary reason for the use of bile acid preparations in Sweden is the dissolution of gall stones but they are also used at primary biliary cirrhosis. Little is known about the use of such drugs during pregnancy.

Table 11.1. Number of women identified who used bile acid preparations

Total:	386
Reported use in early pregnancy	143
Got prescription later in pregnancy	262
Both early and late use	9

Type of drug	ATC code	Early use	Later use
Ursodeoxycholic acid	A05AA02	130	237
Dehydrocholic acid+cholic acid	A05AA00	0	1
Unspecified cholic acid	A05AA	13	4

Because of the low number of women using these drugs (89), only some characteristics could be analyzed.

There is thus a weak trend for a higher use of these drugs with increasing maternal age and parity and a less often use among full time working women than among women working part time or not at all outside home. As only 23 women using these drugs gave birth before 2002, no effort to analyze the effect of maternal education was made.

Table 11.2 Characteristics of women using antiemetics in early pregnancy

Variable	Number of women with drug	OR	95% CI
Maternal age			
<25	16	0.77	0.44-1.35
25-34	86	1.00	reference
≥35	31	1.21	0.78-1.88
Parity			
1	68	1.21	0.84-1.74
≥2	78	1.00	reference
Smoking			
Unknown	9	-	
None	125	1.00	reference
Any smoking	9	0.80	0.28-2.25
Earlier miscarriage			
None	113	1.00	reference
Yes	30	0.99	0.65-1.52
BMI			
Unknown	13	-	
<19.8	7	0.68	0.31-1.50
19.8-25.9	78	1.00	reference
≥26	45	1.38	0.95-2.00
Subfertility			
None	128	1.00	reference
Yes	15	1.23	0.71-2.13
Country of birth			
Unknown	0		
Sweden	128	1.00	reference
Other Nordic country	3	-	-
Non-Nordic country	12	0.49	0.27-0.89
Family situation			
Unkown	3	-	
Co-habiting	133	1.00	reference
Living alone	2	-	-
Other	5	1.16	0.44-2.06
Work outside home			
Unknown	15	-	-
Full time	59	1.00	reference
Part time	42	1.54	1.01-2.36
None	27	1.37	0.86-2.19

Some drugs are used in very strong excess even though the numbers of exposure are low. The only group with a strong excess and based on large numbers is antihistamines, notably . antihistamines mainly used at allergy.

Most numbers are low but some effects appear clear-cut, notably the increased risk for hyperemesis, bleedings in association with delivery, delivery induction, and (less marked) caesarean sections.

Table 11.3. Concomitant drug use (early pregnancy)

Drug group	Number	OR/RR	95% CI
Drugs for stomach ulcer and reflux	7	5.65	2.27-11.6#
Drugs for inflammatory bowel disease	10	26.3	12.6-48.4#
Multivitamins	31	1.05	0.70-1.87
Folic acid	20	1.16	0.72-1.87
Systemic corticosteroids	5	8.62	2.80-20.1#
Thyroid drugs	6	2.91	1.07-6.34#
Antibiotics	10	2.18	1.04-4.01#
Immune suppressants	6	70.6	25.9-154#
Antiasthmatics	6	1.67	0.61-3.63#
Antihistamines	44	7.07	5.14-9.50#
For NVP	17	3.81	1.59-4.38#
For allergy	35	17.1	11.9-23.7#

#observed over expected number with exact Poisson 95% confidence interval.

Table 11.4. Maternal delivery diagnoses associated with the use of bile acid preparations

Diagnosis	Drug in early pregnancy			Drug later in pregnancy		
	Number	OR/RR	95%CI	Number	OR/RR	95% CI
Pre-existing diabetes	5	2.29	0.74-5.35	10	2.53	1.21-4.64
Gestational diabetes	5	3.36	1.09-7.83	9	3.32	1.52-6.30
Chronic hypertension	5	2.27	0.74-5.30	10	2.67	1.28-4.92
Preeclampsia	15	3.36	1.09-7.83	10	1.40	0.86-2.27
Hyperemesis gravidarum	6	3.53	1.30-7.68	9	2.89	1.32-5.49
Placenta previa	5	2.10	0.55-6.08	9	2.62	1.20-4.98
Abruptio placentae	5	2.40	0.78-5.60	9	2.43	1.11-4.61
Antepartum bleeding	5	2.36	0.77-5.50	10	2.67	1.28-4.92
Intrapartum bleeding	5	1.33	0.43-3.10	18	2.69	1.59-4.25
Postpartum bleeding	9	1.11	0.51-2.10	25	1.72	1.14-2.59
Delivery induction	52	4.32	3.18-5.97	90	4.18	3.30-5.30
Caesarean section	31	1.24	0.82-1.87	61	1.38	1.03-1.84

Outcome after Maternal use of Bile Acid Preparations

Infant Sex

After early exposure, there were 80 male and 71 female infants born, sex ratio 1.13 (95% CI 0.82-1.56) and after later exposure 146 male and 139 female infants, sex ratio 1.05 (95% CI 0.83-1.33). The normal sex ratio of 1.06 was thus included in both confidence intervals.

Multiple Birth

After early exposure there were eight twin deliveries (RR = 3.90, 95% CI 1.69-7.69), after later exposure 24 twin deliveries (RR = 6.33, 95% CI 4.06-9.42). There is thus a marked increase in twinnning rate.

Infant Mortality

Only one infant died neonatally, a stillbirth after late exposure.

Table 11.5. Neonatal diagnoses after maternal use of bile acid prepatations

Diagnosis	Drug use in early pregnancy		Drug use later in pregnancy		
	Number	RR 95%CI	Number	RR	95% CI
Hypoglycaemia	10	1.57 0.75-2.88	17	1.79	1.04-2.86
Respiratory diagnoses	12	1.69 0.88-2.96	27	2.16	1.48-3.19
Low Apgar score	3	1.01 0.21-2.94	8	1.60	0.69-3.15
CNS diagnoses	2	1.56 0.19-5.64	4	1.83	0.50-4.68
Jaundice	9	1.26 0.57-2.39	34	2.82	2.00-3.98

Most numbers are low but after exposure in late pregnancies, increased risks for hypoglycaemia, respiratory diagnoses, and jaundice are statistically significant.

Malformation diagnoses were found in ten infants, RR = 1.42 (95% CI 0.68-2.62). Among them three had hip dysplasia and two undescended testicle. The remaining four infants and the drugs used by the mothers were:

1) Atresia of auditory canal, unilateral cervical cyst, pulmonary valve stenosis. Drugs: ursodeoxycholic acid, iron, promethazine.
2) Microcephaly. Drugs: ursodeoxycholic acid, iron, clemastine, nitrofurantoin.
3) Esophageal atresia, eye malformation, VSD, total anomalous pulmonary vein return. Drugs: ursodeoxycholic acid, mycophenolic acid, tacrolimus, prednisolon. (The patient had a liver transplant).
4) Auditory canal atresia, branchial cyst, pulmonary valve stenosis. Drugs; ursodeoxycholic acid, iron, labetalol, alginic acid, omega-3.
5) Pes equinovarus. Drugs: ursodeoxycholic acid, multivitamins, iron.

The complex malformations in case 3 may be related to the exposure for mycophenolic acid which has a suspected teratogenic activity.

Summary

There is a lack of large studies of bile acid preparations during pregnancy. No teratogenic effect can be demonstrated but the small number of exposed women makes it impossible to adequately evaluate the possible risk. Use in later pregnancy is associated with an increased risk for certain maternal complications, e.g., delivery induction, casesarean section, and postpartum bleeding. Also an increased risk for some neonatal outcomes is seen. These may be related to the high twinning rate.

Chapter 12

LAXATIVES

There is no certain ill effects of the use of laxatives during pregnancy. Associations noted with relatively mild cardiac malformations are probably not causal but may be due to undetected confounding.

Laxatives are usually rearded as harmless during pregnancy [1] but little information is available in the literature. No risk for a congenital malformation was noted after maternal use of some laxatives but the number of exposures was low [2].

Table 12.1. Number of women identified reporting the use of laxatives

Total:	7360
Reported us in early pregnancy	2761
Got prescription in pregnancy	5124
Both early and late use	525

Type of drug:	ATC code	Early use	Later use
Softeners	A06AA	2	4
Liquid paraffin	A06AA01	1	4
Docusate sodium	A06AA02	1	0
Contact laxatives	A06AB	203	111
Bisacodyl	A06AB02	91	24
Castor oil	A06AB05	12	8
Senna glycosides	A06AB06	21	6
Sodium picosulfate	A06AB08	76	63
Cascara combination	A06AB57	6	5
Sodium picosulfate combination	A06AB58	1	6
Bulk producers	A06AC	1272	1787
Spaghula	A06AC01	397	611
Ethulose	A06AC03	833	1044
Triticum	A06AC07	30	97
Spaghula combination	A06AC51	7	1
Unspecified bulk producers	A06AC	11	46
Osmotically active laxatives	A06AD	1317	3351
Manesium oxide	A06AD02	55	1
Mineral salts in combination	A06AD10	44	37
Lactulose	A06AD11	1056	2636

Table 12.1 Continued

Type of drug:	ATC code	Early use	Later use
Lactitol	A06AD12	178	711
Macrogol	A06AD15	0	1
Enemas	A06AG	52	32
Bisacodyl	A06AG02	1	0
Sorbitol	A06AG07	0	3
Docusate sodium	A06AG10	7	9
Laurilsulfate	A06AG11	55	29
Other laxatives	A06AX	4	3
Carbon dioxide producing drug	A06AX02	4	4
Unspecified laxatives	A06	6	9

Combined use of laxatives of different types occurred in 86 women in early pregnancy and 180 women later in pregnancy.

Characteristics of Women using Laxatives

Based on women using laxatives in early pregnancy (n=2760, one case lacked maternal age). Each variable is adjusted for all other variables and year of delivery. Comparison with all women who gave birth during the period and with information from the first antenatal care (n= 967 742). The odds ratios for maternal age, parity, smoking in early pregnancy, number of previous miscarriages, BMI, subfertility, and country of birth are adjusted for all other variables and are shown in Figure 12.1.

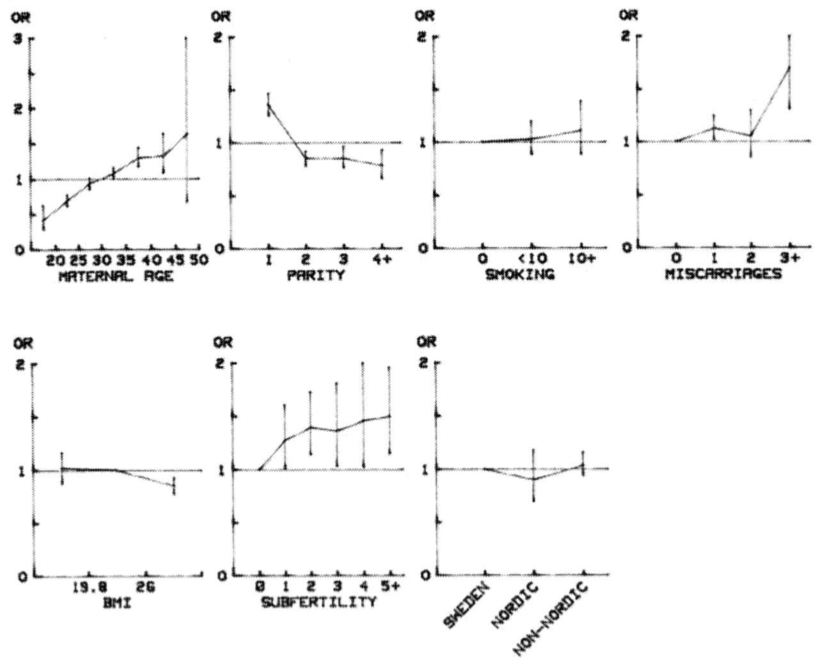

Figure 12.1. Odds ratios for seven maternal characteristics. The odds ratios (OR) for each variable are adjusted for the other variables and year of delivery. Vertical lines mark 95% confidence intervals. For maternal age and parity, each class is compared with all other classes.

Table 12.2. Some further characteristics of women using laxatives in early pregnancy

Variable	Number of women with drug	OR	95%CI
Education (1996-2001, 997 women with laxatives,526 695 in population)			
Unknown	29	-	
<12 years	88	0.96	0.75-1.21
12 years	487	1.00	reference
13-14 years	51	0.89	0.67-1.19
≥14 years	342	1.08	0.93-1.27
Family situation			
Unknown	40	-	
Co-habiting	2598	1.00	reference
Living alone	53	0.86	0.65-1.12
Other family situation	69	0.90	0.70-1.14
Work outside home			
Unknown	336	-	
Full time	1266	1.00	reference
Part time	640	1.14	1.03-1.26
None	518	1.27	1.14-1.41

Some further maternal characteristics were analyzed, adjusting for year of delivery, maternal age, parity, smoking, and BMI (Table 11.2).

Table 12. 3. Concomitant drug use (early pregnancy)

Drug group	Number	OR	95% CI
Drugs for gastric ulcer or gastro-oesophageal reflux	119	5.31	4.49-6.28
Drugs for inflammatory bowel disease	25	3.15	2.04-4.65#
Multivitamins	430	1.73	1.55-1.93
Insulin	9	1.01	0-46-1.92#
Folic acid	302	1.62	1.43-1.83
Antihypertensives	6	0.50	0.23-1.10#
Oral contraceptives	6	0.97	0.36-2.12#
Progestogens	15	1.36	0.82-2.26
Gonadotrophines	5	0.92	0.30-2.14#
Systemic corticoids	20	2.13	1.30-3.30
Thyroid drugs	49	1.33	1.00-1.76
Antibiotics	110	1.32	1.09-1.60
NSAID	56	1.44	1.10-1.87
Opioids	65	4.73	3.77-5.95
Minor analgesics	308	1.91	1.70-2.15
Drugs for migraine	12	1.72	0.89-3.01
Anticonvulsants	13	1.65	0.88-2.82
Neuroleptics, sedatives, hypnotics	31	2.72	1.91-3.87
Antidepressants	46	1.42	1.06-1.90
Drugs for rhinitis	88	2.38	1.94-2.93
Antiasthmatics	118	1.55	1.29-1.86
Cough medicines	33	2.50	1.78-3.49
Antihistamines	281	2.08	1.84-2.35
For NVP	216	2.09	1.82-2.40
For allergy	72	1.83	1.45-2.31

#observed over expected numbers with exact Poisson 95% confidence interval.

Use of laxatives is thus associated with high maternal age, low parity, subfertility, and not working full time.

There are thus many associations between the reporting of laxatives and other drug groups. One explanation is probably that laxatives are usually regarded as harmless for the pregnant woman. Women who report – and midwives who record – laxatives may be more careful in the reporting and recording other drugs which will give a false association. This may be the explanation of the moderately strong association with multivitamins and folic acid, for instance. In other circumstances, the drugs used may increase the risk for constipation and therefore also the use of laxatives. This may be the case with opiates and some cough medicines, for instance. Finally, some gastrointestinal diseases may interact which could explain associations with some drugs.

Whatever the explanation, one should note that a drug with a definite effect on the foetal development and which are associated with the use of laxative could confound the analysis. An example is anticonvulsants with a known teratogenic effect. As only 13 women reported the use of anticonvulsants together with laxatives, this association will have only a marginal effect and statistical significance for the association was not reached.

Table 12.4. Some maternal diagnoses associated with the use of laxatives

Diagnosis	Drug in early pregnancy			Drug later in pregnancy		
	Number	OR	95% CI	Number	OR	95% CI
Pre-existing diabetes	34	0.94	0.68-1.35	64	0.91	0.70-1.21
Gestational diabetes	25	1.03	0.69-1.53	50	1.04	0.83-1.52
Preeclampsia	113	0.86	0.71-1.04	216	0.89	0.79-1.07
Hyperemesis gravidarum	31	1.15	0.81-1.64	56	1.03	0.79-1.34
Chronic hypertension	30	0.92	0.64-1.33	60	0.94	0.72-1.21
Placenta previa	32	1.04	0.73-1.47	69	1.12	0.88-1.43
Abruptio placentae	27	0.80	0.55-1.17	65	0.97	0.75-1.24
Antepartum bleeding	34	0.92	0.65-1.29	78	1.10	0.88-1.40
Intrapartum bleeding	67	1.10	0.86-1.40	139	1.19	1.00-1.41
Postpartum bleeding	148	0.94	0.79-1.11	294	1.03	0.92-1.16
Delivery induction	314	1.05	0.93-1.18	610	1.11	1.01-1.20
Caesarean section	555	1.23	1.12-1.35	923	1.09	1.02-1.18

For most diagnoses there is no significant association with the use of laxatives. The only exception is intrapartum bleeding, probably a result of the increased rate of caesarean section. An increased risk for caesarean section is seen both after early and later use of laxatives.

Outcome after Maternal use of Laxatives

Infant Sex

When the mother had used laxatives in early pregnancy, there were 1476 males and 1331 females (one with unknown sex). The sex ratio was slightly high: 1.11 (95% CI 1.03-1.19) but the confidence interval includes the normal sex ratio (1.06). After later use of laxative, the sex ratio is 1.06 (95% CI 1.01-1.12 based on 2698 males and 2537 females (one with unknown sex).

Multiple Births

There were 46 twin pairs and two triplet sets after maternal use of laxatives in early pregnancy. The odds ratio for twin delivery after exposure in early pregnancy is 1.11 95% CI 0.83-1.49). After maternal use of laxatives in later pregnancy there were 108 twin pairs and two triplet sets. The odds ratio for twin delivery after exposure in late pregnancy is 1.40 (95% CI 1.16-1.70), reasonably due to an increased constipation risk in twin pregnancies.

Table 12.5. Infant mortality after maternal use of laxatives

Age at death	Drug in early pregnancy			Drug later in pregnancy		
	Number	OR/RR	95% CI	Number	OR/RR	95% CI
Stillbirth	13	1.39	0.74-2.38#	14	0.78	0.46-1.33
Early neonatal death	3	0.76	0.16-2.21#	6	0.79	0.29-1.72

No increase in perinatal mortality is thus seen.

Table 12.6. Pregnancy duration and infant birth weight at maternal use of laxatives

Variable studied	Drug use in early pregnancy			Drug use later in pregnancy		
	Number	OR	95% CI	Number	OR	95% C I
<37 weeks	119	0.96	0.80-1.14	233	0.95	0.84-1.09
<2500g	70	0.80	0.63-1.01	132	0.84	0.71-1.01
≥4500g	118	1.13	1.13-1.36	208	1.04	0.88-1.17
SGA	46	0.73	0.55-0.98	93	0.85	0.69-1.05
LGA	179	1.21	1.03-1.41	325	1.09	0.97-1.22

There is a slight excess of LGA infants after exposure in early pregnancy and a decrease in the rate of low birth weight infants after later exposure. These effects may be random.

Table 12.7. Neonatal diagnoses after maternal use of laxatives

Diagnosis	Drug use in early pregnancy			Drug use later in pregnancy		
	Number	OR	95% CI	Number	OR	95% C I
Hypoglycaemia	89	0.84	0.68-1.04	190	1.03	0.89-1.19
Respiratory diagnoses	133	0.95	0.80-1.14	250	1.00	0.88-1.13
Low Apgar score	53	0.97	0.74-1.28	93	0.98	0.80-1.21
CNS diagnoses	27	1.11	0.76-1.63	43	1.11	0.82-1.50
Jaundice	122	0.94	0.78-1.13	239	1.04	0.91-1.18

There are thus no deviations from the expected occurrence of neonatal diagnoses.

There is thus no sign of an increased risk for a congenital malformation after use of laxatices in early preganncy or the main groups of such drugs.

Table 12.8. Congenital malformations in infants whose mothers used laxatives in early pregnancy

Congenital malformations	Number	OR/RR	95% CI
All drugs			
All malformations	141	1.03	0.86-1.24
Relatively severe malformations	105	1.06	0.86-1.31
Chromosome anomalies	7	1.24	0.50-2.55#
Without chromosome anomaly			
Cardiovascular defects	37	1.19	0.84-1.70
Orofacial clefts	6	1.21	0.44-2.63#
Hypospadias	12	1.59	0.88-2.78#
Pes equinovarus	7	1.71	0.69-3.53#
*Exclusion of some concomitant drugs**			
All malformations	138	1.04	0.87-1.25
Relatively severe malformations	102	1.06	0.84-1.70
Cardiovascular defects	37	1.22	0.86-1.74
Hypospadias	12	1.64	0.85-2.86#
Contact laxatives (n=203)			
All malformations	8	0.81	0.35-1.60#
Relatively severe malformations	5	0.72	0.23-1.69#
Bulk producers (n=1291)			
All malformations	60	0.92	0.69-1.21
Relatively severe malformations	47	0.99	0.72-1.37
Cardiovascular defects	19	1.24	0.75-2.07
Hypospadias	6	1.74	0.84-3.79#
Osmotically active laxatives (n=1341)			
All malformations	74	1.17	0.91-1.50
Relatively severe malformations	55	1.21	0.91-1.62
Cardiovascular defects	18	1.29	0.79-2.11
Hypospadias	5	1.40	0.45-3.27#

*Infants exposed to one or more of the following drugs were removed: drugs for inflammatory bowel disease, systemic corticosteroids, opiates, anticonvulsants.
observed over expected number with exact Poisson 95% confidence interval.

Summary

As expected, the use of laxatives seems not to have any major effect on delivery outcome. There is a moderately increased risk for caesarean section.

References

[1] Mahadevan U, Kane S. American Gastroenterological Association Institute technical review on the use of gastrointestinal medications in pregnancy. *Gastroenterology* 2006; 131: 283-311.

[2] Heinonen OP, Slone D, Shapiro S. *Birth Defects and Drugs in pregnancy*. Publishing Sciences Group, Inc. Littleton, Mass. 1977.

Chapter 13

Drugs Used as Antidiarrhoics, Intestinal Anti-Infectives, or at Inflammatory Bowel Disease

Infants born of women who have used drugs belonging to these categories have some deviations in outcome. These are probably to a large extent due to effects of underlying disease, notably Crohn´s syndrom or ulcerative colitis. A moderately increased risk for a congenital malformation, mostly referring to cardiovascular defects, was seen after maternal use of loperamide or mesalazine. These effects could be group specific and not specifically related to these two drugs. If a teratogenic risk is associated with the use of these drugs it is low and of little consequence for an individual and such exposure should not lead to a discussion of a termination of pregnancy.

This group of drugs is usually regarded as low risk drugs [1]. Most studies, however, are based on relatively small materials. Relatively little interest has been paid to loperamide. In a study of Medicaid recipients, six infants among 108 exposed to loperamide during pregnancy were malformed [2]– three of the malformed infants had cardiac defects. In another study from a number of teratology information systems (TIS), 105 women who had used loperamide in early pregnancy were identified and no increased risk of congenital malformations was found [3]. The power of these two studies is low to detect anything but a very strong teratogenic effect. In a review of the use of gastrointestinal medications in pregnancy [1], loperamide was classified as "low risk" with a possibly increased risk for congenital cardiovascular defects. More interest has been shown drugs given for inflammatory bowel disease (IBD), mainly ulcerative colitis or Chron's disease.

The review of the use of gastrointestinal medications in pregnancy [1] included a discussion of drugs used at IBD. Most such drugs were regarded as low risk with the exception of methothrexate which is generally regarded as contraindicated in pregnancy and thalidomide which is a well known strong teratogen. Another literature review [4] also state that except for methotrexate, drugs used in IBD appear safe in pregnancy. An increased risk for premature birth and intrauterine growth retardation was reported when the mother had Crohn's disease but not ulcerative colitis. Disease activity at the time of conception appeared to be the strongest determinant for poor outcome. The use of sulfasalazine or mesalazine was regarded as low risk. The article concluded that there is a need of large, prospective studies.

Most of the studies which these reviews are based on consist of relatively small cohorts of women with IBD from single hospitals or from teratology information systems [5]. The largest cohort study comprised 900 women with Crohn's disease, among which the majority (628) had no drug treatment identified [6]. Data from the Swedish Medical Birth Register on loperamide have been published [7].

Table 13.1. Number of women identified with use of drugs used as antidiarrhoics, intestinal anti-infectives, or at inflammatory bowel disease

Total	3684
Reported use in early pregnancy	3147
Got prescription later in pregnancy	1700
Both early and late use	1163

Type of drug:	ATC code	Early use	Later use
Intestinal antiinfectives	A07A	22	16
Nystatin	A07AA02	20	15
Acetarsol	A07AX02	2	1
Intestinal adsorbents	A07B	11	3
Charcoal	A07BA01	11	3
Antipropulsives	A07D	689	120
Loperamide	A07DA03	677	116
Loperamide oxide	A07DA05	12	5
Intestinal antiinflammatory agents	A07E	2436	1570
Corticosteroids for local use	A07EA	448	427
Prednisolone	A07EA01	314	331
Hydrocortisone	A07EA02	29	22
Budesonide	A07EA06	113	84
Other antiallergic agents	A07EB	12	9
Cromoglicic acid	A07EB01	12	9
5-ASA related drugs	A07EC	2121	1282
Sulfasalazine	A07EC01	937	501
Mesalazine	A07EC02	1023	707
Olsalazine	A07EC03	145	51
Balsalazide	A07EC04	62	51
Antidiarrheal microorganisms	A07F	1	0
Saccharomyces boulardi	A07F02	1	0
Unspecified	A07	15	3

Some women used two categories of drugs:

Intestinal absorbent + antipropulsive: 2 in early pregnancy
Antipropulsive + intestinal antiinflammatory agent: 24 in early, 10 in later pregnancy.

Characteristics for Women using Drugs as Antidiarrhoics, Intestinal Anti-infectives, or at Inflammatory Bowel Disease

Based on women using such drugs in early pregnancy (n=3 147). Each variable is adjusted for all other variables and year of delivery. Comparison with all women who gave birth during the period and with information from the first antenatal care (n=967 742). The odds ratios for maternal age, parity, smoking in early pregnancy, number of previous miscarriages, BMI, subfertility, and country of birth are adjusted for all other variables and are shown in Figure 13.1.

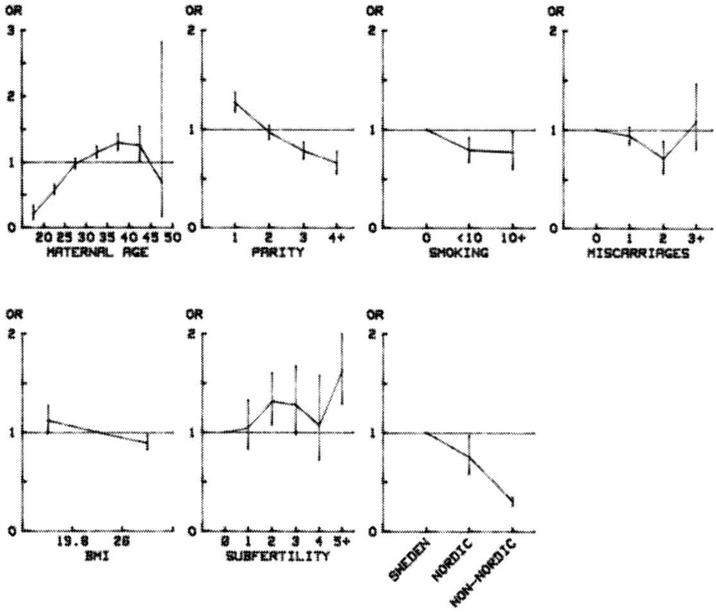

Figure 13.1. Odds ratios for seven maternal characteristics. The odds ratios (OR) for each variable are adjusted for the other variables and year of delivery. Vertical lines mark 95% confidence intervals. For maternal age and parity, each class is compared with all other classes.

Some further characteristics were analyses, adjusting for year of delivery, maternal age, parity, smoking, and BMI (Table 13.2).

Table 13.2. Some further characteristics of women using drugs as antidiarrhoics, intestinal anti-infectives, or at inflammatory bowel disease

Variable	Number of women with drug	OR	95%CI
Education (1996-2001, 1327 women with drugs, 526 695 in population)			
Unknown	15	-	
<12 years	95	0.74	0.59-0.92
12 years	712	1.00	reference
13-14 years	81	0.95	0.75-1.20
≥14 years	424	0.91	0.80-1.03
Family situation			
Unknown	44	-	
Co-habiting	2998	1.00	reference
Living alone	47	0.70	0.52-0.94
Other family situation	58	0.84	0.65-1.10
Work outside home			
Unknown	323	-	
Full time	1564	1.00	reference
Part time	841	1.22	1.11-1.33
None	419	0.90	0.80-1.01

Women using drugs as antidiarrhoics, intestinal anti-infectives, or at inflammatory bowel disease thus differ from other women in many aspects: fewer young women, fewer high parity women, fewer smoking women, a slight overrisk at low BMI, increased fertility problems, and women who more often than expected were born in Sweden. There is an excess of women who work half-time.

Table 13.3. Concomitant drug use (early pregnancy)

Drug group	Number	OR	95% CI
Drugs for gastric ulcer etc.	87	3.41	2.78-4.17
Insulin	16	1.51	0.93-2.47
Multivitamins	217	1.15	0.99-1.33
Folic acid	368	2.62	2.35-2.92
Drugs for hypertension	32	2.46	1.74-3.48
Oral contraceptive	6	0.70	0.26-1.77#
Progestogens	17	1.14	0.70-1.84
Gonadotrophins	6	0.78	0.28-1.69#
Systemic corticosteroids	241	23.6	21.5-26.0
Thyroid drugs	61	1.44	1.11-1.85
Antibiotics	113	1.22	1.01-1.47
NSAID	130	2.42	2.04-2.88
Opioids	52	3.62	2.79-4.69
Minor analgesics	267	1.14	1.00-1.29
Drugs for migraine	15	1.66	1.00-2.76
Anticonvulsants	6	0.69	0.31-1.54
Sedatives, hypnotics	23	1.72	1.14-2.60
Antidepressants	50	1.29	0.97-1.70
Drugs for rhinitis	57	1.26	0.97-1.63
Antiasthmatics	135	1.47	1.24-1.75
Antitussives	18	1.16	0.73-1.84
Antihistamines	143	0.79	0.66-0.93
For NVP	97	0.70	0.57-0.85
For allergy	51	1.06	0.80-1.40
Immunosuppressives	168	158	144-172

observed over expected number with exact Poisson 95% confidence interval.

An increased use of drugs for stomach ulcer and gastro-oesophageal reflux is seen and also use of some other drug categories: drugs for hypertension, systemic corticoids, thyroid drugs, NSAID, opioids and other analgesics, sedatives and hypnotics, antiasthmatics, and immunosuppressives. The associations with systemic corticoids and with immunosuppressive drugs are reasonable when the woman had IBD. Actually one third of all women who reported the use of immunosuppressives had used them together with this drug category.

There is an increased risk for preeclampsia, statistically significant only after late exposure. There is also an increased risk for delivery induction and caesarean section. Related to the latter is the increased risk for intrapartum bleeding. When the study was restricted to infants exposed to drugs for IBD, the risk for caesarean section increased slightly to 1.72 after late exposure. The increased risk for caesarean section existed also for women who had used other drugs than drugs for IBD: after late exposure the OR was 2.15 (95%CI 1.43-3.24).

Table 13.4. Maternal delivery diagnoses associated with the use of drugs used as antidiarrhoics, intestinal anti-infectives, or at inflammatory bowel disease

Diagnosis	Drug in early pregnancy			Drug later in pregnancy		
	Number	OR	95%CI	Number	OR	95% CI
Pre-existing diabetes	36	1.06	0.76-1.48	20	1.13	0.72-1.77
Gestational diabetes	24	1.01	0.68-1.52	15	1.27	0.76-2.12
Preeclampsia	143	1.16	0.98-1.38	84	1.39	1.11-1.73
Chronic hypertension	33	1.07	0.76-1.51	21	1.31	0.85-2.02
Placenta previa	32	1.08	0.76-1.54	19	1.22	0.77-1.93
Abruptio placentae	34	1.02	0.72-1.43	19	1.12	0.71-1.77
Antepartum bleeding	37	1.02	0.73-1.42	23	1.30	0.86-1.97
Intrapartum bleeding	72	1.28	1.01-1.62	40	1.54	1.15-2.06
Postpartum bleeding	164	1.07	0.92-1.26	60	0.81	0.62-1.05
Delivery induction	372	1.43	1.28-1.60	257	1.70	1.47-1.97
Caesarean section	594	1.47	1.34-1.61	315	1.54	1.36-1.75

Outcome after Maternal use of Drugs used as Antidiarrhoics, Intestinal Anti-infectives, or at Inflammatory Bowel Disease

Infant Sex

When the mother had used such drugs in early pregnancy, there were 1387 male and 1335 female infants born (one infant with unknown sex). The sex ratio was 1.04 (95% CI 0.96-1.12). When drug use had occurred later in pregnancy, there were 676 male and 660 female infants. The sex ratio was 1.02 (95% CI 0.92-1.14). Both estimates thus contain the normal sex ratio of 1.06. For infants exposed to drugs for IBD, the sex ratio after early exposure was 1.06 (95% CI 0.97-1.15) and after later exposure 1.05 (95% CI 0.94-1.18). For infants not exposed to drugs for IBD, the sex ratio was 0.98 (95% CI 0.84-1.14) after early exposure and 0.74 (95% CI 0.49-1.09) after later exposure. The latter two sex ratios were thus low but both could be randomly low.

Multiple Births

After drug exposure in early pregnancy, there were 48 twin and one triplet delivery. The odds ratio for twin delivery was 1.16 (95% CI 0.87-1.55). After exposure later in pregnancy, there were 17 twin deliveries, odds ratio 0.84 (95% CI 0.52-1.35). In the latter group, in one twin pair one of the twins was missing in the register. There was no difference between the infants exposed to drugs for IBD and infants not exposed to such drugs (OR = 1.16 and 1.17, respectively). The majority of such non-IBD exposures concerned loperamide.

Table 13.5. Infant mortality at maternal use of drugs as antidiarrhoics, intestinal anti-infectives, or at inflammatory bowel disease

Age at death	Group	Drug in early pregnancy			Drug later in pregnancy		
		Number	OR/RR	95%CI	Number	OR/RR	95% CI
Stillbirth	All	14	1.25	0.74-2.12	5	1.98	0.64-4.62#
	For IBD	10	1.18	0.57-2.17#	5	2.25	0.73-5.25#
Early neonatal death	All	10	2.06	0.99-3.80#	3	2.85	0.59-8.32#
	For IBD	7	2.08	0.84-4.29#	2	2.21	0.24-7.97#

observed over expected number with exact Poisson 95% confidence interval.

There is thus a possibly increased the risk for early neonatal death, apparently associated with the use of drugs for IBD but formal statistical significance is not reached.

Table 13.6. Pregnancy duration and infant birth weight after maternal use of drugs used as antidiarrhoics, intestinal anti-infectives, or at inflammatory bowel disease

Variable studies	Drug	Drug use in early pregnancy			Drug use later in pregnancy		
		Number	OR	95% CI	Number	OR	95% CI
<37 weeks	All	199	1.59	1.38-1.84	113	1.86	1.54-2.25
	For IBD	169	1.80	1.54-2.11	105	1.88	1.54-2.29
	Other	30	0.97	0.67-1.40	8	1.60	0.69-3.15#
<2500g	All	129	1.62	1.36-1.93	70	1.84	1.41-2.33
	For IBD	110	1.85	1.53-1.24	62	1.77	1.38-2.28
	Other	19	0.93	0.59-1.47	8	2.45	1.06-4.84#
≥4500g	All	98	0.92	0.75-1.13	42	0.79	0.58-1.07
	For IBD	72	0.86	0.68-1.09	39	0.78	0.57-1.07
	Other	26	1.12	0.76-1.67	3	0.86	0.18-2.52#
SGA	All	87	1.57	1.26-1.94	43	1.62	1.19-2.20
	For IBD	73	1.78	1.41-2.25	37	1.53	1.10-2.12
	Other	14	0.96	0.56-1.65	6	2.44	0.90-5.31#
LGA	All	167	1.10	0.94-1.29	74	0.95	0.74-1.21
	For IBD	119	0.98	0.81-1.18	69	0.94	0.73-1.21
	Other	48	1.60	1.18-2.17	5	1.02	0.33-2.38#

observed over expected number with exact Poisson 95% confidence interval.

Table 13.7. Neonatal diagnoses after maternal use of drugs as antidiarrhoics, intestinal anti-infectives, or at inflammatory bowel disease

Diagnosis	Drugs	Drug use in early pregnancy			Drug use later in pregnancy		
		Number	OR/RR	95% CI	Number	OR/RR	95% CI
Hypoglycaemia	All	119	1.22	1.02-1.47	64	1.33	1.03-1.71
	Drugs for IBD	99	1.35	1.10-1.66	59	1.34	1.03-1.74
	Other	20	0.83	0.53-1.30	5	1.24	0.40-2.89#
Respiratory diagnoses	All	165	1.21	1.04-1.42	83	1.36	1.09-1.70
	Drugs for IBD	128	1.27	1.06-1.52	74	1.31	1.03-1.65
	Other	37	1.04	0.75-1.46	9	1.91	0.88-6.01#
Low Apgar score	All	68	1.29	1.01-1.65	31	1.33	0.93-1.91
	Drugs for IBD	53	1.36	1.03-1.78	26	1.22	0.82-1.80
	Other	15	1.11	0.66-1.86	1	1.35	0.03-7.53#
CNS diagnoses	All	20	0.92	0.59-1.43	6	1.52	0.56-3.20#
	Drugs for IBD	12	0.74	0.42-1.31	6	1.69	0.62-3.69#
	Other	8	1.42	0.61-2.79#	0	-	-
Jaundice	All	173	1.28	1.10-1.50	48	1.76	1.31-2.35
	Drugs for IBD	133	1.33	1.11-1.56	43	1.78	1.31-1.42
	Other	40	1.15	0.83-1.59	5	1.52	0.49-3.56#

observed over expected number with exact Poisson 95% confidence interval.

When all drugs belonging to this section were analyzed together ("All"), an increased risk for preterm birth, low birth weight, and SGA was seen. These effects were all due to drugs used for IBD. For the other drugs, there was an increased risk for low birth weight after later exposure (based on only eight cases) and an indicated but not statistically significant increase in SGA (based on six cases). There seems to be an increased rate of LGA infants after early (but not later) exposure to other drugs than drugs used for IBD.

All diagnoses with the exception of diagnoses related to CNS problems thus occur in excess but this seems to be restricted to infants exposed to drugs for IBD.

Table 13.8. Congenital malformations in infants whose mothers used drugs used as antidiarrhoics, intestinal anti-infectives, or at inflammatory bowel disease

Congenital malformations	Number	OR/RR	95% CI
All drugs			
All malformations	155	1.25	1.07-1.48
Relatively severe malformations	113	1.28	1.06-1.55
Chromsome anomalies	9	1.25	0.57-2.38#
Without chromosome anomalies:			
Neural tube defects	5	2.84	0.92-6.62#
Cardiovascular defects	47	1.34	1.00-1.79
Orofacial clefts	8	1.20	0.52-2.37#
Anal atresia	3	2.13	0.44-6.22#
Hypospadias	14	1.51	0.83-2.54
Pes equinovarus	5	1.25	0.41-2.91#
Drugs for IBD			
All malformations	115	1.22	1.01-1.48
Relatively severe malformations	82	1.23	0.98-1.53
Chromosome anomalies	7	1.28	0.52-2.64#
Without chromosome anomalies:			
Cardiovascular defects	34	1.28	0.91-1.80
Hypospadias	8	1.14	0.49-2.25#
Drugs not for IBD			
All malformations	40	1.35	0.98-1.86
Relatively severe malformations	31	1.40	1.02-2.10
Without chromosome anomalies:			
Cardiovascular defects	13	1.53	0.81-2.61#
Hypospadias	6	2.68	0.98-5.83#

observed over expected number with exact Poisson 95% confidence interval.

Relatively severe malformations and individual drugs (at least 50 exposures)

Drug	Malformed	Total	Per cent	OR/RR	95% CI
Loperamide	31	616	5.0	1.49	1.04-2.14
Prednisolone locally	7	191	3.7	1.19	0.50-2.46#
Budesonide locally	4	97	4.1	1.23	0.34-3.16#
Sulfasalzine	32	866	3.7	1.13	0.79-2.61
Mesalazine	40	867	4.6	1.48	1.08-2.04
Olsalazine	4	144	2.8	0.82	0.22-2.11#

observed over expected number with exact Poisson 95% confidence interval.

There is no significant difference in the percentages of malformed infants irrespective of which drug had been used ($\chi2=1.77$ at 5 d.f.) but statistically significant effects are only seen after loperamide and mesalazine. The increased rates were mainly due to cardiovascular defects with ORs of the same magnitude for both drugs. For loperamide it was 1.51 (95% CI 0.91-2.70), for mesalazine 1.49 (95% CI 0.91-2.44). The following cardiovascular defects were found:

Table 13.9. Cardiac defects in infants whose mothers used loperamide or mesalazine in early pregnancy

Cardiovacular defect	Number with loperamide	Number with mesalazine
Common arterial trunk	1	0
Transposition of great vessels	1	0
Corrected transposition	0	1
Ventricular septum defect	2	4
Atrium septum defect	2	5
Ventricular+atrium septum defect	1	1
Endocardial cushion defect	0	1
Pulmonary valve atresia with VSD	0	1
Congenital mitral stenosis	1	0
Pulmonary artery anomaly	2	0
Patent ductus arteriosus	1	1
Unspecified cardiac defect	2	2
Total	13	16

Summary

Infants born by mothers using drugs for IBD appear to have a tendency to be born preterm, with low birth weight, and intrauterine growth retardation. Such effects have been associated with underlying disease, Crohn´s disease or ulcerative colitis. There is also an excess of neonatal diagnoses. The same phenomena are not seen for infants whose mothers had used other drugs (mainly loperamide) in this group of drugs. On the other hand, a possibly increased risk for a congenital malformation and notably a cardiovascular defect was seen both after drugs used for IBD and other drugs. These effects were best demonstrated with loperamide and mesalazine but there was no significant difference between the effect of mesalazine and sulfasalazine. The slightly lower OR with sulfasalazine may be related to the use of this drug not only for IBD but also for rheumatic disease. It is doubtful if the noticed effects are due to drug exposure or to underlying disease. It should be noticed that only 22 women used both loperamide and drugs for IBD so a confounding by IBD in the analysis of loperamide seems unlikely. The increased malformation risk is of marginal statistical significance and has not been seen in previous studies which, however, hardly had the power to detect an effect of this magnitude.

References

[1] Mahadevan U, Kane S. American Gastroenterological Association Institute technical review on the use of gastrointestinal medications in pregnancy. *Gastroenterology* 2006; 131: 283-311.

[2] Schwethelm B, Margolis LH, Miller C, Smith S. Risk status and pregnancy outcome among Medicaid recipients, *Am J Prev Med* 1989; 5: 157-163.

[3] Einarson A, Mastroiacovo P, Arnon J, Ornoy A, Addis A, Malm H, Koren G. Prospective, controlled, multicentre study of loperamide in pregnancy. *Can J Gastroenterol* 2000; 14: 185-187.

[4] Heetun Z, Byrnes C, Neary P, O'Morain C. Review article: reproduction in the patient with inflammatory bowel disease. *Aliment Pharmacol Therapeut* 2007; 26: 513-533.

[5] Diav-Citrin O, Park YH, Veerasuntharam G, Polacheck H, Bologa M, Pastuszak A, Koren G. The safey of mesalamine in human pregnancy: a prospective controlled cohort study. *Gastroenterol* 2007; 102: 1406-1413.

[6] Nørgård B, Pedersen L, Christensen LA, Sørensen HT. Therapeutic drug use in women wih Crohn's disease and birth outcomes: a Danish nationwide cohort study. *Am J Gastroenterol* 2007; 102: 1406-1413.

[7] Källén B, Nilsson E, Otterblad Olausson P. Maternal use of loperamide in early pregnancy and delivery outcome. *Acta Paediatr* 2008; 97:541-545.

Chapter 14

ANTI-OBESITY DRUGS

Obesity is in itself associated with an increased risk for certain types of congenital malformations. Use of anti-obesity drugs in early pregnancy could reduce that risk but it is also possible that interference with nutrition in early pregnancy could affect embryonic development. Little is known in the literature on the possible hazards with the two main drugs used in Sweden, orlistat and sibutramine. The present data suggest a difference between the two drugs with the possibility of an increased risk associated with sibutramine. The drug should therefore be avoided in early pregnancy but if exposure already has occurred, the teratogenic risk is so uncertain and weak that a termination of pregnancy is not motivated.

In Sweden, few drugs are registered for use at obesity: sibutramine, orlistat, and rimonabant. There is only little known about possible hazards with these drugs during pregnancy. Orlistat acts locally in the intestines and is unlikely to reach the embryo and cause damage. Sibutramine belongs to the group of SSRI drugs and rimonabant is a cannabinoid-1 receptor blocker. Little information is available on the use of the latter two drugs during pregnancy. Single case reports of sibutramine exist [1,2] and one small study consisting of 10 exposed pregnancies with seven normal live births, two spontaneous and one induced abortion [3]. One further study described outcome of 52 pregnancies with subatramine exposure in the first trimester and no malformed infants [4].

Table 14.1. Number of women identified with use of anti-obesity drugs

Total:	272
Reported use in early pregnancy	264
Got prescription later in pregnancy	10
Both early and later use	2

Type of drug	ATC code	Early use	Later use
Sibutramine	A08AA10	71	1
Orlistat	A08AB01	193	9

Two women reported the use of both sibutramine and orlistat.

Table 14.2. Characteristics of women using anti-obesity drugs

Variable	Number of women with drug	OR	95% CI
Maternal age			
<25 years	28	0.79	0.53-1.18
25-34 years	173	1.00	reference
≥35 years	63	1.09	0.81-1.46
Parity			
1	97	1.00	0.76-1.32
2	71	0.67	0.51-0.87
3	65	1.65	1.24-2.20
≥4	31	1.10	0.74-1.63
Smoking			
Unknown	8		
No	214	1.00	reference
Yes	42	1.35	0.95-1.90
Earlier miscarriages			
No	206	1.00	reference
Yes	58	0.89	0.66-1.20
BMI			
Unknown	15		
<19.8	1*	0.58	-
19.8-25.9	14	1.00	reference
≥26	234	34.5	24.8-48.0
Subfertility (years of unwanted childlessness)			
No	224	1.00	reference
Yes	40	2.66	1.92-3.70
Education (1996-2001, 147 women with anti-obesity drugs, 526 695 in population)			
Unknown	0	-	-
<12 years	29	1.25	0.81-1.93
12 years	97	1.00	reference
>12 years	26	0.43	0.27-0.66
Country of birth			
Unknown	0	-	-
Sweden	215	1.00	reference
Other Nordic country	9	1.34	0.69-2.61
Non-Nordic country	40	0.91	0.66-1.27
Family situation			
Unknown	3	-	-
Co-habiting	279	1.00	reference
Living alone	11	1.60	0.86-2.97
Other family situation	11	1.63	0.88-3.01
Variable	Number of women with drug	OR	95% CI
Work outside home			
Unknown	34	-	-
Full time	111	1.00	reference
Part time	60	0.96	0.70-1.33
None	59	1.17	0.85-1.63

Characteristics of Women Using Anti-Obesity Drugs

Based on women reporting anti-obesity drugs in early pregnancy (n=264). Comparison with all women who gave birth during the period and with information from the antenatal care. The odds ratios for maternal age, parity, smoking in early pregnancy, number of previous miscarriages, BMI, subfertility, and country of birth are adjusted for all other variables and for year of birth. The odds ratios for education, family situation, and work outside home are adjusted for year of delivery, maternal age, parity, smoking, and BMI (Table 14.2).

The most remarkable characteristics – except the high odds ratio for high BMI – are an increased risk for subfertility and a decreased use of the drugs at high education. There is also a clear-cut effect of parity with a U-form with a minimum for parity 2. Other ORs are also increased (e.g., maternal smoking in early pregnancy) but the limited size of the material makes these estimates uncertain.

Table 14.3. Concomitant drug use (early pregnancy)

Drug group	Number	OR/RR	95%CI
Drugs for stomach ulcer and reflux	10	3.09	1.48-5.68#
Insulin	5	1.32	1.23-1.81#
Multivitamins	8	0.92	0.40-1.81#
Folic acid	8	0.78	0.38-1.60#
Thyroid drugs	11	2.32	1.16-4.15#
Antibiotics	12	1.35	0.70-2.35#
NSAID	14	1.89	1.04-3.18#
Minor analgesics	25	0.86	0.57-1.29
Antidepressants	14	2.80	1.53-4.70#
Drugs for rhinitis	6	1.37	0.50-2.98#
Antihistamines	19	1.09	0.68-1.73
For NVP	9	0.67	0.34-1.29
For allergy	12	2.55	1.46-4.44#

#observed over expected number with exact Poisson 95% confidence interval.

Table 14.4. Some maternal diagnoses associated with the use of anti-obesity drugs. As only few exposures occurred during late pregnancy, only early pregnancy exposures could be analyzed

Diagnosis	Number	OR/RR	95%CI
Preexisting diabetes	16	2.29	1.31-3.72#
Gestationaldiabetes	9	1.73	0.79-3.28#
Chronic hypertension	14	2.06	1.13-3.46#
Preeclampsia	10	1.62	0.78-2.98#
Hyperemesis gravidarum	9	1.60	0.77-3.04#
Placenta previa	10	1.62	0.78-2.98#
Abruptio placenta	10	1.53	0.74-2.82#
Antepartum bleeding	11	1.77	0.89-3.17#
Intrapartum bleeding	14	1.46	0.80-2.44#
Postpartum bleeding	24	1.45	0.95-2.21
Delivery induction	49	1.31	0.96-1.80
Caesarean section	62	1.19	0.89-1.60

A clear excess is seen of concomitant use of drugs for stomach ulcer and reflux, of insulin, thyroid drugs, NSAID (but not analgesics), antidepressants, and antihistamines used for allergy (but not for NVP).

All odds ratios are above 1.0 but for most statistical significance is not reached. Pre-existing diabetes and hypertension are the only conditions which show significant excess.

Outcome after Maternal use of Anti-Obesity Drugs

Infant Sex

When the mother had used anti-obesity drugs in early pregnancy, 150 of the 266 children were male and 116 female. Sex ratio is then 1.29 (95% CI 1.02-1.66) which is somewhat high but the normal sex ratio (1.06) lies within the confidence interval.

Multiple Births

After maternal use of anti-obesity drugs in early pregnancy, only two twin deliveries occurred and no higher order multiple births.

Infant Mortality

Only one infant died – a stillbirth after early exposure for an anti-obesity drug.

Table 14.5. Pregnancy duration and infant birth weight after maternal use of anti-obesity drugs in early pregnancy

Variable studied	Number	OR	95%CI
<37 weeks	23	1.67	1.09-2.56
<2500g	10	1.19	0.63-2.34
≥4500g	23	1.37	0.90-2.11
SGA	7	1.29	0.52-2.65#
LGA	30	1.21	0.81-1.80

#observed over expected number with exact 95% Poisson confidence interval.

Table 14.6. Neonatal diagnoses in infants whose mothers used anti-obesity drugs in early pregnancy

Diagnosis	Number	OR	95% CI
Hypoglycaemia	24	2.07	1.37-3.13
Respiratory diagnoses	12	0.78	0.44-1.40
Low Apgar score	4	0.74	0.20-1.90#
CNS-diagnoses	2	0.88	0.11-3.18#
Jaundice	17	1.37	0.83-2.26

#observed over expected number with exact 95% Poisson confidence interval.

There was thus a significantly increased risk for preterm birth but effects on birth weight and intrauterine growth were not statistically significant.

The increased risk for hypoglycaemia is probably an effect of the association with maternal diabetes (see above).

Table 14.7. Congenital malformations in infants whose mothers used anti-obesity drugs

Congenital malformations	Number	OR	95% CI
All infants			
Any congenital malformation	12	0.82	0.26-2.58
Relatively severe malformations	11	1.08	0.52-1.99
Exposed to orlistat			
Any congenital malformation	5	0.66	0.16-2.70
Relatively severe malformations	4	0.58	0.16-1.48
Exposed to sibutramine			
Any congenital malformation	7	2.29	0.92-4.71
Relatively severe malformations	7	3.01	1.21-6.21

The following congenital malformations were present:

Exposed to orlistat	
Anencephaly + unstable hip	1
Pylorostenosis	1
Undescended testicle	1
Unspecified male genital organ malformation	1
Congenital bowing of tibia and fibula	1
Exposed to sibutramine	
Ear and skull malformation	1
Ventricular septum defect	1
Atrium septum defect	1
Hypospadias	1
Hydronephrosis	1
Accessory hallux	1
Trisomy 18	1 (stillbirth)

The majority of the registered malformations were thus relatively severe and formal statistical significance was reached for sibutramine while no increase in malformation risk was seen after orlistat. As obesity itself may be a risk factor for at least some malformations, the proportion of women with a BMI above 26 was compared between the two exposure groups. For orlistat this percentage was 88%, for sibutramine 92% but these two proportions did not differ significantly (Fisher exact test $p=0.77$). The mean BMI in the orlistat group was 33.0 ± 0.4 and in the subatramine group 35.0 ± 0.7 – these two means did not differ significantly ($p=0.34$).

Against a causal association between the use of sibutramine and the occurrence of congenital malformations in the infants speaks the variability in malformation type even though two infants had cardiac septal defects.

Summary

The reason for the use of these drugs is obesity, a condition which in itself carries an increased risk for a congenital malformation. Adjustment was made for BMI in the analysis, but BMI was not always known and the highest BMI group is open (≥26) and within it women with anti-obesity drugs probably had a higher mean BMI than women who did not use such drugs. There is, however, a striking difference between orlistat and sibutramine in malformation risk but only a small difference in mean BMI. This favours a specific effect of sibutramine but the formally significant risk increase is based on only seven cases. A larger material will be needed in order to definitely define the possible teratogenic risk with sibutramine.

References

[1] Ramzi F, Elias D, Mona S, Zreik TG. Sibutramine in pregnancy. *Europ J Obst Gynecol Reprod Biol* 2005; 122: 243-244.

[2] Kadioglu M, Ulku C, Yaris F, Kesim M, Kalyoncu NI, Yaris E. Sibutramine use in pregnancy: report of two cases. *Birth Def Research (A)* 2004; 70: 545-546.

[3] Einarson A, Bonari L, Sarkar M, McKenna K, Koren G. Exposure to sibutramine during pregnancy: case series. *Europ J Obst Gynecol Reprod Biol* 2004; 116: 142.

[4] De Santis M, Straface G, Cavaliere B, Caruso A. Early first-trimester sibutramine exposure: pregnancy outcome and neonatal follow-up. *Drug Saf* 2006; 29: 255-259.

Chapter 15

DIGESTIVES, INCLUDING ENZYMES

Use of digestives, including enzymes, is associated with co-morbidity which may explain an increased risk for pregnancy complications. One such association is with diabetes and among infants born an excess of hypoglycaemia is seen. In the limited material available, no signs of teratogencity is found but even a marked teratogenic effect cannot be excluded. If possible it may be wise to avoid use of these drugs in early pregnancy but if exposure has occurred, there is no reason to discuss a termination of the pregnancy.

In Sweden, digestive enzyme preparations are mainly used at pancreatic insufficiency with malabsorption and glutamic acid is used at achylia or hypochylia. Little is known about the use of these drugs during pregnancy. In one study, 21 patients using peroral enzyme preparations were included – none of the infants had a congenital malformation [1].

Table 15.1. Number of women identified with use of digestive drugs

Total	112
Reported use in early pregnancy	95
Got prescription later in prgnancy	46
Both early and later use	30

Type of drug	ATC code	Early use	Later use
Enzyme preparations	A09AA02	88	44
Glutamic acid	A09AB01	4	1
Unspecified	A09A000	3	1

CHARACTERISTICS OF WOMEN USING DIGESTIVE DRUGS

Based on women reporting digestive drugs in early pregnancy (n= 95). Comparison with all women who gave birth during the period and with information from the antenatal care (n=967 742). The odds ratios for maternal age, parity, smoking in early pregnancy, number of previous miscarriages, BMI, subfertility, and country of birth are adjusted for all other variables and for year of birth. The odds ratios for education, family situation, and work outside home are adjusted for year of delivery, maternal age, parity, smoking, and BMI (Table 15.2).

Table 15.2. Characteristics of women using digestive drugs in early pregnancy

Variable	Number of women with drug	OR	95% CI
Maternal age			
<25 years	11	0.60	0.32-1.14
25-34 years	63	1.00	Reference
≥35 years	21	1.52	0.91-2.53
Parity			
1	57	2.34	1.56-3.53
2+	38	1.00	Reference
Smoking			
Unknown	2	-	-
No	79	1.00	Reference
Yes	14	3.63	1.38-9.55
Earlier miscarriages			
No	74	1.00	Reference
Yes	21	1.20	0.74-1.95
BMI			
Unknown	11	-	-
<19.8	14	2.02	1.12-3.64
19.8-25.9	53	1.00	Reference
≥26	17	0.77	0.44-1.33
Subfertility (years of unwanted childlessness)			
No	85	1.00	Reference
Yes	10	1.07	0.56-2.08
Education (1996-2001, 45 women with digestive drugs, 526 695 in population)			
Unknown	2	-	-
<12 years	6	1.59	0.59-4.29
12 years	17	1.00	Reference
>12 years	20	1.57	0.81-2.02
Country of birth			
Unknown	0	-	-
Sweden	77	1.00	Reference
Other Nordic country	6	2.63	1.16-5.97
Non-Nordic country	12	0.90	0.49-1.64
Family situation			
Unknown	2	-	-
Co-habiting	84	1.00	Reference
Living alone	7	2.86	1.32-6.20
Other family situation	2	0.96	0.26-3.82
Work outside home			
Unknown	13	-	-
Full time	45	1.00	Reference
Part time	19	1.27	0.68-2.37
None	10	1.70	0.93-3.10

There is thus a trend of increasing drug use with maternal age and an excess at first parity. Smoking seems associated with the use of this drug category.

Most outcomes occur in excess but due to the relatively low number of exposures, many do not reach statistical significance. The increased risk of preexisting diabetes (and use of insulin, see above) is statistically significant and so is the increased risk for preeclampsia and placenta previa and also of having a caesarean section.

Table 15.3. Concomitant drug use (early pregnancy)

Drug group	Number	RR	95%CI
Drugs for stomach ulcer and reflux	5	5.68	1.84-13.3
Insulin	3	9.09	1.87-26.6
Multivitamins	14	2.73	1.49-4.58
Folic acid	6	1.38	0.51-3.00
Antibiotics	6	2.13	0.78-4.63
Minor analgesics	9	1.28	0.59-2.43
Antidepressants	4	3.20	0.87-8.19
Antihistamines	9	1.73	0.79-3.28

There is thus an association with insulin use but this is based on only three cases.

Table 15.4. Maternal delivery diagnoses associated with the use digestive drugs. As only few exposures occurred during late pregnancy, only early pregnancy exposures could be analyzed

Diagnosis	Number	OR/RR	95%CI
Preexisting diabetes	6	5.30	1.95-11.6#
Gestationaldiabetes	3	4.05	0.84-11.8#
Chronic hypertension	3	3.13	0.64.0.13#
Preeclampsia	11	2.44	1.22-4.37#
Hyperemesis gravidarum	3	3.80	0.78-11.1#
Placenta previa	4	4.08	1.11-10.5#
Abruptio placenta	3	2.65	0.55-7.76#
Antepartum bleeding	4	3.39	0.92-8.68#
Intrapartum bleeding	3	1.62	0.33-4.74#
Postpartum bleeding	8	1.49	0.64-2.94#
Delivery induction	17	1.71	0.99-2.73#
Caesarean section	30	2.25	1.47-3.44

#observed over expected number firh exact Poisson 95% confidence interval.

Outcome after Maternal use of Digestive Drugs

Infant Sex

When the mother had used digestive drugs in early pregnancy, 50 of the children were male and 46 female. Sex ratio is then 1.09 (95% CI 0.73-1.64) which is close to the normal sex ratio (1.06).

Multiple Births

After maternal use of digestive drugs in early pregnancy, only one twin delivery occurred.

Infant Mortality

No infant died perinatally.

Table 15.5. Pregnancy duration and infant birth weight after maternal use of digestive drugs in early pregnancy

Variable studied	Number	RR	95%CI
<37 weeks	14	2.77	1.51-4.64
<2500g	6	1.78	0.65-3.86
≥4500g	1	0.33	0.01-1.86
SGA	5	1.85	0.60-4.32
LGA	2	0.50	0.06-1.80

The increased risk for preterm birth is also seen among infants born after drug exposure later in pregnancy: RR =2.58, 95% CI 1.04-5.32.

Table 15.6. Neonatal diagnoses in infants whose mothers used digestive drugs in early pregnancy

Diagnosis	Number	OR	95% CI
Hypoglycaemia	9	2.37	1.08-4.50#
Respiratory diagnoses	5	0.94	0.30-2.19#
Low Apgar score	1	0.49	0.01-2.73#
CNS-diagnoses	1	1.01	0.03-5.63#
Jaundice	7	1.53	0.62-3.17#

#observed over expected number with exact 95% Poisson confidence interval.

The increased risk for hypoglycaemia was indicated also among infants exposed during late pregnancy: RR = 2.20, 95% CI 0.60-5.63 and is reasonably associated with the excess of maternal diabetes.

Two infants whose mothers used digestive drugs had a diagnosis of a congenital malformation. One had an atrium septum defect and the mother reported the use of an unspecified enzyme preparation. The second had an ileum atresia/stenosis and the mother had used glutamic acid. The malformation rate is thus low (2.1%) but the 95% CI is wide (0.3-7.3%) and can hide a marked teratogenicity,

Summary

Co-morbidity is apparent among women who used digestive drugs, including enzymes. Pregnancy complications appear to occur at an increased rate, reasonably due to co-morbidity. The number of studied pregnancies is relatively small but there are no signs of an increased risk for a congenital malformation in the offspring.

References

[1] Heinonen OP, Slone D, Monson RR, Hook EB, Shapiro S. *Birth Defects and Drugs in Pregnancy*. Publishin Sciences Group, Inc. Littleton, MA.

Chapter 16

DRUGS FOR DIABETES

Preexisting maternal diabetes type 1 and probably also type 2 are associated with a number of pregnancy and neonatal complications, including a marked increased risk for a congenital malformation. There is no strong specificity in malformation type but malformations in the central nervous system, cardiovascular malformations, and hypospadias all show significant risk increases. It is possible that intensive pre-pregnancy diabetes regulation can reduce the malformation risk. Intense supervision of the diabetic woman will increase the probability for a good pregnancy outcome but in spite of extensive efforts in this direction, intrauterine death and other serious complications occur at an increased frequency in such pregnancies.

Numerous studies have shown that maternal diabetes is associated with various pregnancy and delivery complications, including an increased risk for congenital malformations [1-5]. As diabetes type 1 is always treated with insulin, these associations will remain when outcome after maternal use of insulin is studied. The possible teratogenic effect of diabetes type 2 is less well known but has repeatedly been demonstrated. Diabetes type 2 may be treated with insulin but oral hypoglycaemic drugs are often used. The possible teratogenic effect of such drugs is still an open question. In this text, the two main groups of drugs for diabetes will be treated separately. Gestational diabetes arises during pregnancy and is sometimes treated with drugs. A teratogenic effect of gestational diabetes has been thought to be due to undetected pre-existing diabetes type 2.

Only one third of women who reported the use of insulin in early pregnancy were identified as having insulin in later pregnancy in spite of the fact that practically all will have had it. The reason to this is that drug prescription to diabetic women during pregnancy will in most instances be recorded in separate medical records and will therefore often not be recorded in the MV2 form.

Table 16.1. Number of women identified with drugs for diabetes

	Insulin	Oral
Total	4136	248
Reported in early pregnancy	3162	217
Got prescription later in pregnany	2028	80
Both early and late use	1054	49

Type of insulin	ATC code	Early use	Later use
Unspecified	A10A	889	442
Fast-acting insulin			
Human	A10AB01	889	388
Insulin lispro	A10AB04	873	622
Insulin aspart	A10AB05	450	520
Intermedium- acting insulin			
Human	A10AC01	1661	942
Intermedium-acting, rapid onset insulin			
Human	A10AD01	35	28
Insulin lispro	A10AD04	67	4
Long acting insulin			
Unspecified	A10AE00	299	275
Insulin glargine	A10AE04	17	20
Insulin detemir	A10AE05	17	14

Type of oral antidiabetic drugs	ATC code	Early use	Later use
Biagunides			
Metformin	A10BA02	183	71
Sulfonamides			
Glibenclamide	A10BB01	20	4
Glipizide	A10BB07	13	1
Combinations			
Metformin+rosiglitazone	A10BD03	1	0
Alpha glucosidase inhibitor			
Acarbose	A10BF01	1	0
Tiazolidindiones			
Rosiglitazone	A10BG02	10	5
Pioglitazone	A10BG03	1	0
Other			
Repaglinide	A10BX02	4	1

Information on the use of antidiabetic drugs in early pregnancy can be compared with delivery diagnoses of diabetes. Among 3347 women who had reported the use of an antidiabetic drug, 350 (=10.5%) had no delivery diagnosis of diabetes. Among those who had such a diagnosis, 2509 (83.7) had a diagnosis of preexisting diabetes type 1 and 42 (2.7%) a diagnosis of pre-existing diabetes type 2. A (mis)diagnosis of gestational diabetes existed in 193 cases (6.4%) and in 203 (7.1%) instances an other or unspecific diabetes diagnosis was given.

Characteristics of Women using Antidiabetic Drugs

Based on women reporting the drug in early pregnancy (n=7913, one missing maternal age). Each variable is adjusted for all other variables and year of delivery. Comparison with all women who gave birth during the period and with information from the first antenatal care (n=967 742). The odds ratios for maternal age, parity, smoking in early pregnancy, number of previous miscarriages, BMI, subfertility, and country of birth are adjusted for all other variables and are shown in Figure 16.1. The unbroken graphs refer to women using insulin, the dashed graphs to women using oral antidiabetics.

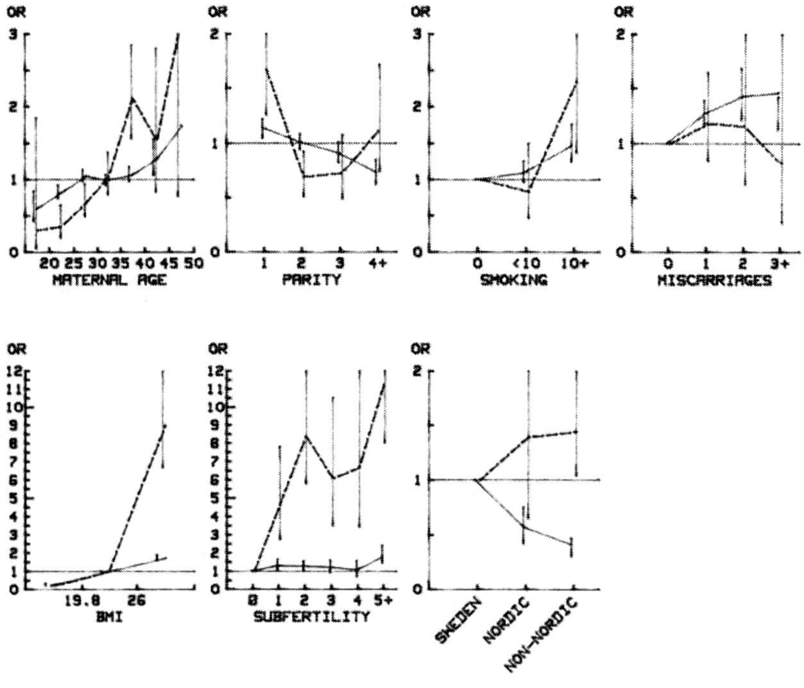

Figure 16.1. Odds ratios for seven maternal characteristics. The odds ratios (OR) for each variable are adjusted for the other variables and year of delivery. Vertical lines mark 95% confidence intervals. For maternal age and parity, each class is compared with all other classes.

Some further maternal characteristics were analyzed, adjusting for year of delivery, maternal age, parity, smoking, and BMI (Table 16.2).

Table 16.2. Some further characteristics of women using antidiabetic drugs during pregnancy

Variable	With insulin			With oral antidiabetic		
	Number of women with drug	OR	95%CI	Number of women with drug	OR	95% CI
Education (1996-2001 ,1 472 women with insulin, 57 with oral antidiabetics,526 695 inpopulation)						
Unknown	29	-		2	-	-
<12 years	160	0.90	0.75-1.08	7	1.22	0.51-2.96
12 years	831	1.00	reference	32	1.00	reference
13-14 years	62	0.70	0.52-0.88	16	0.59	0.31-1.11
≥14 years	390	0.80	0.71-0.91			
Family situation						
Unknown	21	-	-	2	-	-
Cohabiting	2963	1.00	reference	205	1.00	reference
Living alone	62	0.76	0.59-0.98	9	1.51	0.77-2.96
Other family situation	74	0.91	0.71-1.15	1	-	-
Work outside home						
Unknown	396	-	-	23	-	-
Full time	1438	1.00	reference	100	1.00	reference
Part time	795	1.11	1.02-1.22	44	0.98	0.67-1.43
None	531	1.04	0.93-1.15	50	1.32	0.91-1.91

There is an increased use with maternal age, more evident for oral antidiabetic drugs than for insulin. There is an excess of first parity women in both groups and an increased percentage of heavy smokers. There is an association with previous miscarriages in women using insulin but no certain such association for women using oral antidiabetics. High BMI and subfertility occur strongly associated with use of oral antidiabetics but only weakly with insulin. The pattern of country of birth differs markedly between the two groups. Women using antidiabetic drugs have a shorter education than expected. Use of insulin occurs more often than expected among co-habiting women than among women in other family situations and they more often than expected work only part time.

Table 16.3. Concomitant drug use (early pregnancy)

Drug group	Insulin			Oral antidiabetics		
	Number	OR	95% CI	Number	OR	95% CI
Drugs used for stomach ulcer and reflux	27	0.97	0.66-1.43	6	2.39	0.88-5.20#
Drugs for inflammatory bowel disease	15	1.80	1.01-2.97	2	2.82	0.34-10.2#
Multivitamins	126	0.68	0.56-0.82	9	0.62	0.31-1.21#
Folic acid	148	0.98	0.82-1.16	13	0.98	0.55-1.74
Drugs for hypertension	139	10.7	9.30-12.4	17	9.19	5.35-14.8#
Oral contraceptive	7	0.72	0.29-1.50#	0	0.00	0.00-7.10#
Progestogens	8	0.59	0.30-1.17	6	5.04	1.85-11.6#
Gonadotrophins	9	1.23	0.56-2.34#	6	12.2	4.49-26.7#
Systemic corticosteroids	15	1.25	0.75-2.08	2	2.56	0.31-9.26#
Thyroid drugs	280	7.26	6.52-8.08	11	2.51	1.25-4.49#
Antibiotics	66	0.66	0.52-0.85	7	1.25	0.50-2.58#
NSAID	30	0.52	0.36-0.74	7	1.34	0.54-2.58#
Opioids	17	0.95	0.59-1.54	1	0.52	0.02-2.90#
Minor analgesics	89	0.34	0.28-0.41	9	0.45	0.24-0.86#
Drugs for migraine	2	0.22	0.03-0.81#	1	1.20	0.03-6.71#
Anticonvulsants	16	1.63	0.93-2.65	1	1.25	0.03-7.53#
Sedatives, hypnotics	14	0.88	0.51-1.50	4	2.23	0.61-5.72#
Antidepressants	49	1.17	0.88-1.56	11	2.08	1.04-3.73#
Drugs for rhinitis	21	0.46	0.30-0.69	3	0.86	0.18-2.53#
Antiasthmatics	92	0.89	0.72-1.10	13	1.56	0.83-2.67#
Antitussives	7	0.42	0.21-0.87	1	0.88	0.02-4.93#
Antihistamines	80	0.44	0.31-0.54	9	0.71	0.37-1.38
For NVP	56	0.41	0.31-0.52	4	0.43	0.12-1.10#
For allergy	28	0.56	0.39-0.81	5	1.44	0.47-3.35#

#observed over expected numbers with exact Poisson 95% confidence interval.

The number of women using oral antidiabetics is low and therefore numbers with concomitant drug use very low for most classes. Women using insulin report less use than expected of many common drug groups but a strong association with drugs for hypertension and thyroid drugs (both also seen for women using oral antidiabetics), indicating co-morbidity. Also for drugs for inflammatory bowel disease, an excess use of insulin in seen.

In the further discussion, only exposures during early pregnancy will be analyzed. These are to be looked upon as proxies for maternal diabetes. If a woman actually used insulin in later but not early pregnancy, this would indicate the development of severe gestational diabetes but such women are difficult to identify because some use of insulin in early pregnancy have probably not been recorded.

The association between diabetes and chronic hypertension is evident with both types of antidiabetic drugs. There is a markedly increased risk for pregnancy complications for both types of drugs leading to an increased use of delivery inductions and caesarean sections, more marked for users of insulin than for users of oral antidiabetic drugs.

Table 16.4. Maternal delivery diagnoses associated with the use of antidiabetic drugs in early pregnancy

Diagnosis	Insulin			Oral antidiabetics		
	Number	OR	95%CI	Number	OR	95% CI
Chronic hypertension	262	6.03	5.37-6.77	26	4.60	3.01-6.74#
Preeclampsia	701	4.97	4.60-5.37	39	4.68	2.86-7.23#
Hyperemesis gravidarum	194	5.20	4.54-5.95	19	4.33	2.61-6.62#
Placenta previa	197	4.73	4.13-5.41	19	3.89	2.34-5.94#
Abruptio placentae	216	4.80	4.22-5.46	20	4.02	2.45-6.20#
Antepartum bleeding	199	4.11	3.59-4.71	20	4.02	2.45-6.20#
Intrapartum bleeding	314	4.35	3.89-4.85	30	3.74	2.52-5.33#
Postpartum bleeding	309	1.64	1.46-1.85	30	2.17	1.48-3.18#
Delivery induction	1166	6.19	5.77-6.64	75	3.47	2.52-6-20
Caesarean section	1708	5.22	4.90-5.56	92	2.57	1.97-3.34

#observed over expected numbers with exact Poisson 95% confidence interval.

Outcome after Maternal use of Antidiabetic Drugs

Infant Sex

Among infants born of women treated with insulin in early pregnancy, 1 680 were male and 1 526 female, sex ratio 1.10 (95% CI 1.03-1.18) and among infants born of women treated with oral antidiabetics in early pregnancy, 111 were male and 109 female, sex ratio 1.03 (95% CI 0.78-1.33). The normal sex ratio (1.06) is thus contained in both confidence intervals.

Multiple Births

After maternal use of insulin in early pregnancy, there were 41 twin deliveries and two triplet deliveries. The odds ratio for a twin delivery was 0.84 (95% CI 0.62-1.15). After maternal use of oral antidiabetics, there were three twin deliveries, risk ratio 0.78 (exact Poisson 95% CI 0.10-2.28). Even though twinning rates were lower than expected, this could well be random.

Table 16.5. Infant mortality (including multiple births)

	Insulin			Oral antidiabetics		
Variable studied	Number	OR	95% CI	Number	OR	95%CI
Stillbirth	43	3.62	2.70-4.84	0	-	-
Early neonatal death	9	1.83	0.84-3.46#	0	-	-

#observed over expected numbers with exact Poisson 95% confidence interval.

There is thus a clear-cut increased perinatal mortality after early use of insulin, that is, mainly diabetes type 1. After oral antidiabetics no deaths occurred.

Table 16.6. Pregnancy duration and birth weight at maternal use of antidiabetics

Variable studied	Insulin			Oral antidiabetic		
	Number	OR	95% CI	Number	OR/RR	95% CI
<37 weeks	689	5.48	5.08-5.92	29	2.53	1.73-3.69
<2500g	164	1.74	1.49-2.04	11	1.47	0.73-2.63#
≥4500g	404	3.16	2.86-3.50	18	1.53	0.92-2.49
SGA	51	0.75	0.57-1.00	3	0.61	0.13-1.78#
LGA	1117	8.55	8.01-9.11	36	2.24	1.57-3.18

#observed over expected numbers with exact Poisson 95% confidence interval.

For both types of drugs, an increased risk for preterm birth is seen but also for LGA and for heavy infants (not significant for oral antidiabetics).

Table 16.7. Neonatal diagnoses in infants whose mothers used antidiabetics in early pregnancy

Variable studied	Insulin			Oral antidiabetic		
	Number	OR	95% CI	Number	OR/RR	95% CI
Hypoglycaemia	1566	23.8	22.7-25.0	62	7.67	5.92-9.94
Respiratory diagnoses	475	3.22	2.93-3.53	21	1.65	1.05-2.61
Low Apgar score	110	1.74	1.44-2.10	4	0.74	0.20-1.89#
CNS diagnoses	76	3.74	3.01-4.64	2	0.94	0.11-3.41#
Jaundice	480	3.99	3.64-4.37	19	1.72	1.07-2.74

#observed over expected numbers with exact Poisson 95% confidence interval.

The high risk for hypoglycaemia is expected among infants born of women with diabetes but also the other neonatal diagnoses studied show marked overrisks. After use of oral antidiabetics, risk estimates are lower but have wide confidence intervals.

Table 16.8. Congenital malformations in infants whose mothers used insulin in early pregnancy

Congenital malformations	Number	OR/RR	95% CI
All malformations	263	1.69	1.46-1.94
Relatively severe malformations	213	1.86	1.59-2.17
Chromosome anomalies	8	1.16	0.50-2.29#
Without chromosome anomalies			
CNS malformations	10	2.39	1.15-4.40
Ear malformations	13	1.67	0.89-2.86#
Orofacial clefts	7	1.14	0.46-2.35#
Cardiovascular defects	101	2.91	2.34-3.62
Among them VSD or ASD	56	3.12	2.37-4.12
Among them unspecified defects	11	3.18	1.59-5.69#
Hypospadias	21	2.05	1.26-3.34#
Severe kidney malformations	3	1.52	0.31-4.45#
Limb reduction defects	3	1.49	0.31-4.37#
Poly/syndactyly	11	1.69	0.84-3.03#
Unstable hip	12	0.66	0.36-1.18

#observed over expected number with exact Poisson 95% confidence interval.

The CNS malformations consisted of: one infant with microcephaly, three with hydrocephaly, one with holoprosencephaly, one with brain substance reduction, two with spina bifida, and two with another spinal cord malformation. Eleven of the 13 ear malformations were preauricular appendices. A three times increased risk for a cardiovascular defect appears to occur both for severe, mild, and unspecified defects. There is an increased risk for hypospadias. - Some of these infants were multimalformed.

The total malformation rate varies slightly according to type of insulin used but partly these variations can be random, partly the interpretation is complex because many patients use a mixture of different insulins.

Table 16.9. Malformations after maternal use of different types of insulin in early pregnancy

Insulin used	Number malformed	OR	95% CI
Fast acting	183	1.73	1.46-2.05
Intermedium acting	140	1.71	1.41-2.07
Intermedium acting, fast onset	7	1.53	0.66-3.02#
Long acting	24	1.40	0.85-2.30
Insulin lispro	68	1.31	0.97-1.70
Insulin aspart	36	1.88	1.28-2.78

observed over expected number with exact Poisson 95% confidence interval.

The lower risk after insulin lispro compared with insulin aspart can be random ($z=1.45$, $p=0.14$). Among 17 infants exposed to insulin glargine, none was malformed. Among 17 infants exposed to insulin detemir, one had a malformation (ventricular septum defect).

Only nine malformed infants were observed after maternal use of oral antidiabetics in early pregnancy. Two malformations were mild: tongue tie and hip (sub)luxation, respectively. The OR for a relatively severe malformation was 0.89 (95% CI 0.31-1.83).

Table 16.10. Specification of congenital malformations after use of oral antidiabetics

Congenital malformation	Antidiabetic drug used	Other drugs
Atrium septum defect	glibenclamide	terbutaline+diclofenac+ibuprofen+ paracetamol
Pulmonary valve stenosis	metformin+acarbose	valproic acid+lamotrigine+iron
Cleft lip	metformin	-
Pes equinovarus	metformin	-
Pes calcaneovalgus	glibenclamide+insulin lispro	enalapril+metoprolol
Chest deformity	metformin	iron
Unspecified malformation	metformin	furosemide+metoprolol+isradipine+ amlodipine+captopril

It can be noted that one of the mothers with a malformed infant had used two anticonvulsants and two had used antihypertensive drugs.

SUMMARY

Women with diabetes type 1 or type 2 and therefore using antidiabetic drugs have an increased risk for pregnancy complications. Infants born of these women also have an increased risk for neonatal complications and – after insulin – of stillbirth. The risk of congenital malformations is markedly increased after maternal use of insulin but not after use of oral antidiabetics but numbers are low and estimates uncertain. Three groups of malformations are especially increased in rate: CNS malformations, cardiovascular defects, and hypospadias. According to the literature an increased risk also exists for other types of malformations [5] but numbers in the present study are not large enough to study rare malformations. Everything speaks in favour of the idea that these deviations are linked to preexisting diabetes and especially to diabetes type 1 and are no effect of treatments.

References

[1] Åberg A, Westbom L, Källén B. Congenital malformations among infants whose mothers had gestational diabetes or preexisting diabetes. *Early Hum Dev* 2001; 61: 85-95.

[2] Correa A, Gilboa SM, Besser Lm, Botto LD, Moore CA, Hobbs CA, Cleves MA, Riehle-Colarusso TJ, Waller DK, Reece EA. Diabetes mellitus and birth defects, *Am J Obst Gynecol* 2008; 199: 237.el-9.

[3] Bell R, Bailey K, Cresswell T, Hawthorne G, Critchley J, Lewis-Barned N, on behalf of the Northern Diabetic Pregnancy Survey Steering Group. BJOG. Trends in prevalence and outcomes of pregnancy in women with pre-existing type I and type II diabetes. 2008; E-publication before print: DOI: 10,1111/j.1471-0528.2007.01644.x. 445-452.

[4] Allen VM, Armson BA, Wilson RD Allen VM, Blight C, Gagnon A, Johnson JA, Langlois S, Summers A, Wyatt P, Farine D, Armson BA, Crane J, Delisle MF, Keenan-Lindsay L, Morin V, Schneider CE, Van Aerde J: Teratogenicity associated with preexisting and gestational diabetes. *J Obstet Gynaecol Can* 2007; 29: 927-944.

[5] Frías JL, Frías JP, Frías PA, Martínez.Frías ML. Infrequently studies congenital anomalies as clues to the diagnosis of maternal diabetes mellitus. *Amer J Med Genet Part* A. 2007; 143A: 2904-2909.

Chapter 17

VITAMINS AND MINERALS

Use of multivitamin preparations in early pregnancy and still more later in pregnancy is common and may have beneficial effects for the woman and child but the described positive effects on the rate of congenital malformations are not verified in Swedish studies. It is possible that in populations with wide-spread vitamin deficiency, vitamin supplementation may decrease malformation risk but most studies are based on retrospective interviews with a risk for recall bias. High doses of vitamin A (50,000 IU or more) should be avoided but possible risks involved are uncertain and hardly motivate a discussion of pregnancy termination.

Table 17.1. Number of women identified using vitamins or minerals

Total	200 612
Reported use in early pregnancy	57 419
Got prescription later in pregnancy	169 801
Both early and later use	26 608

Type of drug	ATC code	Early use	Later use
Vitamins	A11	55 491	164 453
Multivitamins	A11A,B,J	53 154	160 695
Vitamin A	A11CA	12	4
Vitamin B	A11D,AH,HA02	135	121
Vitamin C	A11GA	1 435	3 326
Vitamin D	A11CC	133	96
Vitamin E	A11HA03	197	222
Minerals	*A12*	3 352	9 475
Calcium	A12A	2 916	8 668
Potassium	A12B	54	58
Zink	A12CB	183	164
Magnesium	A12CC	224	448

Use of vitamins and minerals are generally regarded as beneficial. Notably the use of multivitamin preparations has often been linked to a reduced risk of various congenital malformations [1-6]. On the other hand, high doses of vitamin A (even as low as 10,000 IU) has been regarded as teratogenic in analogy with some retinoic acid derivates [7-8] but other studies have not found such an effect [9-10]. One TIS study identified 120 infants exposed to 50,000 IU of vitamin A or more without finding an excess of congenital malformotions [11]. A recent study even suggested a protective effect of vitamins for isolated cleft palate [12].

Among women reporting the use of vitamins in early pregnancy, 1374 also reported the use of minerals (2.5%) and among the women who reported the use of minerals, 41% reported also the use of vitamins

Characteristics of Women using Vitamins or Minerals

Based on women reporting only vitamins (n=54 064, three missing maternal age, unbroken graphs) or only minerals (n=1 978, dashed graphs) in early pregnancy. Each variable is adjusted for all other variables and year of delivery. Comparison with all women who gave birth during the period and with information from the first antenatal care (n=967 742). The odds ratios for maternal age, parity, smoking in early pregnancy, number of previous miscarriages, BMI, subfertility, and country of birth are adjusted for all other variables and are shown in Figure 17.1.

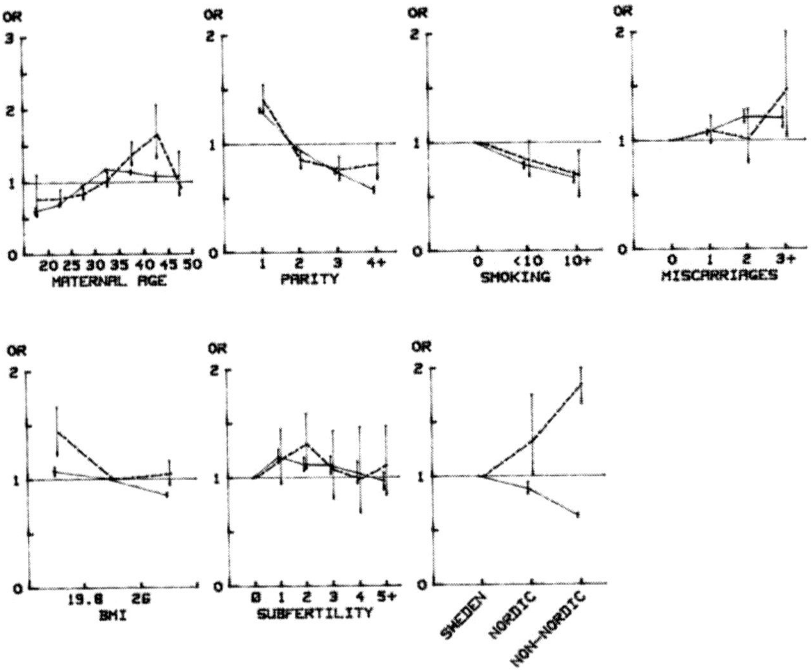

Figure 17.1. Odds ratios for seven maternal characteristics. The odds ratios (OR) for each variable are adjusted for the other variables and year of delivery. Vertical lines mark 95% confidence intervals. For maternal age and parity, each class is compared with all other classes. Unbroken graphs show vitamin users, dashed graphs mineral users.

Some further maternal characteristics were analyzed, adjusting for year of delivery, maternal age, parity, smoking, and BMI (Table 17.2).

Table 17.2. Some further characteristics of women using vitamins or minerals

Variable studied	Vitamins only			Minerals only		
	Number	OR	95% CI	Number	OR	95% CI
Education (1996-2001, women withonly vitamins, 485 with only mineral , 526 695 in population)						
Unknown	176	-	-	23	-	-
<12 years	480	0.83	0.75-0.91	47	0.92	0.66-1.29
12 years	2973	1.00	reference	227	1.00	reference
13 years	442	1.23	1.11-1.37	32	1.25	0.86-1.82
≥14 years	2352	1.18	1.16-1.25	156	1.11	0.89-1.38
Family situation						
Unknown	775	-	-	33	-	-
Co-habiting	51243	1.00	reference	1822	1.00	reference
Living alone	651	0.71	0.65-0.77	41	1.04	0.76-1.43
Other family situation	1395	0.78	0.74-0.83	82	1.29	1.03-1.62
Work outside home						
Unknown	4537	-	-	232	-	-
Full time	27872	1.00	reference	850	1.00	reference
Part time	12677	1.02	1.00-1.05	412	1.08	0.95-1.22
None	8978	0.96	0.93-0.98	484	1.63	1.45-1.83

Table 17.3. Concomitant drug use (early pregnancy)

Drug group	Vitamins only			Minerals only		
	Number	OR	95% CI	Number	OR/RR	95% CI
Drugs for stomach ulcer and reflux	480	1.06	0.96-1.17	37	2.19	1.58-3.00
Drugs for inflammatory bowel disease	210	1.30	1.12-1.51	65	10.7	8.28-13.7#
Insulin	130	0.68	0.56-0.81	12	1.80	0.93-3.15#
Folic acid	5467	0.96	0.95-0.98	589	4.64	4.24-5.08
Antihypertensives	215	0.82	0.71-0.96	24	2.60	1.67-2.89#
Oral contraceptives	73	0.83	0.65-1.04	6	1.55	0.57-3.37#
Progestogens	183	1.08	0.92-1.26	9	1.24	0.57-2.36#
Gonadotrophines	57	0.76	0.58-0.99	2	0.60	0.07-2.17#
Systemic corticosteroids	146	0.87	0.73-1.03	91	13.7	11.0-16.8#
Thyroid drugs	914	1.16	1.08-1.35	81	2.94	2.37-3.64
Antibiotics	1459	0.94	0.88-0.99	71	1.12	0.97-1.56
NSAIDs	568	0.87	0.80-0.95	27	1.05	0.72-1.55
Opioids	245	0.81	0.71-0.92	29	2.82	1.97-4.01
Minor analgesics	3018	1.15	1.11-1.20	126	1.17	0.97-1.40
Drugs for migraine	66	0.58	0.48-0.75	9	2.13	0.98-4.05#
Anticonvulsants	151	1.04	0.88-1.23	11	2.03	1.01-3.64#
Neuroleptics	30	1.12	0.77-1.65	2	1.63	0.20-5.87#
Sedatives, hypnotics	169	0.84	0.72-0.99	12	1.51	0.78-2.64#
Antidepressants	604	0.91	0.89-1.00	29	1.21	0.84-1.74
Drugs for rhinitis	813	1.15	1.07-1.25	39	1.47	1.06-1.71
Cough medicines	291	0.90	0.85-0.96	122	1.42	1.18-1.70
Antiasthmatics	1271	1.23	1.08-1.40	13	1.46	0.78-2.50#
Antihistamines	2541	0.94	0.90-0.99	103	1.03	0.85-1.26
For NVP	1967	0.97	0.92-1.02	67	0.88	0.69-1.12
For allergy	652	0.87	0.80-0.95	40	1.46	1.07-1.99

#observed over expected number with exact Poisson 95% confidence interval

Maternal characteristics of the two groups resemble each other except for country of birth (women born outside Sweden use less vitamins and more minerals than women born in Sweden), family situation and work outside home. Use of vitamins and minerals increased with maternal age, decreased with parity, was less prevalent among smokers, and slightly more prevalent among women who had previous miscarriages. Minerals but not vitamins were used more often among women with low than high BMI.

There is thus a very strong association between use of minerals and drugs for immunological bowel disease and systemic corticosteroids. Thyroid drugs are associated both with vitamin and mineral use. The associations, for instance, with minor analgesics and drugs for rhinitis could be an expression of an unusually detailed reporting or recording of drug use.

Table 17.4. Some maternal diagnoses associated with the use of vitamins or minerals The analysis is restricted to use in early pregnancy

Diagnosis	Only vitamins			Only minerals		
	Number	OR/RR	95% CI	Number	OR/RR	95% CI
Pre-existing diabetes	533	0.73	0.67-0.80	35	1.30	0.93-1.82
Chronic hypertension	537	0.81	0.74-0.89	33	1.27	0.90-1.80
Gestational diabetes	393	0.85	0.76-0.94	19	1.02	0.65-1.61
Preeclampsia	2198	0.85	0.81-0.89	94	0.97	0.79-1.19
Hyperemesis gravidarum	441	0.80	0.73-0.89	24	1.14	0.76-1.70
Placenta previa	546	0.89	0.81-0.97	22	0.93	0.61-1.41
Abruptio placentae	570	0.86	0.78-0.94	29	1.13	0.78-1.63
Antepartum bleeding	621	0.88	0.81-0.96	32	1.12	0.79-1.60
Intrapartum bleeding	1272	0.99	0.93-1.05	46	0.95	0.71-1.27
Postpartum bleeding	3155	1.04	1.00-1.08	95	0.83	0.68-1.02
Delivery induction	5945	0.95	0.93-0.98	260	1.20	1.05-1.37
Caesarean section	9518	0.99	0.97-1.02	422	1.26	1.12-1.40

#observed over expected number with exact Poisson 95% confidence interval.

The only significant excess concerns delivery induction and caesarean section after use of minerals and postpartum bleeding after the use of vitamins.

Outcome after Maternal use of Vitamins and Minerals

Infant Sex

After early use of vitamins, there were 28 344 male infants and 26 552 female infants (6 with unknown sex) which gives a sex ratio of 1.07 (95% CI 1.05-1.09). After early use of minerals, there were 1032 male and 987 female infants, sex ratio 1.05 (95% CI 0.96-1.14). There is thus no deviation from the normal sex ratio of 1.06.

Multiple Births

After use of vitamins in early pregnancy, there were 831 twin deliveries and 6 triplet deliveries. The odds ratio for twinning was 1.09 (95% CI 1.01-1.17). After exclusion of women who reported a period of unwanted childlessness from the analysis, 614 twin deliveries remained with an odds ratio of twinning 1.07 (0.98-1.17). The remaining slight increase in twinning rate is thus not statistically significant.

After early use of minerals, there were 39 twin and one triplet delivery. The odds ratio for twinning was 1.34 (95% CI 0.97-1.84). After exclusion of women with unwanted childlessness, the odds ratio (based on 25 twins) went down to 1.18 (9%% CI 0.78-1.74). One triplet delivery remained.

Table 17.5. Infant mortality after maternal use of minerals or vitamins

Variable studied	Vitamin use			Mineral use		
	Number	OR	95% CI	Number	RR	95% CI
Stillbirth	155	0.90	0.76-1.07	8	0.70	0.30-1.38
Early neonatal death	64	0.93	0.72-1.21	6	1.34	0.59-3.02#

There is thus no significant deviation from expected rates of perinatal mortality.

Table 17.6. Pregnancy duration and infant birth weight at maternal use of vitamins and minerals

Variable studied	Vitamins			Minerals		
	Number	OR/RR	95% CI	Number	OR/RR	95% CI
<37 weeks	2357	0.90	0.86-0.94	126	1.33	1.11-1.60
<2500g	1443	0.85	0.80-0.90	97	1.57	1.28-1.93
≥4500g	2206	1.12	1.01-1.17	60	0.78	0.60-1.01
SGA	1049	0.87	0.82-0.93	67	1.53	1.19-1.95
LGA	3111	1.09	1.04-1.13	95	0.86	0.70-1.06

After early vitamin use, the risk for preterm birth, low birth weight, and SGA is slightly reduced while after early mineral use there is a clear-cut excess of preterm birth, low birth weight, and SGA.

In order to see to what extent the latter phenomena could be effects of concomitant drugs, used in excess, the analysis was repeated after exclusion of women who reported also the use of the following drugs: drugs for immunological bowel disease, systemic corticosteroids, thyroid drugs, antihypertensives, opiates and antiasthmatic drugs. The odds ratio for preterm birth then decreased to 1.07 (95% CI 0.86-1.33) and for SGA to 1.31 (95% CI 0.98-1.75). It is likely that these effects were mainly the result of confounding from concomitant drug use.

Table 17.7. Neonatal diagnoses after maternal use of vitamins or minerals in early pregnancy

Diagnosis	Vitamin use			Mineral use		
	Number	OR/RR	95% CI	Number	OR/RR	95% CI
Hypoglycaemia	1922	0.92	0.88-0.97	89	1.17	0.94-1.45
Respiratory diagnoses	2432	0.94	0.90-0.98	126	1.31	1.10-1.58
Low Apgar score	882	0.87	0.81-0.94	51	1.33	1.00-1.76
CNS diagnoses	349	0.83	0.74-0.93	25	0.99	0.66-1.47
Jaundice	2386	1.00	0.95-1.04	201	1.37	1.19-1.58

Infants born of mothers who took vitamins in early pregnancy thus consistently have lower risk than expected for neonatal complications while the opposite is seen after mineral use. After exclusion from the analysis of women who had used some drugs which occurred in excess (see above), the odds ratios declined and only two remained statistically significant: respiratory diagnoses (OR = 1.26, 95% CI 1.02-1.54) and CNS diagnoses (OR = 1.72 (95% CI 1.13-2.61). The latter OR thus actually increased somewhat.

Table 17.8. Congenital malformations in infants whose mothers had used vitamins or minerals in early pregnancy

Congenital malformation	Number	OR	95% CI
Vitamin use			
All malformations	2443	1.02	0.99-1.06
Relatively severe malformations	1702	1.00	0.95-1.06
Chromosome anomalies	110	1.13	0.91-1.39
Without chromosome anomalies			
Any CNS malformation	39	0.84	0.59-1.20
Neural tube defects	10	0.69	0.34-1.39
Eye malformations	32	1.05	0.71-1-54
Ear malformations	95	0.97	0.78-1.21
Any cardiovascular defect	577	1.04	0.94-1.14
VSD and/or ASD	368	1.09	0.97-1.23
Unspecified cardiac defect	44	1.09	0.77-1.54
Orofacial cleft	84	0.90	0.71-1.15
Oesophageal atresia	13	1.11	0.59-2.08
Small gut atresia	17	1.39	0.78-2.49
Anal atresia	14	0.82	0.46-1.46
Pylorostenosis	35	0.91	0.62-1.32
Hypospadias	145	1.02	0.85-1.23
Abdominal wall defect	6	0.43	0.19-0.97
Diaphragmatic hernia	18	1.50	0.80-2.61
Kidney a/dysgenesis	9	0.77	0.39-1.54
Cystic kidney	16	0.68	0.37-1.24
Pes equinovarus	75	0.93	0.71-1.21
Poly/syndactyly	112	0.95	0.77-1.17
Limb reduction defects	26	0.87	0.56-1.34
Hip (sub)luxation, unstable hip	373	1.04	0.92-1.16
Craniostenosis	34	1.12	0.76-1.15
Mineral use			
All malformations	96	1.07	0.86-1.32
Relatively severe malformations	68	1.09	0.84-1.40
Chromosome anomalies	4	0.94	0.26-2.41#
Without chromosome anomalies			
Ear malformations	3	0.82	0.26-5.53#
Any cardiovascular defect	20	1.10	0.71-1.71
VSD and/or ASD	9	0.82	0.42-1.57#
Hypospadias	7	1.28	0.51-2.63#
Limb reduction defect	3	2.94	0.61-8.60#
Hip (sub)luxation, unstable hip	16	1.12	0.66-1.90

#observed over expected number with exact Poisson 95% confidence interval.

There is thus no convincing reduction in the risk of getting an infant with a congenital malformation after use of vitamins (mainly multivitamins) or minerals. Only for one condition, abdominal wall defects, a risk ratio significantly less than 1.0 was seen but this was based on only 6 cases (two omphalocele, three gastroschisis and one other abdominal wall defect). This apparent protective effect can well be a result of multiple testing.

Only 13 infants had been exposed to vitamin A in high dosage (50,000 IU) – none had a congenital malformation. None of the 135 infants born of women who had taken D vitamin preparations in early pregnancy had a congenital malformation. The risk for a congenital malformation was non-significantly low after maternal use of C vitamin (OR = 0.85, 95% CI 0.65-1.11) or E vitamin preparations (OR = 0.88, 95% CI = 0.45-1.71) and slightly but non-significantly high after the use of vitamin B preparations (RR = 1.08, 95% CI 0.50-2.33).

Summary

Women who reported use of vitamin preparations in early pregnancy had slightly better delivery outcome than other women but no protective effect was seen on congenital malformations. The slight positive effects could be the result of residual confounding, notably of a socioeconomic nature. After maternal use of mineral supplements, there was an excess of pregnancy and neonatal complications which seemed largely explainable by effects of concomitantly used drugs and maternal pathology associated with those. No increase in the risk for a congenital malformation was seen.

References

[1] Mulinare J, Cordero JF, Erickson JD, Berry RS. Periconceptional use of multivitamins and the occurrence of neural tube defects. *JAMA* 1988;260:3141-5.

[2] Milunsky A, Jick H, Jick SS, Bruell CJ, Maclaughlin DA, Rothman KJ, Willett W. Multivitamin/folic acid supplementation in early pregnancy reduces the prevalence of neural tube defects. *JAMA* 1989;262:2847-52.

[3] Shaw GM, Schaffer D, Velie EM, Morland K, Harris JA. Periconceptional vitamin use, dietary folate, and the occurrence of neural tube defects. *Epidemiology* 1995;6:219-26.

[4] Botto LD, Khoury MJ, Mulinare J, Erickson JD. Periconceptional multivitamin use and the occurrence of conotruncal heart defects: results from a population-based, case-control study. *Pediatrics* 1996;98:911-7.

[5] Werler MM, Cragan JD, Wasserman CR,Shaw GM, Erickson JD, Mitcell AA. Multivitamin supplementation and multiple births. *Am J Med Genet* 1997;71:93-6.

[6] Botto LD, Mulinare J, Erickson JD. Occurrence of congenital heart defects in relation to maternal mulitivitamin use. *Am J Epidemiol* 2000;151:878-84.

[7] Rothman KJ, Moore LL, Singer MR, Nguyen US, Mannino S, Milunsky A. Teratogenicity of high vitamin A intake. *N Engl J Med* 1995;333:1369-73.

[8] Botto LD, Loffredo C, Scanlon KS, Ferencz C, Khoury MJ, David Wilson P, Correa A. Vitamin A and cardiac outflow tract defects. *Epidemiology* 2001;12:491-6.

[9] Mills JL, Simpson JL, Cunningham GC, Conley MR, Rhoads GG. Vitamin A and birth defects. *Am J Obstet Gynecol* 1997;177:31-6.

[10] Miller RK, Hendrickx AG, Mills JL, Hummler H, Wiedand UW. Periconceptional vitamin A use: how much is teratogenic? *Reprod Toxicol* 1998;12:75-88.

[11] Mastroiacovo P, Mazzone T, Addis A, Elephant E, Carlier P, Vial T, Gaarbis H, Robert E, Ornoy A, Finardi A, Schaffer C, Caramelli L, Rodrígues-Pinilla E, Clementi M. High vitamin A intake in early pregnancy and major malformations: a multicenter prospective controlled study. *Teratology* 1999;59:7-11.

[12] Johansen AM, Lie RT, Wilcox AJ, Andersen LF, Drevon CA. Maternal dietary intake of vitamin A and risk of orofacial clefts: A population-based case-control study in Norway. *Amer J Epidemiol* 2008; 167: 1164-1170.

Chapter 18

ANABOLIC STEROIDS

Anabolic steroids have androgenic properties and use or mis-use of such drugs can result in masculinization of a female embryo. This was not evident in the material presented here but it only involved five female infants and it is not certain that a moderate masculinization with an enlarged clitoris would be recorded. Such a masculinization can usually be corrected by plastic surgery and exposure to anabolic steroids does not necessarily mean that a termination of pregnancy should be discussed.

In Sweden, there is only one anabolic steroid, nandrolone, among official drugs. The indication for its use is anemia at uremia and osteoporosis in the elderly. Anabolic steroids are also used illegally, e.g., by bodybuilders, but the reporting of illegal drug use is probably very incomplete. Such steroids have androgenic properties and can therefore affect sex differentiation, notably by masculinization of a female embryo. Few data on the use of anabolic steroids during pregnancy exist in the literature but an early summary descibed cases of female masculinization after use of drugs with androgenic properties, including anabolic steroids [1].

Table 18.1. Number of women identified with use of anabolic steroids

Total	20
Reported in early pregnancy	15
Got prescription later in pregnancy	5
Both early and late use	0

All exposures except one referred to nandrolone (A14AB01) which is an estren derivative. There was one early exposure to an unspecified anabolic steroid.

The maternal age distribution is approximately normal (10 of the 15 women using anabolic steroids in early pregnancy were between 25-34 years), 10 were of first parity, only two smoked (≥10 cigarettes per day), three had a BMI ≥26. Two of the women used clomipramine and one haloperidol.

Among the 15 infants born after early exposure to anabolic drugs, 10 were male and 5 female. There were no indications that any masculinization had occurred among the female infants but it is not certain that a mild such effect had been recorded. None of the 15 deliveries was a twin delivery. Two infants had congenital malformations: one had an undescended testicle, one had a ventricular septum defect. None of the infants had other serious neonatal diagnoses.

Among maternal delivery diagnosis there was none which could indicate a medical reason why anabolic steroids had been given.

Summary

Very few exposures to anabolic steroids were identified and no ill effects on the exposed infants could be seen. The expected effect, a masculinization of a female embryo, was not identified but mild such effects could be unrecorded.

References

[1] Schardein JL. Congenital abnormalities and hormones during pregnancy: A clinical review. *Teratology* 1980; 22: 251-270.

Chapter 19

ANTICOAGULANTS

Maternal use of K-vitamin antagonists in early pregnancy (week 6-12) carries a risk for severe congenital malformations in the child. The effect seems to be dose-dependent. Therapy with heparin group drugs or with low dose acetylsalicylic acid seems to carry no significant risk for a congenital malformation. Anticoagulant therapy is associated with an increased risk for maternal and neonatal complications, probably mainly due to underlying maternal pathology. An excess risk for foetal bleeding may exist, however, as a direct effect of the therapy.

Anticoagulation therapy during pregnancy may be caused by a temporary or chronic pre-pregnancy condition where maternal congenital heart defects or prosthetic heart valves represent important groups. In other instances, anticoagulants are given because of coagulopathy of pregnancy which increases the risk for thromboembolic complications. Low doses of acetylsalicylic acid are given as thrombosis prophylaxis.

Coumarine derivates, notably warfarin, are generally regarded as one of the rather few strongly teratogenic drugs [1-5]. Use of these drugs in early pregnancy may cause a typical embryopathy which is dominated by skeletal malformations of a type resembling a genetic condition, chondrodystrophia calcificans or Conradi´s syndrome. Nasal hypoplasia is common and so is choanal atresia but other malformations are sometimes present. The effect appears to be dose dependent [6,7] and doses above 5 mg/day increases the risk. Use of these drugs after the first trimester may cause bleedings in the foetus with CNS damage, blindness or psychomotor retardation [8] and give other long time sequeles [9,10]. Among 71 cases analyzed [6], there were 23 foetal deaths and embryopathy was present in four. It is often suggested that if a woman plans a pregnancy or becomes pregnant during coumarine treatment, the drug should be stopped and anticoagulation should continue with heparin or equivalent drugs. The risk for foetal bleeding is regarded as smaller with these drugs than with coumarine derivates but the risk for maternal complications may be higher [11].

Table 19.1. Number of women identified who used anticoagulants

Total	6492
Reported use in early pregnancy	2950
Got prescription later in pregnancy	4869
Both early and late use	1327

Type of drug	ATC code	Early use	Later use
Vitamin K antagonists	B01AA	88	16
Dicoumarol	B01AA01	2	0
Warfarin	B01AA03	85	16
Phenprocoumon	B01AA04	2	0
Heparin group	B01AB	1593	2561
Heparin	B01AB01	101	89
Antithrombin III	B01AB02	5	2
Dalteparin	B01AB04	1410	2347
Enoxaparin	B01AB05	36	55
Nadroparin	B01AB06	1	0
Danaparoid	B01AB09	0	7
Tinzaparin	B01AB10	64	104
Unspecified	B01AB	2	0
Platelet aggregation inhibitors, excl. heparin	B01AC	1489	2536
Clopidogrel	B01AC04	2	2
Ticlopidine	B01AC05	0	1
Acetylsalicylic acid	B01AC06	1482	2531
Dipyridamol	B01AC07	8	4
Epoprostenol	B01AC09	1	0
Anagrelide	B01AC14	1	0
Eptifibatide	B01AC16	1	0
Enzymes	B01AD	0	0
Direct thrombin inhibitors	B01AE	0	0
Other antithrombic drugs	B01AX	0	0

Some women used two or more drugs of this category

	Heparin group	Platelet aggregation inhibitors excl. heparin
Early pregnancy us		
Vitamin K antagonists	53	4
Heparin group		152
Later pregnancy use		
Vitamin K antagonists	10	1
Heparin group		227

Five women used drugs from all three groups.

Characteristics of Women using Anticoagulant Drugs

Based on women reporting the drug in early pregnancy (n=2948, two missing maternal age). Each variable is adjusted for all other variables and year of delivery. Comparison with all women who gave birth during the period and with information from the first antenatal care (n=967 742). The odds ratios for maternal age, parity, smoking in early pregnancy, number of previous miscarriages, BMI, subfertility, and country of birth are adjusted for all other variables and are shown in Figure 19.1.

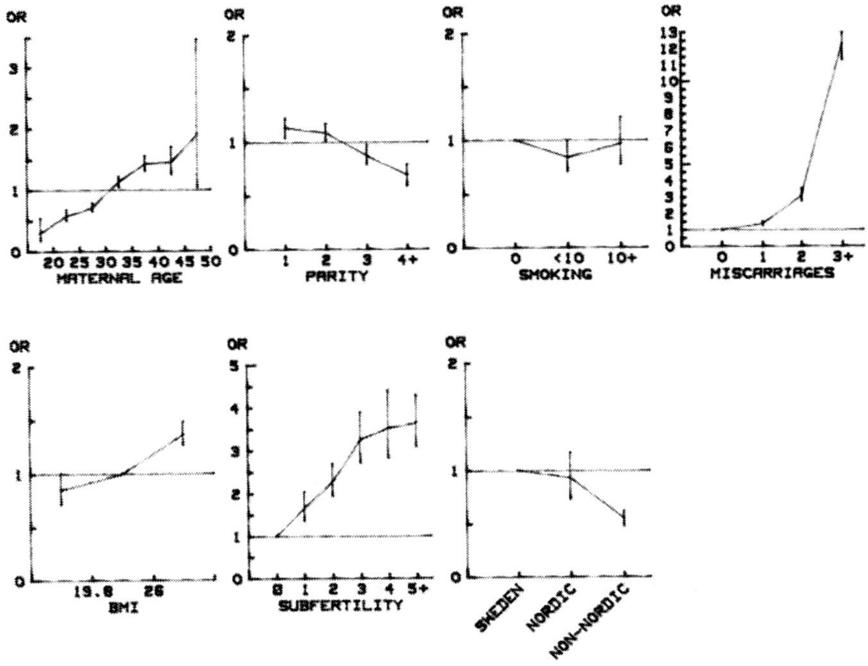

Figure 19.1. Odds ratios for seven maternal characteristics. The odds ratios (OR) for each variable are adjusted for the other variables and year of delivery. Vertical lines mark 95% confidence intervals. For maternal age and parity, each class is compared with all other classes.

Some further maternal characteristics were analyzed, adjusting for year of delivery, maternal age, parity, smoking, and BMI (Table 19.2).

Table 19.2. Some further characteristics of women using anticoagulant drugs in early pregnancy

Variable studied	Number	OR	95% CI
Education (1996-2001, 789 women with drugs, 526 695 in population)			
Unknown	6	-	
<12 years	84	1.04	0.81-1.33
12 years	399	1.00	reference
13-14 years	44	0.95	0.70-1.30
≥14 years	256	0.96	0.82-1.14
Family situation			
Unknown	55	-	
Co-habiting	2784	1.00	reference
Living alone	52	0.86	0.64-1.14
Other family situation	57	0.74	0.56-0.97
Work outside home			
Unknown	302	-	
Full time	1363	1.00	reference
Part time	760	1.13	1.03-1.24
None	523	1.10	0.99-1.23

Women using anticoagulants thus have a number of different characteristics compared with other women. An increasing use with age but decreasing with parity is seen. The risk for previous miscarriage and for subfertility is markedly increased and an association with high BMI is also apparent. Women from non-Nordic countries show a lower usage of these drugs than Nordic women.

Table 19.3. Concomitant drug use (early pregnancy)

Drug group	Number	OR	95% CI
Drugs for stomach ulcer and reflux	51	1.88	1.43-2.48
Drugs for inflammatory bowel disease	37	4.21	3.11-5.69
Insulin	24	2.09	1.40-3.14
Multivitamins	290	0.95	0.84-1.09
Folic acid	390	1.90	1.71-2.17
Drugs for hypertension	79	2.23	1.79-2.12
Progestogens	190	16.7	14.8-18.9
Gonadotrophins	64	10.2	7.82-13.0#
Systemic corticosteroids	106	11.5	9.79-13.4
Thyroid drugs	87	1.81	1.46-2.24
Antibiotics	108	1.26	1.04-1.53
NSAIDs	30	0.64	0.45-0-92
Opioids	42	2.47	1.84-3.32
Minor analgesics	144	0.71	0.60-0.84
Drugs for migraine	7	0.92	0.37-1.89#
Anticonvulsants	18	2.15	1.36-3.39
Sedatives, hypnotics	21	1.52	0.98-2.36
Antidepressants	46	1.14	0.85-1.53
Drugs for rhinitis	47	1.10	0.82-1.46
Antiasthmatics	114	1.36	1.13-1.64
Antitussives	12	0.76	0.43-1.36
Antihistamines	151	0.97	0.77-1.13

risk ratio with exact Poisson 95% confidence interval.

There is thus a very strong concomitant use of some drug categories: drugs for inflammatory bowel disease, insulin, drugs for hypertension, drugs given in association with fertility treatments, systemic corticosteroids, thyroid drugs, anticonvulsants, and antiasthmatics. This mirrors that women using anticoagulants is a group with complex pathology.

Table 19.4. Maternal delivery diagnoses associated with the use of anticoagulants

Diagnosis	Drug in early pregnancy			Drug later in pregnancy		
	Number	OR	95%CI	Number	OR	95% CI
Pre-existing diabetes	124	1.05	0.88-1.26	87	1.09	0.87-1.35
Gestational diabetes	102	1.21	0.99-1.48	53	0.93	0.70-1.23
Chronic hypertension	125	1.14	0.95-1.36	85	1.15	0.91-1.41
Preeclampsia	474	1.21	1.10-1.33	303	1.29	1.14-1.45
Placenta previa	125	1.22	1.02-1.46	70	0.99	0.78-1.27
Abruptio placentae	134	1.20	1.01-1.42	75	0.96	0.76-1.22
Hyperemesis	134	1.48	1.24-1.75	97	1.57	1.28-1.92
Antepartum bleeding	145	1.20	1.01-1.41	75	0.96	0.76-1.21
Intrapartum bleeding	208	1.12	0.97-1.29	141	1.12	0.94-1.33
Postpartum bleeding	462	1.01	0.92-1.11	274	1.02	0.91-1.16
Delivery induction	1055	1.21	1.13-1.30	726	1.39	1.28-1.51
Caesarean section	1628	1.27	1.20-1.34	1019	1.28	1.20-1.38

There is an excess of pregnancy complications leading to an excess of delivery inductions and caesarean sections after maternal use of anticoagulants. Also later use of anticoagulants is associated with pregnancy complications – sometimes (e.g., preeclampsia) the use of anticoagulants may be because of the complication.

OUTCOME AFTER MATERNAL USE OF ANTICOAGULANTS

Infant Sex

Among 3049 infants born after maternal use of anticoagulants in early pregnancy, 1 540 were male and 1 509 female, a sex ratio of 1.02 (95% CI 0.95-1.10). After use in late pregnancy, there were 2 550 male and 2 422 female infants (sex unknown for two) with a sex ratio of 1.05 (95% CI 1.00-1.11). The normal sex ratio (1.06) is thus contained within both confidence intervals.

Multiple Births

After maternal use of anticoagulants in early pregnancy, there were 97 twin and one triplet delivery which gives an odds ratio for twinning of 2.04 (95% CI 1.68-2.50). After later use of anticoagulants, there were 100 twin and two triplet deliveries, odds ratio for twinning 1.31 (95% CI 1.07-1.80). A reasonable explanation to the high twinning rate is the association between subfertility and use of anticoagulants in early pregnancy (see above). After exclusion of women who reported earlier miscarriages or any period of unwanted childlessness, the odds ratio for twinning (based on 30 twin pairs) went down to 1.62 (95% CI 1.12-2.32) but is still statistically significantly increased. Also exclusion of women who reported the use of folic acid (which has been associated with twinning) reduced the odds ratio only little to 1.56 (95% CI 1.06-2.30). Unregistered subfertility or previous miscarriages could explain the remaining about 60% over-risk for twins but in order to explain that overrisk, the lack of registration of miscarriages or subfertility must be around 50% which does not seem likely.

Table 19.5. Infant mortality after maternal use of anticoagulant drugs

Variable studied	Drug use in early pregnancy			Drug use later in pregnancy		
	Number	OR	95% CI	Number	OR	95% CI
Stillbirth	25	2.35	1.60-3.45	29	1.75	1.22-2.52
Early neonatal death	9	1.87	0.80-3.55#	16	2.12	1.21-3.45#

observed over expected ratio with exact Poisson 95% confidence interval.

The stillbirth risk is thus increased. Among 90 infants exposed to vitamin K antagonists in early pregnancy, one was stillborn. The stillborn risk among 1647 infants exposed to heparin in early pregnancy was non-significantly increased: risk ratio 1.91 (95% CI 0.95-3.41), slightly lower than after maternal use of platelet aggregation inhibitors other than heparin: odds ratio 2.65 (95% CI 1.40-4.29). Similar results were seen after later exposure. After heparin use in late pregnancy 18 infants were stillborn with a risk ratio of 1.98, 95% CI 1.18-3.14, and after use of other platelet aggregation inhibitors there were 11 stillborns, risk ratio 1.28, 95% CI 0.64-2.29. The stillbirth rates after heparin and after other platelet aggregation inhibitors did not differ significantly (p=0.35). Also the rate of early neonatal death was increased, significantly so after later exposure.

Table 19.6. Pregnancy duration and infant birth weight at maternal use of anticoagulants

Variable studied	Drug use in early pregnancy			Drug use later in pregnancy		
	Number	OR	95% CI	Number	OR	95% CI
< 37 weeks	333	2.61	2.34-2.92	518	2.51	2.29-2.74
<2500g	249	3.09	2.73-3.51	405	3.23	2.93-3.56
≥4500g	92	0.69	0.56-0.85	158	0.67	0.57-0.78
SGA	119	2.17	1.80-2.60	221	2.80	2.46-3.20
LGA	167	0.81	0.69-0.95	293	0.78	0.69-0.87

There is a clear-cut effect with an increased risk for preterm birth and SGA, of similar magnitude after early and later exposure. Late effects may be explained by conditions like preeclampsia, treated with anticoagulants, early effects perhaps by underlying maternal morbidity.

Table 19.7. Neonatal diagnoses after maternal use of anticoagulants

Diagnosis	Drug use in early pregnancy			Drug use later in pregnancy		
	Number	OR	95% CI	Number	OR	95% CI
Hypoglycaemia	215	1.90	1.66-2.19	324	1.90	1.70-2.12
Respiratory daignoses	245	1.71	1.50-1.95	377	1.69	1.52-1.88
Low Apgar score	90	1.58	1.28-1.95	138	1.62	1.37-1.92
CNS diagnoses	42	1.68	1.24-2.29	58	1.71	1.32-2.22
Intracranial bleeding	35	1.62	1.16-2.27	56	1.78	1.36-2.32
Jaundice	251	2.08	1.82-2.36	358	1.90	1.15-2.12

All studied neonatal diagnoses thus occur in excess, probably the result of underlying pathology. A more direct effect could exist between maternal use of anticoagulants during pregnancy and infant intracranial bleeding but against this speaks the fact that effects are similar after early and later exposure.

There are thus no indication of an increased malformation risk among infants whose mothers had used anticoagulants in early pregnancy. K-vitamin antagonists are regarded as clear teratogenic drugs. Among the 90 infants exposed to such drugs in early pregnancy, there were only five with a congenital malformation.

Table 19.8. Congenital malformations in infants whose mothers used anticoagulants

Congenital malformation	Number	OR/RR	95% CI
All anticoagulants			
All malformations	134	0.89	0.83-1.09
Relatively severe malformations	93	0.84	0.67-1.08
Chromosome anomalies	3	0.43	0.09-1.24#
Without chromosome anomalies			
Any CNS malformation	4	1.32	0.36-3.37#
Any cardiovascular malformation	43	1.25	0.88-1.77

Table 19.8. Cotninued

Congenital malformation	Number	OR/RR	95% CI
Ear malformation	7	1.16	0.47-2.40#
Orofacial cleft	6	1.11	0.41-2.42#
Hypospadias	7	0.82	0.33-1.68#
Pes equinovarus	5	1.08	0.35-2.52#
Poly/syndactyly	6	0.95	0.35-2.07#
(Sub)luxation of hip, clicking hip	17	0.91	0.55-1.51
K vitamin antagonists			
All malformations	5	0.95	0.31-2.22#
Relatively severe malformations	5	1.23	0.40-2.88#
Heparin group			
All malformations	77	0.96	0.74-1.24
Relatively severe malformations	52	0.88	0.64-1.21
Any cardiovascular malformation	24	1.32	0.83-2.11
Platelet aggregation inhibitors other than heparin group			
All malformations	70	0.91	0.69-1.19
Relatively severe malformations	47	0.84	0.60-1.18
Any cardiovascular malformation	23	1.28	0.79-2.07

risk ratio with exact Poisson 95% confidence interval.

Table 19.9. Malformations among infants exposed to K-vitamin antagonists in early pregnancy

Malformation diagnosis	Anticoagulants	Other drugs
Hydrocephaly (stillborn) Cleft palate+nose malformation+ aorta malformation+pectus excavatum+	dicoumarol+dipyridamol	-
Syndactyly	dicoumarol+dalteparin	-
Oesophageal atresia	warfarin+enoxaparin	atenolol+tetracycline+ paracetamol
Hypospadias	warfarin	-
Unspec. musculoskeletal anomaly	warfarin+dalteparin	sertraline+paracetamol

The first three malformations listed are rather severe but of different nature.

Table 19.10. Malformations in infants exposed to some specific anticoagulants

Anticoagulant	Malformed	OR/RR	95% CI
Heparin (n=104)			
All malformations	9	1.79	0.82-3.40#
Relatively severe malformations	6	1.64	0.60-3.57#
Dalteparin (n=1454)			
All malformations	66	0.94	0.71-1.24
Relatively severe malformations	46	0.87	0.62-1.22
Any cardiovascular defect	24	1.49	0.93-2.37
VSD and/or ASD	12	1.38	0.71-2.40#
Tinzaparin (n=68)			
All malformations	2	0.73	0.09-2.63#
Acetylsalicylic acid (n=1528)			
All malformations	68	0.89	0.68-1.18
Relatively severe malformations	46	0.82	0.58-1.15
Any cardiovascular defect	23	1.28	0.80-2.07

Only four further specific drugs were represented by 50 or more exposed infants: The six relatively severe malformations after heparin exposure were:

Table 19.11. Relatively severe malformations in infants exposed to heparin

Malformation diagnosis	Anticoagulants	Other drugs
Encephalocele	heparin	ranitidine+lymecycline+ immunoglobulin+epinephrine
Congenital cataract	heparin	-
Congenital cataract	heparin	chorionic gonadotropin
Ventricular septum defect + penis malformation	heparin+dalteparin	-
Uterine malformation	heparin+dalteparin	-
Down syndrome	heparin+acetyl-salicylic acid	progesterone+chorionic gonadotropin

Two cases of congenital cataract after heparin exposure are astonishing but may still be random.

Summary

There are numerous complications during pregnancy and for the neonate when the mother has used anticoagulants. Most of these associations are probably due to underlying pathology, either presence of various diseases which have motivated the use of anticoagulants and which are associated with a complication risk (e.g., high blood pressure) or use of anticoagulants at the therapy of pregnancy complications (e.g., preeclampsia). The only complication which may be a direct consequence of the use of anticoagulants is the increased risk for an intracranial bleeding in the neonate. This was seen also after use in early pregnancy but many of these women have probably continued with anticoagulants during the rest of the pregnancy. There is no clear teratogenicity seen but as expected, a few severe conditions were observed after early use of K vitamin antagonists, including warfarin which is a known teratogen.

References

[1] Kerber IJ, Warr OS 3rd, Richardson C. Pregnancy in a patient with a prosthetic mitral valve. Associated with a foetal anomaly attributed to warfarin sodium. *JAMA* 1968: 203:223-225.

[2] Barr M, Burdi AR. Warfarin-associated embryopathy in a 17-week-old abortus. *Teratology* 1976;14:129-34.

[3] Hall JG, Pauli RM, Wilson KM. Maternal and fetal sequelae of anticoagulation during pregnancy. *Am J Med* 1980;68:122-40.

[4] Iturbe-Alessio I, Fonseca MC, Mutchinik O, Santos MA, Zajarías A, Salazar E. Risks of anticoagulant therapy in pregnant women with artificial heart valves. *N Engl J Med* 1986;315:1390-3.

[5] van Driel D, Wesseling J, Sauer PJ, Touwen BC, van de Veer E, Heymans HS. Teratogen update: Foetal effects after in utero exposure to coumarins, overview of cases, follow-up findings, and pathogenesis. *Teratology* 2002;66:127-40.

[6] Cotrufo M, De Feo M, De Santo LS, Romano GP, Della Corte A, Renzulli A, Gallo C. Risk of warfarin during pregnancy with mechanical valve prostheses. *Obstet Gynecol* 2002;99:35-40.
[7] Vitale, N, de Feo M, de Santo LS, Pollice A, Tedesco N, Cotrufo M. Dose-dependent fetal complications of warfarin in pregnant women with mechanical heart valves. *J Am Coll Cardiol* 1999; 33: 1637-1641.
[8] Stevenson RE, Buron OM, Ferlauto GJ, Taylor HA. Hazards of oral anticoagulants during pregnancy. *JAMA* 1980; 243: 1549-1551.
[9] Wesseling J, van Driel D, Smrkovsky M, ven der Veer E, Geven-Boere LM, Sauer PJ, van der Veer E. Neurological outcome in school-age children after in utero exposure to coumarins. *Early Hum Dev* 2001;63:83-95.
[10]van Driel D, Wesseling J, Rosendaal FR, Odlink RJ, van der Veer E, Gerver WJ, Geven-Boere LM, Sauer PJ. Growth until puberty after in utero exposure to coumarins. *Am J Med Genet* 2000; 95: 438-443.
[11]Oakley CM. Anticoagulation and pregnancy. *Europ Heart J* 1995; 16: 1317-1319.

Chapter 20

HAEMOSTATICS

Haemostatics are often used by women with coagulopathies which by themselves may represent a risk for pregnancy complications and possibly also a risk for a disturbance of embryonic development. Use of tranexamic acid in early pregnancy is associated with a near doubled risk for a relatively severe malformation, including a cardiovascular defect. If this is a drug effect or a result of the underlying pathology cannot be decided. There was an unexpected association with infant craniostenosis – this may be random and more data are needed in order to accept or reject the association which was based on only four cases.

Table 20.1. Number of women identified using haemostatics

Total	1522
Reported use in early pregnancy	684
Got prescription later in pregnancy	935
Both early and later use	97

Type of drug:	ATC code	Early use	Later use
Fibrinolytic agent	B02A	638	661
Tranexamic acid	B02AA01	638	661
Vitamin K and other coagulation factors	B02B	46	270
Vitamin K	B02BA01	38	242
Coagulation factor VIII	B02BD02	7	32
Activated prothrombin complex against antibodies against factor VIII	B02BD03	1	0
Unspecific	B02	0	1

To this group of drugs belong fibrinolytic drugs among which tranexamic acid is used perorally and vitamin K (phytomenadione) and other coagulation factors, among which only vitamin K is used perorally. Fibrinolytic drugs are mainly used for menorrhagia, often associated with inherited bleeding disorders [1], but also at bleeding complications during pregnancy and delivery or in order to prevent such complications. Treatment in early pregnancy is not recommended but women may become pregnant during treatment with tranexamic acid, resulting in early pregnancy exposure. Little is known about possible effects of such exposure on the embryo but in animal experiments no teratogenicity was identified. Vitamin K therapy is especially relevant as an adjunct to other drug treatments which may affect the activity of the vitamin, notably anticonvulsant drugs. Other haemostatic drugs are specific for distinct coagulation defects and are administered parentally.

Characteristics of Women using Haemostatics

Based on women using laxatives in early pregnancy (n=694). Each variable is adjusted for all other variables and year of delivery. Comparison with all women who gave birth during the period and with information from the first antenatal care (n= 967 742). The odds raatios for maternal age, parity, smoking in early pregnancy, number of previous miscarriages, BMI, subfertility, and country of birth are adjusted for all other variables and are shown in Figure 1.

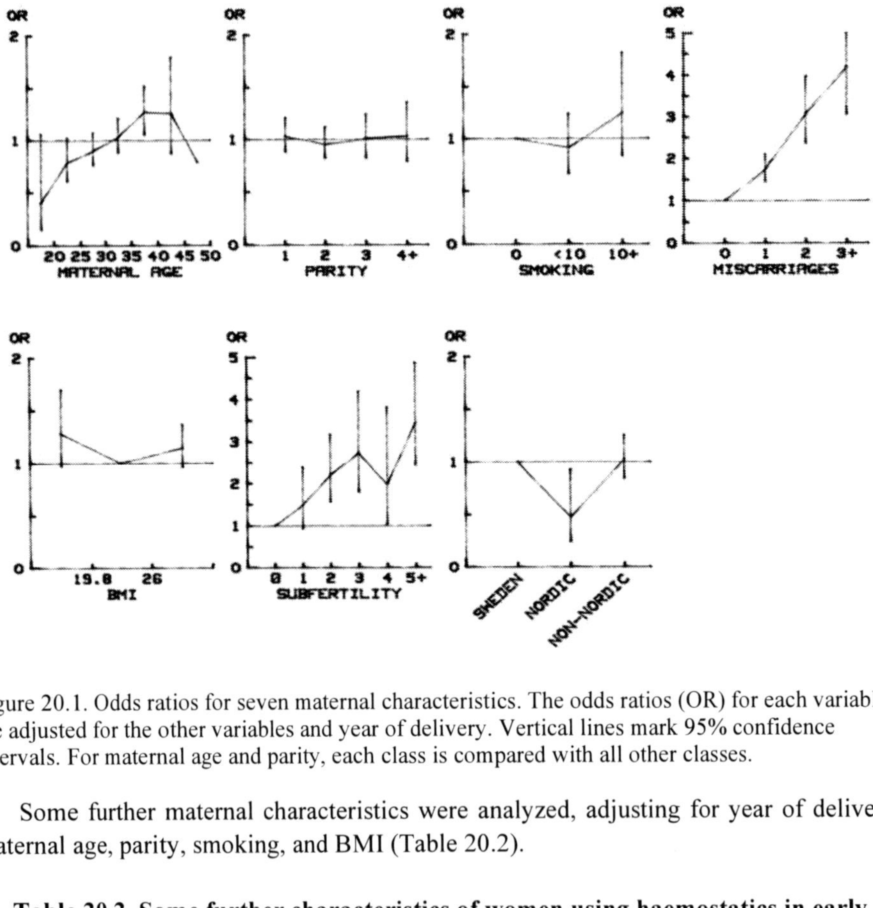

Figure 20.1. Odds ratios for seven maternal characteristics. The odds ratios (OR) for each variable are adjusted for the other variables and year of delivery. Vertical lines mark 95% confidence intervals. For maternal age and parity, each class is compared with all other classes.

Some further maternal characteristics were analyzed, adjusting for year of delivery, maternal age, parity, smoking, and BMI (Table 20.2).

Table 20.2. Some further characteristics of women using haemostatics in early pregnancy

Variable studied	Number	OR	95% CI
Education (1996-2001, 340 women with drugs, 526 695 in population)			
Unknown	8		
<12 years	51	1.42	1.01-2.00
12 years	160	1.00	Reference
≥13 years	121	1.08	0.85-1.38

Family situation			
Unknown	9	-	
Co-habiting	640	1.00	Reference
Living alone	18	0.96	0.60-1.55
Other family situation	17	1.08	0.66-1.76
Work outside home			
Unknown	76	-	
Full time	291	1.00	Reference
Part time	185	1.22	1.00-1.49
None	132	1.21	1.97-1.50

Women using these drugs are thus characterized by a higher age than expected and notably by a high risk of having previous miscarriages and a period of unwanted childlessness. They worked less often than expected outside home.

Table 20.3. Concomitant drug use (early pregnancy)

Drug group	Number	OR/RR	95% CI
Drugs for stomach ulcer and reflux	10	1.63	0.78-3.00#
Drugs for inflammatory bowel disease	6	3.42	1.25-7.46#
Insulin	4	1.76	0.48-4.53#
Multivitamins	46	1.01	0.75-1.37
Folic acid	81	2.67	2.09-3.41
Oral contraceptives	5	2.54	0.82-5.92#
Progestogens	21	6.69	4.14-10.2#
Gonadotropins	11	6.51	3.25-11.6#
Systemic corticosteroids	9	3.67	1.68-6.97#
Thyroid drugs	14	1.53	0.84-2.53#
Antibiotics	45	2.20	1.63-2.96
NSAIDs	16	1.50	0.92-2.47
Opioids	11	2.87	1.43-5.14#
Minor analgesics	70	1.48	1.16-1.90
Anticonvulsants	24	12.1	7.77-18.0#
Sedatives, hypnotics	3	0.90	0.19-2.64#
Antidepressants	5	0.57	0.18-1.32#
Drugs for rhinitis	9	0.97	0.44-1.84#
Antiasthmatics	23	1.15	0.76-1.74
Antihistamines	59	1.68	1.29-2.19
For NVP	43	1.59	1.17-2.16
For allergy	20	2.05	1.32-3.17

#observed over expected number with exact Poisson 95% confidence interval.

The high rate of folic acid usage and of antiasthmatics is seen both for tranexamic acid and vitamin K. The excess usage of oral contraceptives, progestogens, and gonadotrophines is restricted to transexamic acid and of anticonvulsants to vitamin K (23 of the 24 anticonvulsant users).

Some conditions related to bleedings thus occur in excess also after early exposure to haemostatics – the associations in late pregnancy can be explained by the use of haemostatics therapeutically. An excess of delivery inductions and caesarean sections is seen both after early and later exposures.

Table 20.4. Some maternal diagnoses associated with the use of haemostatics

Diagnosis	Drug use in early pregnancy			Drug use later in pregnancy		
	Number	OR/RR	95% CI	Number	OR/RR	95% CI
Pre-existing diabetes	10	1.07	0.51-1.97#	16	1.18	0.72-1.94
Chronic hypertension	8	0.92	0.40-1.81#	14	1.15	0.68-1.95
Gestational diabetes	5	0.72	0.23-1.69#	12	1.28	0.66-2.23
Preeclampsia	33	1.05	0.74-1.49	51	1.23	0.92-1.63
Hyperemesis gravidarum	7	0.97	0.39-2.00#	13	1.25	0.72-2.16
Placenta previa	14	1.68	0.92-2.82#	57	5.07	3.97-6-47
Abruptio placentae	22	2.24	1.40-3.39#	36	2.85	2.07-3.93
Antepartum bleeding	19	1.98	1.27-3.09#	42	3.24	2.41-4.36
Intrapartum bleeding	24	1.60	1.06-2.42	32	1.48	1.03-2.11
Postpartum bleeding	53	1.36	1.03-1.80	85	1.71	1.37-2.14
Delivery induction	97	1.42	1.14-1.76	142	1.61	1.34-1.92
Caesarean section	190	1.90	1.61-2.24	249	1.87	1.62-2.16

#observed over expected number with exact Poisson 95% confidence interval.

Outcome after Maternal use of Haemostatics

Infant Sex

Among infants born after maternal use of haemostatics in early pregnancy, 370 were boys and 342 girls, sex ratio 1.08 (95% CI 0.93-1.25). The confidence interval thus contains the normal sex ratio of 1.06. After exposure in late pregnancy, there is a just statistically significant excess of boys: 526 boys and 437 girls (one unknown sex), sex ratio 1.20 (95% CI 1.06-1.37).

Multiple Births

There is an excess of multiple births both after early and later exposure to haemostatics. After early exposure 26 twin and one triplet delivery occurred. The odds ratio for twinning was 2.38 (95% CI 1.62-3.49) but after removal of women with subfertility (where therapy can result in twinning) and women using folic acid (which has been suggested to increase twinning rate), the risk ratio for twinning decreased only slightly to 1.83 but lost statistical significance (95% CI 0.97-3.13). The risk ratio for twinning after late use of haemostatics remained high and statistically significant: RR = 2.62, 95% CI 1.58-4.09. This is probably due to an increased bleeding risk in twin pregnancies. The possibly increased risk for twinning after early exposure resembles that seen after anticoagulants (see Chapter19).

There is thus an excess of prematurity, low birth weight, and SGA both after early and later exposures and the odds ratio estimates are of the same order of magnitude.

Table 20.5. Pregnancy duration and infant birth weight at maternal use of haemostatics

Variable studied	Drug use in early pregnancy			Drug use later in pregnancy		
	Number	OR	95% CI	Number	OR	95% CI
<37 weeks	100	3.34	2.85-4.28	143	3.75	3.17-4.43
<2500g	77	4.09	3.27-5.11	97	3.94	3.23-4.80
≥4500g	21	0.74	0.48-1.14	34	0.86	0.61-1.21
SGA	22	1.59	1.04-2.44	28	1.65	1.12-2.41
LGA	47	1.07	0.79-1.45	54	0.86	0.65-1.14

Infant Mortality

After early exposure for haemostatics, there was only one stillbirth and four early neonatal deaths, numbers which agree well with the expected numbers. After later exposure, there were two stillbirths but five early neonatal deaths (risk ratio = 3.58, 95% CI 0.98-9.17). One of the latter had a trisomy 18, one was born preterm after premature rupture of the membranes and died in an infection, one had asphyxia with cerebral bleeding, convulsions, and disseminated intravascular coagulation, one had an intrauterine asphyxia with adrenal haemorrhage and the mother had placenta previa, one was born preterm because of amnionitis.

Table 20.6. Neonatal diagnoses after maternal use of haemostatics

Diagnosis	Drug use in early pregnancy			Drug use later in pregnancy		
	Number	OR/RR	95% CI	Number	OR/RR	95% CI
Hypoglycaemia	47	1.75	1.31-2.35	54	1.64	1.25-2.16
Respiratory diagnoses	76	2.25	1.78-2.85	97	2.30	1.88-2.83
Low Apgar score	28	1.96	1.35-2.86	36	2.16	1.56-2.99
CNS diagnoses	8	1.75	0.76-3.46#	12	1.97	1.02-3.44#
Jaundice	79	2.93	2.34-3.68	105	3.01	2.48-3.66

#observed over expected number with exact Poisson 95% confidence interval.

All diagnoses thus occur in excess also after early exposures and there are no major differences between the odds ratios after early and later exposures.

A total of 60 infants with congenital malformations were identified, five of them after maternal use of K vitamin and 55 after the use of tranexamic acid.

K-Vitamin

The expected number of infants with any malformation is only 1.67 and the RR = 3.50 with a 95% CI of 0.97-6.99. Four of them were relatively severe (the fifth had an unstable hip). The mothers of all four had used carbamazepine, a known teratogen. The four malformations were:

1. Hydrocephaly
2. Ventricular septum defect
3. Hypospadias
4. Congenital syndrome associated with short status.

Table 20.7. Congenital malformations in infants after maternal use of tranexamic acid

Congenital malformation	Number	OR	95% CI
All malformation	54	1.93	1.45-2.57
Relatively severe malformation	35	1.82	1.29-2.57
Chromosome anomalies	0	-	-
Without chromosome anomalies			
Any cardiovascular defect	15	2.19	1.23-3.61#
Specified cardiovascular defect	12	1.95	1.05-3.41#
VSD and/or ASD	7	1.86	0.75-3.84#
Without cardiovascular defect	20	1.56	0.99-2.45
Craniostenosis	4	9.52	2.59-24.4#

There is thus an approximately doubled risk for a cardiac defect. The risk ratio for craniostenosis is high and statistically significant but based on only four cases. Mothers of two of them had only used tranexamic acid, one mother had also taken iron and folic acid, and one had used chorion gonadotropin before pregnancy. This association may well be random in spite of statistical significance as there was no prior hypothesis of an association. – Among other serious malformations can be mentioned one infant with Arnold-Chiari malformation, one with cleft lip and palate, one with oesophageal atresia, one with pylorostenosis, two with hypospadias, and one with polycystic kidneys.

Summary

Maternal use of haemostatics in early pregnancy is usually due to the presence of coagulation defects and menorrhagia. Later use is associated with pregnancy complications and notably bleedings where the drugs have been given as therapy. Previous miscarriages and a period of unwanted childlessness are strongly associated with the use of haemostatics in early pregnancy. The early use of haemostatics is associated with an increased risk for twinning but this is partly – but not completely – explained by the association with therapy for subfertility. Infants born of women who used haemostatics in early pregnancy had a tendency to be born preterm, have low birth weight, and be small for gestational age. The infants had an excess of neonatal diagnoses also after early exposure. A high rate of congenital malformations is seen after vitamin K use in early pregnancy, explainable by the use of vitamin K together with anticonvulsants. Also after tranexamic acid, a moderately increased risk for congenital malformations is seen, perhaps stronger for cardiovascular defects than for other malformations. An association with craniostenosis is seen which may be random.

References

[1] Demers C, Derzko C, David M, Douglas J. Society of Obstetricians and Gynaecologists of Canada. Gynaecological and obstetric management of women with inherited bleeding disorders. *Int J Gynaecol Obstet* 2006; 95: 75-87.

Chapter 21

Vitamin B12 and Folic Acid

The preconceptional use of vitamin B12 and notably of folic acid is generally regarded as a certain way to reduce the risk for a congenital malformation and also to have other beneficial effects. This may well be true in many populations but it is difficult to detect these effects in Sweden. On the contrary a weak risk increase for certain malformations is seen after early use of folic acid which may be the result of undetected confounding. An increased risk for dizygotic twinning has been postulated in some earlier studies and is indicated also here – in some other populations this effect has not been observed.

In most scientific and popular articles, it is stated that it has been shown that preconceptional use of folic acid will reduce the risk for a neural tube defect in the infant; usually a 50% risk reduction is mentioned. This conclusion is based on a number of studies in different countries using different methodologies. A critical review of the early studies which resulted in this conclusion was published in 2000 [1]. Some of these studies were retrospective case-control studies with a risk for recall and sometimes interviewer bias [2], a few were prospective studies [3-4]. Two randomized studies exist. One concerned the possibility to prevent recurrence of neural tube defects with a high dose of folic acid (4-5 mg/day) [5], the other which was of limited size concerned occurrence [6]. A large study performed in China [7] had some uncertainties in data analysis. The studies resulted in recommendations of folic acid supplementation preconceptionally (usually 0.4 mg/day) and later as food additive. Follow-up studies of the result of such preventive measures in most cases have shown a reduction in neural tube rate but it is uncertain to which extent this is part of a long-time downward trend in neural tube rate [8]. An international study compared changes in neural tube rates in different populations with different strategies of folate supplementation without being able to demonstrate a relationship [9]. The beneficial effect of folic acid is not only said to exist for neural tube defects but also for many other types of congenital malformations [10].

Less interest has been paid to the importance of vitamin B12. There seems to be a moderate association between low B12 status and the risk of a neural tube defect [11,12]. A similar relationship with congenital heart defects has also been suggested [13].

Vitamin B12 is in Sweden available as a prescription drug as 1 mg tablets. Folic acid is available as a prescription drug with 5 mg folic acid and also as a number of OTC drugs containing 0.4 mg and supposed to be used for congenital malformation prophylaxis. A study indicated that about 70% of early folic acid use had started preconceptionally [14].

Table 21.1. Women identified using vitamin B12 or folic acid

	B12	Folic acid
Total	8 854	127 858
Reported use in early pregnancy	3 926	43 212
Got prescription later in pregnancy	6 588	108 211
Both early and later use	1 660	24092

Characteristics of Women using Vitamin B12 or Folic Acid

Based on women reporting vitamin B12 in early pregnancy (n=3 925, one missing maternal age) or folic acid (n=43 210, two missing maternal age). Each variable is adjusted for all other variables and year of delivery. Comparison with all women who gave birth during the period and with information from the first antenatal care (n=967 742). The odds ratios for maternal age, parity, smoking in early pregnancy, number of previous miscarriages, BMI, subfertility, and country of birth are adjusted for all other variables and are shown in Figure 21.1.

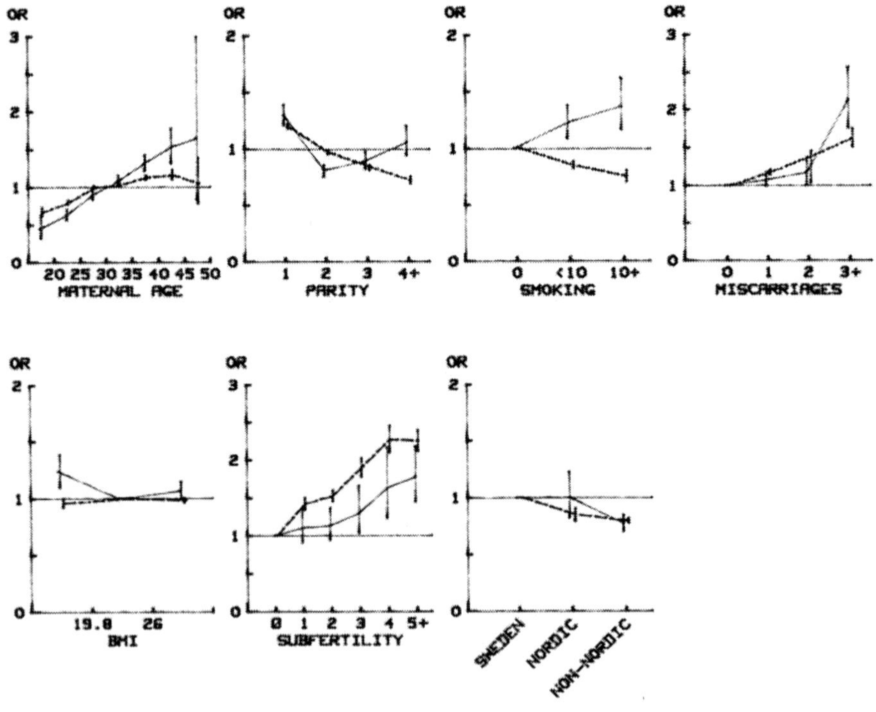

Figure 21.1. Odds ratios for seven maternal characteristics. Unbroken graph refers to vitamin B12, dashed graph to folic acid. The odds ratios (OR) for each variable are adjusted for the other variables and year of delivery. Vertical lines mark 95% confidence intervals. For maternal age and parity, each class is compared with all other classes.

Some further maternal characteristics were analyzed, adjusting for year of delivery, maternal age, parity, smoking, and BMI (Table 21.2).

Table 21.2. Some further characteristics of women using B12 or folic acid in early pregnancy

Variable studied	Vitamin B12			Folic acid		
	Number	OR	95% CI	Number	OR	95% CI
Education (1996-2001, 1 149 women with B12, 2 597 with folic acid, 526 695 in population)						
Unknown	8	-	-	123	-	-
<12 years	127	0.93	0.76-1.14	472	0.73	0.66-0.81
12 years	646	1.00	reference	3358	1.00	reference
13-14 years	53	0.72	0.55-0.96	433	1.07	0.97-1.19
≥14 years	315	0.77	0.66-0.88	2435	1.08	1.02-1.15
Family situation						
Unknown	62	-	-	659	-	-
Co-habiting	3467	1.0	reference	36345	1.00	reference
Living alone	104	1.18	0.97-1.45	803	0.70	0.64-0.77
Other family situation	112	0.95	0.78-1.15	5759	0.75	0.70-0.80
Work outside home						
Unknown	478	-	-	3799	-	-
Full time	1753	1.00	reference	21283	1.00	reference
Part time	907	1.17	1.07-1.27	10877	1.12	1.09-1.14
None	787	1.31	1.20-1.44	7251	0.96	0.94-0.99

High maternal age is a stronger determinant for B12 use than for folic acid use. The relation between B12 use and parity is U-formed but the use of folic acid declines with increasing parity. B12 use is associated with smoking while the opposite is seen for folic acid. The relationship with subfertility is similar but more marked for folic acid than B12. High education is associated with a lower use of B12 but with a higher use of folic acid. Family situation and work outside home also differ.

After maternal use of vitamin B12, concomitant drug use indicates the presence of various chronic maternal diseases like inflammatory bowel disease, diabetes, hypertension, thyroid disease, epilepsy, psychiatric problems, and allergy. For most of these conditions, no similar association is seen with the use of folic acid. Exceptions are inflammatory bowel disease, thyroid disease, and epilepsy. Odd ratio estimates are lower for folic acid than for vitamin B12 for the first two types of drugs while the association with anticonvulsants is very strong for folic acid and weaker for vitamin B12. For both vitamins the association with subfertility can be seen in the concomitant use of progestogens and (partly) gonadotropines.

In spite of the excess morbidity suggested from the analysis of concomitant drug use, the use of vitamin B12 seems not to be associated with maternal pregnancy complications and this is also true for the use of folic acid. For both early and later vitamin use, there is an excess of delivery inductions and caesarean sections which are thus not explainable by the pregnancy complications studied.

Table 21.3. Concomitant drug use (early pregnancy)

Drug group	Vitamin B12			Folic acid		
	Number	OR/RR	95% CI	Number	OR/RR	95% CI
Drugs for stomach ulcer and reflux	83	2.36	1.90-2.93	394	1.05	0.95-1.17
Drugs for inflammatory bowel disease	153	14.6	12.8-16.6	344	3.03	2.71-3.39
Insulin	25	1.78	1.20-2.65	148	0.98	0.83-1.17
Multivitamins	514	1.43	1.30-1.57	4994	0.87	0.84-0.89
Folic acid	1690	10.8	10.2-11.3	-	-	-
Vitamin B12	-	-	-	1690	10.8	10.2-11.3
Antihypertensive	43	2.25	1.66-3.05	208	1.05	0.91-1.22
Oral contraceptives	11	1.17	0.59-2.10#	64	0.70	0.55-0.90
Progestogens	27	1.72	1.18-2.50	502	3.76	3.43-4.12
Gonadotropins	10	1.27	0.61-2.33#	107	1.55	1.27-1.89
Systemic corticosteroids	60	4.52	3.56-5.73	205	1.55	1.34-1.80
Thyroid drugs	306	5.69	5.11-6.32	804	1.28	1.18-1.37
Antibiotics	120	1.04	0.87-1.25	1078	0.85	0.80-0.91
NSAIDs	62	0.96	0.74-1.24	470	0.73	0.66-0.80
Opioids	47	2.09	1.57-2.79	236	0.97	0.85-1.11
Minor analgesics	259	0.98	0.86-1.11	2325	0.89	0.80-0.93
Drugs for migraine	14	1.40	0.83-2.37	79	0.79	0.63-0.99
Anticonvulsants	48	4.36	3.34-5.71	1185	22.3	21.0-23.6
Antipsychotics	7	2.31	0.93-4.76#	24	1.00	0.66-1.52
Sedatives, hypnotics	50	2.68	2.03-3.53	167	0.95	0.81-1.12
Antidepressants	129	2.33	1.96-2.77	517	0.90	0.82-0.99
Drugs for rhinitis	57	1.06	0.82-1.38	548	0.92	0.84-1.00
Antiasthmatics	154	1.36	0.63-1.57	1063	0.88	0.83-0.94
Cough medicines	19	1.00	0.63-1.57	186	0.91	0.78-1.05
Antihistamines	284	1.39	1.24-1.57	2443	1.08	1.03-1.12
For NVP	223	1.44	1.26-1.65	1963	1.14	1.09-1.20
For allergy	75	1.31	1.04-1.65	548	0.88	0.80-0.96

#observed over expected number with exact Poisson 95% confidence interval.

Table 21.4. Some maternal diagnoses associated with the use of vitamin B12

Diagnosis	Drug use in early pregnancy			Drug use later in pregnancy		
	Number	OR	95% CI	Number	OR	95% CI
Pre-existing diabetes	69	1.23	0.95-1.59	96	1.01	0.82-1.24
Chronic hypertension	60	1.11	0.84-1.47	89	1.02	0.82-1.26
Gestational diabetes	38	0.89	0.62-1.28	66	1.00	0.78-1.28
Preeclampsia	205	1.05	0.90-1.23	309	0.99	0.88-1.11
Hyperemesis gravidarum	34	0.91	0.65-1.27	80	1.08	0.87-1.35
Placenta previa	54	0.94	0.72-1.24	87	1.04	0.84-1.29
Abruptio placentae	52	0.91	0.67-1.23	91	0.99	0.80-1.22
Antepartum bleeding	60	1.03	0.80-1.33	94	0.98	0.80-1.20
Intrapartum bleeding	98	1.00	0.82-1.22	168	1.10	0.94-1.28
Postpartum bleeding	211	0.93	0.81-1.07	402	1.10	0.99-1.22
Delivery induction	493	1.11	1.01-1.22	832	1.16	1.09-1.25
Caesarean section	834	1.25	1.16-1.35	1284	1.22	1.14-1.29

Table 21.5. Some maternal diagnoses associated with the use of folic acid

Diagnosis	Drug use in early pregnancy			Drug use later in pregnancy		
	Number	OR	95% CI	Number	OR	95% CI
Pre-existing diabetes	555	0.92	0.84-1.00	1173	0.76	0.72-0.81
Chronic hypertension	508	0.91	0.84-1.00	1109	0.80	0.76-0.86
Gestational diabetes	379	0.95	0.85-1.05	813	0.78	0.73-0.84
Preeclampsia	2043	0.99	0.94-1.03	4786	0.93	0.90-0.96
Hyperemesis gravidarum	419	0.90	0.81-0.99	1014	0.86	0.81-0.92
Placenta previa	516	0.99	0.91-1.09	1115	0.84	0.79-0.90
Abruptio placentae	536	0.95	0.87-1.04	1229	0.84	0.79-0.89
Antepartum bleeding	578	0.98	0.90-1.07	1281	0.84	0.80-0.89
Intrapartum bleeding	1082	1.02	0.96-1.09	2334	0.94	0.90-0.99
Postpartum bleeding	2357	0.96	0.92-1.00	5990	1.01	0.98-1.04
Delivery induction	4986	1.01	0.98-1.04	12181	1.03	1.01-1.05
Caesarean section	7803	1.03	1.01-1.06	17981	1.02	1.00-1.04

Very small and uncertain deviations from the expected outcome are seen after folic acid use but there is a tendency for odds ratios slightly below 1.0 after early use and the odds ratios after later use are more markedly reduced.

OUTCOME AFTER MATERNAL USE OF VITAMIN B12 OR FOLIC ACID

Infant Sex

After maternal use of vitamin B12, the sex ratio was slightly low. After use in early pregnancy, there were 1991 male and 2017 female infants with a sex ratio of 0.99 (95% CI 0.93-1.05) and after later use there were 3292 males and 3440 females (two with unknown sex) and a sex ratio of 0.96 (9%% CI 0.91-1.00). Both confidence intervals exclude the normal sex ratio of 1.06. A low sex ratio is associated with an increased risk for nausea and vomiting and antihistamines used for this condition were also used in excess.

After maternal use of folic acid in early pregnancy, there were 22 665 male and 21 499 female (6 with unknown sex) infants, sex ratio 1.05 (95% CI 1.03-1.07 which thus contains the normal sex ratio). After later use there were 56 540 male and 54 375 female infants (31 with unknown sex) and a sex ratio of 1.04 (95% CI 1.03-1.05), thus slightly low.

Multiple Births

After maternal use of vitamin B12 in early pregnancy, there were 82 twin pairs and no higher order births. The odds ratio for twinning was 1.39 (9%% CI 1.11-1.73). After exclusion from the analysis of women who reported a period of unwanted childlessness, the odds ratio decreased to 1.17 (95% CI 0.91-1.52) and was thus no longer statistically significant. After later use of vitamin B12, there were 144 twin and one triplet delivery. Odds ratio for twinning was 1.46 (95% CI 1.24-1.72). After exclusion of women reporting a period of unwanted childlessness, the odds ratio decreased to 1.24 but remained statistically significant (95% CI 1.02-1.50).

After maternal use of folic acid in early pregnancy, there were 957 twin and 5 triplet deliveries. The odds ratio for twinning was 1.61 (95% CI 1.51-1.73). After exclusion of women who reported unwanted childlessness or who reported the use of any of the following concomitant drugs which occurred in excess: drugs for inflammatory bowel disease, progestogens, gonadotropines, systemic corticosteroids, or thyroid drugs, the odds ratio declined but remained statistically significant: OR = 1.30 (95% CI 1.19-1.42). After later use of folic acid, there were 2 717 twin and 27 triplet deliveries and one quadruplet delivery. The odds ratio for twinning was 1.89 (95% CI 1.81-1.97). After the exclusions mentioned above, the odds ratio decreased only little: OR = 1.80 (95% CI 1.72-1.90).

The increased odds ratios after late use of vitamin B12 or folic acid may be due to a high use of the vitamins in twin pregnancies which cannot explain the possibly increased twinning risk after folic acid use in early pregnancy. Either this is due to residual confounding, notably of undetected treatments of subfertility like IVF, or it is actually a folic acid effect as has been suggested in the literature.

Table 21.6. Infant mortality after maternal use of B12 or folic acid

Variable studied	Drug use in early pregnancy			Drug use later in pregnancy		
	Number	OR/RR	95% CI	Number	OR/RR	95% CI
Vitamin B12						
Stillbirth	9	0.65	0.30-1.23	2	0.42	0.05-1.52#
Early neonatal death	5	0.82	0.27-1.92	7	0.67	0.27-1.38
Folic acid						
Stillbirth	147	1.06	0.90-1.26	288	0.92	0.82-1.04
Early neonatal death	67	1.14	0.89-1.47	142	0.88	0.74-1.04

#observed over expected number with exact Poisson 95% confidence interval.

There is one odds ratio which is slightly high (although not statistically significant), early neonatal death after early folic acid use.

Table 21.7. Pregnancy duration and infant birth weight after maternal use of vitamin B12 or folic acid

Variable studied	Drug use in early pregnancy			Drug use later in pregnancy		
	Number	OR	95% CI	Number	OR	95% CI
Vitamin B12						
<37 weeks	211	1.09	0.95-1.25	295	0.91	0.81-1.02
<2500g	148	1.16	0.99-1.37	190	0.90	0.78-1.04
≥4500g	163	1.04	0.89-1.22	290	1.11	0.98-1.25
SGA	96	1.07	0.87-1.32	153	1.06	0.90-1.24
LGA	258	1.13	1.00-1.29	456	1.19	1.08-1.31
Folic acid						
<37 weeks	2085	1.02	0.98-1.07	4782	0.91	0.89-0.94
<2500g	1329	1.02	0.96-1.08	2918	0.87	0.84-0.91
≥4500g	1785	1.06	1.01-1.12	4523	1.05	1.01-1.08
SGA	887	0.97	0.90-1.04	2113	0.93	0.88-0.97
LGA	2587	1.05	1.01-1.10	6023	1.05	1.02-1.08

There is thus a tendency of an increased rate of LGA infants both after the use of vitamin B12 and folic acid, both in early pregnancy and later. Later use of folic acid seems associated with a slightly decreased risk for preterm birth, low birth weight, and SGA. If this is a drug effect or due to confounding (e.g., from socioeconomic level) is uncertain.

Table 21.8. Neonatal diagnoses after maternal use of B12 or folic acid

Diagnosis	Drug use in early pregnancy			Drug use later in pregnancy		
	Number	OR	95% CI	Number	OR	95% CI
Vitamiin B12						
Hypoglycaemia	167	1.09	0.92-1.27	283	1.17	1.04-1.32
Respiratory diagnoses	223	1.13	0.98-1.29	352	1.10	0.98-1.22
Low Apgar score	75	0.97	0.77-1.22	111	0.90	0.74-1.08
CNS diagnoses	34	1.19	0.85-1.67	56	1.32	1.01-1.72
Jaundice	172	1.01	0.86-1.18	271	0.98	0.87-1.11
Folic acid						
Hypoglycaemia	1739	1.07	1.02-1.13	1739	1.07	1.02-1.13
Respiratory diagnoses	2217	1.09	1.04-1.14	2217	1.09	1.04-1.14
Low Apgar score	878	1.12	1.05-1.21	878	1.12	1.05-1.21
CNS diagnoses	365	1.14	1.02-1.27	772	1.11	1.02-1.27
Jaundice	2038	1.10	1.05-1.15	4682	1.04	1.01-1.08

Table 21.9. Congenital malformations in infants whose mothers had used vitamin B12 or folic acid in early pregnancy

Congenital malformation	Vitamin B12			Folic acid		
	Number	OR	95% CI	Number	OR	95% CI
All malformations	201	1.04	0.90-1.22	2088	1.06	1.01-1.11
Relatively severe malformations	138	1.07	0.89-1.29	1395	1.05	0.99-1.12
Chromosome anomalies	7	0.84	0.34-1.73#	68	0.80	0.61-1.03
Without chromosome anomalies						
Any CNS malformation	1	0.21	0.01-1.18#	47	1.11	0.80-1.54
Neural tube defects	1	0.53	0.01-2.93#	17	1.40	0.83-1.34
Eye malformations	4	1.37	0.51-3.64#	29	0.98	0.66-1.47
Ear malformations	7	0.84	0.34-1.73#	72	0.90	0.70-1.15
Orofacial clefts	10	1.37	0.51-3.64#	78	0.99	0.77-1.28
Any cardiovascular defect	43	1.00	0.72-1.40	479	1.05	0.95-1.16
VSD and/or ASD	34	1.39	0.96-2.01	286	1.01	0.89-1.15
Unspecified cardiovascular defects	4	1.19	0.32-3.04#	42	1.29	0.92-1.81
Oesophageal atresia	2	2.01	0.24-7.27#	10	1.05	0.56-1.97
Small gut atresia	1	0.98	0.02-5.46#	11	1.06	0.55-2.06
Anal atresia	4	2.60	0.71-6.65#	17	1.10	0.64-1.89
Pylorostenosis	5	1.97	0.64-4.59#	35	1.13	0.83-1.71
Hypospadias	11	0.93	0.48-1.78	144	1.21	1.01-1.46
Kidney a/dysgenesis	2	2.31	0.28-8.34#	14	1.60	0.91-2.81#
Cystic kidneys	0	0.00	0.00-2.44#	13	0.84	0.47-1.48
Abdominal wall defects	2	2.08	0.25-7.51#	11	0.96	0.48-1.92
Diaphragmatic hernia	1	1.15	0.03-6.42#	10	1.01	0.48-1.46#
Pes equinovarus	8	1.30	0.56-1.56#	67	1.12	0.86-1.47
Poly/syndactyly	8	0.97	0.42-1.91#	83	0.89	0.70-1.13
Craniostenosis	1	0.43	0.01-2.38#	27	1.07	0.71-1.62

#observed over expected number with exact Poisson 95% confidence interval.

No neonatal ill effects are seen of maternal use of B12 in early pregnancy but later use may be associated with hypoglycaemia and possibly CNS diagnoses. All risk estimates for neonatal diagnoses after early use of folic acid were slightly increased but after exclusion from the analysis of women who reported the use of unwanted childlessness or had used one of the above-listed drugs, the odds ratios decreased and lost statistical significance.

After early use of B12 there is thus no significant increase or decrease in the rate of congenital malformations. After early use of folic acid, the total malformation rate is slightly increased and for specific types this is seen for hypospadias. If the analyses are made after exclusion of women who had reported unwanted childlessness or had used an anticonvulsant (which is strongly associated with folic acid use and is teratogenic) the risk for any congenital malformation (based on 1661 malformed infants) even increased marginally and remained significantly increased: OR = 1.13, 95% CI 1.07-1.19. This is true also for relatively severe malformations: OR = 1.10, 95% CI 1.03-1.18, while the risks for any cardiac defect and for hypospadias remain increased but just lost statistical significance: OR =1.11, 95% CI 0.99-1.24 and OR = 1.20, 95% CI 0.97-1.48. The weak increase in the risk for a congenital malformation seems not to be due to these confounders even if they were incompletely ascertained.

Summary

Both vitamin B12 and folic acid are used at certain maternal pathology, the most obvious being folic acid use together with anticonvulsants. Also other diseases are reasons for supplementation, usually with high dose of folic acid, e.g., immunological bowel disease. B12 is also given at these and other pathologies. Extra folic acid and vitamin B12 is often given to women who undergo treatment for subfertility, notably IVF, and a period of subfertility may itself increase the use of folic acid. The majority of early pregnancy users of folic acid, however, have taken it in order to reduce the risk for a congenital malformation, notably a neural tube defect. The reporting/registration of folic acid is with certainty far from complete which will bias the estimated odds ratio towards 1. Pregnancy and neonatal characteristics are little affected by early use of vitamin B12 or folic acid but a clear tendency to an increased occurrence of LGA infants is seen. No certain effects on the risk of a congenital malformation were found. There was an increased risk for twinning after early use of folic acid which is partly explained by the association with fertility treatments but a remaining risk increase after exclusion from the analysis of women with fertility problem indicates that folic acid may facilitate implantation and therefore increase the risk for twinning.

References

[1] Kalter H. Folic acid and human malformations: a summary and evaluation. *Reprod Toxicol* 2000; 14: 463-476.

[2] Shaw GM, Schaffer D, Velie EM, Morland K, Harris JA. Periconceptional vitamin use, dietary folate, and the occurrence of neural tube defects. *Epidemiology* 1995; 6: 219-226.

[3] Källén B, Otterblad Olausson P. Use of folic acid and delivery outcome: a prospective registry study. *Reprod Toxicol* 2002; 16: 327-332.

[4] Källén B. Congenital malformations in infants whose mothers reported the use of folic acid in early pregnancy in Sweden. A prospective population study. *Cong Anomal* 2007; 47: 119-124.

[5] MRC Vitamin Study Research Group.Prevention of neural tube defects: results of the Medical Research Council Vitamin Study. *Lancet* 1991; 338: 131-137.

[6] Czeizel AE, Dudás I. Prevention of the first occurrence of neural tube defects by periconceptional vitamin supplementation. *N Engl J Med* 1992; 327: 1832-1835.

[7] Berry RJ, Zi Z, Erickson JD, Li S, Moore CA, Wang H, Mulinare J, Zhao P, Wong LY, Gindler J, Hong SX, Correa A. Prevention of neural tube defects with folic acid in China. *N Engl J Med* 199; 341: 1485-1490.

[8] Besser LM, Williams LJ, Cragan JD. Interpreting changes in the epidemiology of anencephaly and spina bifida following folic acid fortification of the U.S. grain supply in the setting of long-term trends, Atlanta, Georgia, 1968-2003. *Birth Def Res (Part A)* 2007; 79: 730-736.

[9] Rosano A, Smithells D, Cacciani L, Botting B, Castilla E, Cornel M, Erickson D, Goujard J, Irgens I, Merlob P, Robert E, Siffel C, Stoll C, Sumivochi Y. Time trends in neural tube defects prevalence in relation to preventive strategies: an international study. *J Epidemiol Comm Health* 1999; 53: 630-635.

[10] Botto LD, Olney RS, Erickson JD. Vitamin supplements and the risk for congenital anomalies other than neural tube defects. *Amer J Med Genet Part C* 2004;125C: 12-21.

[11] Molloy AM, Kirke PN, Brody LC, Scott JM, Mills JL. Effects of folate and vitamin B12 deficiencies during pregnancy on fetal, infant and child development. *Food Nutr Bull* 2008; 29 (2 Suppl): 101-111.

[12] Ray JG, Blom HJ. Vitamin B12 insufficiency and the risk of fetal neural tube defects. *Q J Med* 2003; 96: 289-295.

[13] Verkleij-Hagoort AC, van Driel LMJW, Lindemans J, Isaacs A, Steegers EAP, Helbing WA, Uittrlinden AG, Steegers-Theunissen RPM. Genetic and lifestyle factors related to the periconception vitamin B12 status and congenital heart defects: A Dutch case-control study. *Mol Genet Metabol* 2008; 94: 112-119.

[14] Källén B, Lundberg G, Åberg A. Relationship between vitamin use, smoking, and nausea and vomiting of pregnancy. *Acta Obst Gynecol Scand* 2003; 82: 916-920.

Chapter 22

DRUGS FOR CARDIAC DISEASES

> Even though maternal heart disease is associated with an increased risk for pregnancy complications, there is no evidence to indicate that drugs used for cardiac disease have an effect of their own and notably not a teratogenic effect, even though the number of analyzed pregnancies is low. Exposure in early pregnancy probably does not carry such a high risk that it can motivate a discussion of termination of pregnancy for fear of teratogenesis.

Women with heart disease will have an increased risk for cardiac and pregnancy complications [1]. Women with congenital heart malformations represent a subgroup of them [2]. Women with valvular stenosis have a higher risk profile than women with regurgitant valve disease [3]. Relatively little information is available on the possible teratogenic effect of cardiac drugs. One study described a small material with 52 women who used digitalis glycosides and 39 women who used vasodilators with 6 and 5 malformed infants, respectively [4].

Most drugs are thus represented by only few exposures. It is probable that the majority of the exposures for epinephrine occurred in a treatment for allergic reactions (Anapen® or EpiPen®) or at acute asthma attacks (Adrenalin Merck®) and not because of cardiac problems. These 52 women were therefore removed from the analysis but the presence of congenital malformations after maternal use of this drug is described separately.

CHARACTERISTICS OF WOMEN USING DRUGS FOR CARDIAC DISEASES

Based on women reporting the drug in early pregnancy (n=257). Each variable is adjusted for all other variables and year of delivery. Comparison with all women who gave birth during the period and with information from the first antenatal care (n=967 742). The odds ratios for maternal age, parity, smoking in early pregnancy, number of previous miscarriages, BMI, subfertility, and country of birth are adjusted for all other variables.

Table 22.1. Number of women identified using

Total	714
Reported use in early pregnancy	309
Got prescription later in pregnancy	475
Both early and later use	70

Type of drug	ATC code	Early use	Later use
Digitalis glycosides	C01A	21	40
Acetyldigoxin	C01AA01	1	0
Digoxin	C01AA05	20	40
Antiarrhythmics	C01B	9	16
Quinidine	C01BA01	2	0
Procainamide	C01BA02	0	2
Disopyramide	C01BA03	2	5
Lidocaine	C01BB01	1	2
Mexiletine	C01BB02	3	2
Flecainide	C01BC04	0	4
Amiodarone	C01BD01	0	1
Cardiac stimulants excl. glycosides	C01C	242	396
Etilefrine	C01CA01	183	366
Dopamine	C01CA04	2	5
Norfenefrine	C01CA05	1	0
Dobutamine	C01CA07	1	0
Dopexamine	C01CA14	1	0
Epinephrine	C01CA24	52	23
Amrinone	C01CE01	1	2
Unspecified	C01C	1	0
Vasodilators	C01D	31	21
Glyceryl nitrate	C01DA02	28	20
Isosorbide dinitrate	C01DA08	1	0
Isosorbide mononitrate	C01DA14	5	1
Other cardiac drugs	C01E	1	0
Alprostadil	C01EA01	0	2
Adenosine	C01EB10	1	0

Some further maternal characteristics were analyzed, adjusting for year of delivery, maternal age, parity, smoking, and BMI (Table 22.3).

Women using drugs for cardiac diseases are thus older than expected, are less often than expected of first parity, may smoke more than expected, are less often over-weight, and are more often than expected born outside Sweden.

The strongest association is thus seen with antihypertensives but relatively strong associations also exist with drugs for stomach ulcer and reflux, thyroid drugs, opioids, psychoactive drugs, and antihistamines.

There is no certain increase in the risk for pregnancy complications but the rates of delivery induction and caesarean section are increased, both after early and later drug use. Most numbers are low and confidence intervals wide.

Table 22.2. Some characteristics of women using drugs for cardiac diseases

Variable studied	Number	OR	95% CI
Maternal age			
<25 years	36	1.21	0.82-1.77
25-34 years	151	1.00	reference
≥35 years	70	1.57	1.18-2.09
Parity			
1	85	0.72	0.55-0.94
≥2	172	1.00	reference
Smoking			
Unknown	10	-	-
No	204	1.00	reference
Yes	43	1.81	0.88-3.73
Previous miscarriage			
No	202	1.00	reference
Yes	55	0.91	0.67-1.24
BMI			
Unknown	27	-	-
<19.8	24	1.13	0.73-1.75
19.8-25.9	158	1.00	reference
≥26	48	0.64	0.46-0.90
Subfertility (period of unwanted childlessness)			
No	239	1.00	reference
Yes	18	0.93	0.56-1.54
Country of birth			
Unknown	3	-	-
Sweden	180	1.00	reference
Other Nordic	15	2.44	1.46-4.07
Non-Nordic	59	1.68	1.26-2.25

Table 22.3. Some further characteristics of women using drugs for cardiac disease in early pregnancy

Variable studied	Number	OR	95% CI
Education (1996-2001, 156 women with drugs, 526 695 in population)			
Unknown	6		
<12 years	25	1.13	0.70-1.83
12 years	90	1.00	reference
≥13 years	11	0.55	0.37-0.82
Family situation			
Unknown	6	-	- -
Co-habiting	229	1.00	reference
Living alone	15	1.76	1.05-2.97
Other family situation	7	1.09	0.50-2.35
Work outside home			
Unknown	37	-	
Full time	101	1.00	reference
Part time	69	1.22	0.88-1.70
None	50	1.36	0.95-1.95

Table 22.4. Concomittant drug use (early pregnancy)

Drug group	Number	OR/RR	95% CI
Drugs for stomach ulcer and reflux	11	4.58	2.29-8.20#
Multivitamins	14	0.93	0.54-1.61
Folic acid	15	1.35	0.78-2.34
Antihypertensives	16	11.7	6.68-19.0#
Thyroid drugs	9	3.07	1.40-5.83#
Antibiotics	13	1.53	0.82-2.63#
NSAIDs	6	1.42	0.52-3.08#
Opioids	10	7.63	3.66-14.0#
Minor analgesics	21	1.14	0.73-1.80
Sedatives, hypnotics	8	4.88	8.11-9.61#
Antidepressants	15	5.00	2.80-8.25#
Drugs for rhinitis	4	1.31	0.36-3.36#
Antiasthmatics	11	1.42	0.71-2.55#
Antihistamines	35	2.92	2.07-4.11

#observed over expected number with exact Poisson 95% confidence interval.

Table 22.5. Some maternal diagnoses associated with the use of cardiac drugs

Diagnosis	Drug use in early pregnancy			Drug use later in pregnancy		
	Number	OR/RR	95% CI	Number	OR/RR	95% CI
Pre-existing diabetes	5	1.13	0.50-3.58#	3	0.55	0.11-1.62
Chronic hypertension	4	1.38	0.38-3.53#	5	1.03	0.33-2.40#
Gestational diabetes	4	1.72	0.47-4.41#	3	0.78	0.16-2.28#
Preeclampsia	12	1.17	0.65-2.09	6	1.12	0.41-2.44#
Hyperemesis gravidarum	5	1.67	0.54-3.89#	5	1.13	0.37-2.64#
Placenta previa	4	1.36	0.37-3.47#	5	1.02	0.33-2.38#
Abruptio placentae	7	2.14	0.86-4.41#	6	1.12	0.41-2.47#
Antepartum bleeding	5	1.42	0.46-3.31#	4	0.67	0.18-1.72#
Intrapartum bleeding	9	1.71	0.78-3.25#	14	1.67	0.91-2.81#
Postpartum bleeding	10	0.69	0.36-1.31	21	0.86	0.55-1.33
Delivery induction	33	1.40	0.95-2.05	58	1.39	1.05-1.85
Caesarean section	61	1.65	1.22-2.22	87	1.46	1.15-1.86

#observed over expected number with exact Poisson 95% confidence interval.

Outcome after Maternal use of Cardiac Drugs

Infant Sex

After early exposure for cardiac drugs, there were 139 male and 122 female infants born, sex ratio 1.14 (95% CI 0.89-1.46). After later exposure, there were 250 male and 217 female infants, sex ratio 1.15 (95% CI 0196-1.38). Both sex ratios are slightly high but the normal sex ratio (1.06) is included in the confidence intervals.

Multiple Births

After early exposure for cardiac drugs, there was only 4 twin deliveries (RR = 0.91, 95% CI 0.25-2.34) while after later exposure the twinning rate was increased: 14 twins

(RR = 2.23, 95% CI 1.22-3.74) and there was one triplet birth. This is probably the result of an increased use of such drugs in twin pregnancies.

Infant Mortality

After maternal use of cardiac drugs in early pregnancy there was no stillbirth but one early neonatal death. The mother had used etilefrine and antacids. There was a placental anomaly, foetal distress with intrauterine hypoxia and severe birth asphyxia, and an emergency caesarean section was performed.

After maternal use of cardiac drugs later in pregnancy there was one stillbirth. The mother had used etilefrine and multivitamins. There was no maternal delivery diagnosis. Two infants died within the first week of life. Both mothers had used etilefrine, one of them had also used folic acid and the other one had got a bladder X-ray examination with amidotrizoine acid contrast. One mother had a delivery diagnosis of hypotension and the infant a cause of death diagnosis of maternal placenta previa. The other mother had a diagnosis of placenta anomaly and an emergency caesarean section and the infant had intrauterine hypoxia and severe birth asphyxia.

Thus all four mothers to the dead infants had used etilefrine. The expected number of deaths after maternal use of this drug is 2.8 and the RR is 1.45 (95% CI 0.40-3.70).

Table 22.6. Pregnancy duration and infant birth weight at maternal use of cardiac drugs

Variable studied	Drug use in early pregnancy			Drug use later in pregnancy		
	Number	OR/RR	95% CI	Number	OR/RR	95% CI
<37 week	19	1.54	0.97-2.43	21	0.98	0.63-1.51
<2500g	11	1.33	0.66-2.38#	14	1.02	0.60-1.72
≥4500g	2	0.19	0.06-0.67#	17	0.92	0.56-1.51
SGA	6	1.12	0.41-2.43#	8	0.96	0.42-1.90#
LGA	7	0.41	0.20-0.85#	29	1.00	0.68-1.47

#observed over expected number with exact Poisson 95% confidence interval.

After early exposure, signs of a reduction of the occurrence of large infants and LGA infants are seen but after later exposure, no deviations from the expected values are noticed.

Table 22.7. Neonatal diagnoses after maternal use of drugs for cardiac diseases

Diagnosis	Drug use in early pregnancy			Drug use later in pregnancy		
	Number	OR/RR	95% CI	Number	OR/RR	95% CI
Hypoglycaemia	19	2.07	1.25-3.24#	16	1.03	0.62-1.69
Respiratory diagnoses	22	1.83	1.18-2.83	23	1.06	0.70-1.60
Low Apgar score	5	1.04	0.34-2.42#	8	0.96	0.42-1.90#
CNS diagnoses	1	0.52	0.01-2.92#	3	1.20	0.25-3.51#
Jaundice	23	1.90	1.25-2.90	22	1.22	0.80-1.88

#observed over expected number with exact Poisson 95% confidence interval.

There are thus signs of increased neonatal problems when the mother had used cardiac drugs in early pregnancy while no deviations in neonatal outcome are seen after later use.

Table 22.8. Congenital malformations in infants whose mothers had used cardiac drugs in early pregnancy

Congenital malformation	Number	RR	95% CI
All malformation	8	0.69	0.34-1.19
Relatively severe malformation	7	0.80	0.32-1.65
Chromosome anomalies	2	2.94	0.36-10.6

There was one infant with an unspecified cardiac defect, one with a syndrome diagnosis affecting the skull, one with pylorostenosis, one with polydactyly, one with syndactyly, one with unstable hip, and two with Down syndrome. All women had used etilefrine except two: one had used glyceryl nitrate (infant had Down syndrome) and one had used adenosine (infant had polydactyly).

Among the 52 infants whose mothers used epinephrine in early pregnancy, one had a congenital malformation: coarctatio aortae.

No malformations were observed in infants whose mothers had use digitalis (n=21) or antiarrythmics (n=10).

Summary

Relatively few women had used cardiac drugs in early pregnancy. The majority had got cardiac stimulants excluding digitalis, and notably etilefrine. There are no certain ill effects on pregnancy outcome except for an increased risk for some neonatal diagnoses: hypoglycaemia, respiratory diagnoses, and jaundice. There are no signs of teratogenicity of these drugs.

Use later in pregnancy seems not to be associated with any ill effects and especially not neonatal diagnoses. It is likely that there is a difference in case mix: women using these drug in early pregnancy may have a pre-existing cardiovascular disease while use later in pregnancy may be associated with pregnancy complications and notably low blood pressure.

References

[1] Siu SC, Colman JM, Alvarez AN, Mercier L-A, Morton BC, Kells CM, Beergin L, Kiess MC, Marcotte F, Taylor DA, Gordon EP, Spears JC, Tam JW, Amankwah KS, Smallhorn JF, Farine D, Sørensen S. Prospective multicenter study of pregnancy outcomes in women with heart disease. *Ciculation* 2001; 104: 515-421.

[2] Ford AA, Wylie BJ, Waksmonski CA, Simpson LL. Maternal congenital cardiac disease. Outcomes of pregnancy in a single tertiary care center. *Obstet Gynecol* 2008; 112: 828-833.

[3] Iung B. The valve patient and pregnancy. *Expert Rev Cardiovasc Ther* 2008; 6: 1249-1258.

[4] Heinonen OP, Slone D, Shapiro S. *Birth Defects and Drugs in Pregnancy*. Publishing Sciences Group, Littleton, Mass. 1977.

Chapter 23

ANTIHYPERTENSIVES

Maternal chronic hypertension increases the risk for severe pregnancy and neonatal complications. Adequate treatment can reduce the risk for the hypertension to get aggravated but other complications are difficult to prevent. Infants born of women who use antihypertensives in early pregnancy have an increased risk for a cardiovascular defect. It is difficult to say if this is an effect of the maternal disease or a group specific drug effect but in contrast to what has been described in the literature, no clear differences between different antihypertensive drug categories are seen. Most of the cardiac defects seen were relatively mild and the risk increase is moderate so an exposure to this type of drugs should hardly result in a discussion of a termination of the pregnancy.

Women with chronic hypertension have various severe complications including a worsening of the hypertension, and increased risk for preeclampsia, eclampsia, and HELLP syndrome, liver or renal failure, placental abruption, miscarriage or foetal death, preterm birth and intrauterine growth restriction, and neonatal complications [1-4]. Pregnancies in women with mild or moderate hypertension are therefore carefully monitored and treated and in this way the risk for severe hypertension can be reduced but little effect is seen on maternal and neonatal complications [5]. It is not clear whether maternal chronic hypertension can increase the risk for a congenital malformation in the infant and relatively little information is available [6]. In a study of maternal drug use and infant cardiovascular defects [7], a doubled risk for such a defect was seen after maternal use of antihypertensives and another study [8] linked maternal use of ACE-inhibitors (but not other antihypertensives) to infant cardiac defects. A recent study of calcium channel blockers, based on 29 pregnancies, found no signs of teratogenicity [9].

Table 23.1. Number of women identified using antihypertensives

Total	5963
Reported use in early pregnancy	3644
Got prescription later in pregnancy	3747
Both early and later use	1428

Type of drug	ATC code	Early use	Later use
Centrally acting agents	C02	124	223
Methyldopa	C02AB01	33	55
Clonidine	C02AC01	15	5
Doxazozin	C02CA04	6	4
Terazosin	C02CA05	1	0
Diazoxide	C02DA01	2	0
Hydralazine	C02DB02	67	157
Nitroprusside	C02DD01	0	2
Unspecified	C02	2	1
Beta blocking agents	C07	3163	3326
Pindolol	C07AA03	281	562
Propanolol	C07AA05	794	290
Timolol	C07AA06	9	2
Sotalol	C07AA07	54	22
Metoprolol	C07AB02	827	637
Metoprolol+felodipin	C07FB02	10	2
Atenolol	C07AB03	669	427
Betaxolol	C07AB05	5	2
Bisoprolol	C07AB07	30	19
Nebilovol	C07AB52	0	1
Labetalol	C07AG01	533	1564
Carvediol	C07AG02	16	7
Alprenolol+diuretics	C07BA01	0	3
Unspecified	C07	2	1
Calcium channel blockers		342	466
Amlodipine	C08CA01	41	21
Felodipine	C08CA02	101	58
Isradipine	C08CA03	68	143
Nicardipine	C08CA04	2	3
Nifedipine	C08CA05	69	218
Verapamil	C08DA01	62	27
Diltiazem	C08DB01	4	1
ACE-inhibitors	C09A-B	194	43
Captopril	C09AA01	10	2
Enalapril	C09AA02	124	30
Enalapril+diuretics	C09BA02	1	0
Lisinopril	C09AA03	17	2
Lisinopril+diuretics	C09BA03	2	0
Ramipril	C09AA05	17	6
Ramipril+diuretics	C09BA05	3	0
Quinapril	C09AA06	3	0
Quinapril+diuretics	C09BA06	2	0
Cilazapril	C09AA08	9	0
Cilazapril+diuretics	C09BA08	4	3
Fosinopril	C09AA09	1	0
Trandolapril+diuretics	C09BB10	1	0
Angiotensin II antagonists	C09C-D	73	21
Losartan	C09CA01	30	10
Losartan+diuretics	C09DA01	2	1
Valsartan	C09CA03	6	1
Irbesartan	C09CA04	9	3
Irbesartan+diuertics	C09DA04	4	0
Candesartan	C09CA06	23	5
Telmisartan	C09CA07	0	1

Some women used two drugs of different categories (table 23.2). More than two antihypertensive drug categories were used by 18 women in early pregnancy. Eleven of them used a combination of beta-blocking agent, calcium channel blocker and ACE inhibitor. In later pregnancy, 21 women used more than two antihypertensive drug categories. Sixteen of them used a combination of centrally acting agent, beta-blocking agent and calcium channel blocker.

Table 23.2. Use of two antihypertensives

	Beta blockers	Calcium channel blocker	ACE-inhibitor	Angiotensin II antagonist
Early pregnancy use				
Centrally acting agent	41	5	4	2
Beta-blocking agent	-	107	33	18
Calcium channel blocker	-	-	6	0
Later pregnancy use				
Centrally acting agent	102	3	0	1
Beta-blocking agent	-	164	8	9
Calcium channel blocker	-	-	1	0
ACE-inhibitor	-	-	-	1

Characteristics of Women using Drugs for Antihypertensives

Based on women reporting the drug in early pregnancy (n=3644). Each variable is adjusted for all other variables and year of delivery. Comparison with all women who gave birth during the period and with information from the first antenatal care (n=967 742). The odds ratios for maternal age, parity, smoking in early pregnancy, number of previous miscarriages, BMI, subfertility, and country of birth are adjusted for all other variables and are shown in Figure 23.1.

Some further maternal characteristics were analyzed, adjusting for year of delivery, maternal age, parity, smoking, and BMI (Table 23.3).

Women using antihypertensive drugs are thus older than expected, more often of first parity, smokers, over-weight and with an excess of previous miscarriages and subfertility. Long education is associated with a low use and so is to be born outside the Nordic countries.

Many drug groups have thus been used in excess. The strongest associations are seen with insulin, systemic corticosteroids, and antidepressants, but also drugs used for stomach ulcer and gastro-oesophageal reflux and for inflammatory bowel disease, thyroid drugs, NSAIDs, and opioids are used in statistically significant excess.

There is thus an excess of pre-existing diabetes and of all pregnancy complications studied, resulting in a high rate of delivery inductions and caesarean sections.

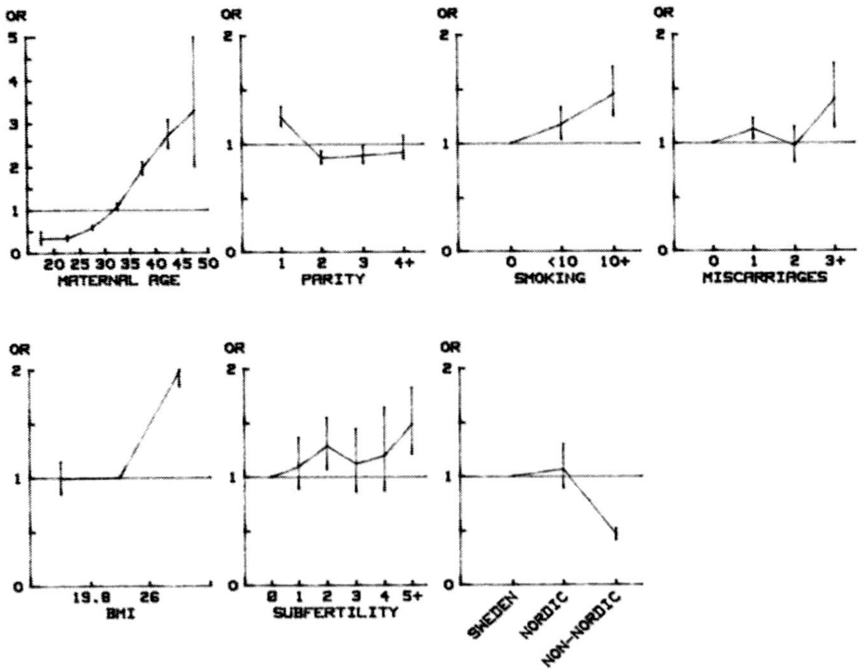

Figure 23.1. Odds ratios for seven maternal characteristics. The odds ratios (OR) for each variable are adjusted for the other variables and year of delivery. Vertical lines mark 95% confidence intervals. For maternal age and parity, each class is compared with all other classes.

Table 23.3. Some further characteristics of women using antihypertensives in early pregnancy

Variable studied	Number	OR	95% CI
Education (1996-2001, 1 677 women with drugs, 526 695 in population)			
Unknown	25		
<12 years	171	0.85	0.71-1.00
12 years	903	1.00	reference
13-14 years	77	0.73	0.58-0.93
≥14 years	501	0.82	0.73-0.92
Family situation			
Unknown	80	-	
Co-habiting	3385	1.00	reference
Living alone	110	1.12	0.93-1.37
Other family situation	69	0.76	0.60-0.97
Work outside home			
Unknown	465	-	
Full time	1682	1.00	reference
Part time	921	1.15	1.05-1.25
None	576	0.98	0.88-1.08

Table 23.4. Concomitant drug use (early pregnancy)

Drug group	Number	OR/RR	95% CI
Drugs for stomach ulcer and reflux	79	2.23	1.79-2.79
Drugs for inflammatory bowel disease	28	2.80	1.95-4.02
Insulin	138	10.7	9.26-12.3
Multivitamins	210	0.83	0.72-0.97
Folic acid	208	1.05	0.91-1.22
Oral contraceptives	6	0.65	0.24-1.41#
Progestogens	13	0.68	0.40-1.17
Gonadotropins	11	1.19	0.60-2.14
Systemic corticosteroids	62	4.73	3.74-5.97
Thyroid drugs	136	2.41	2.03-2.85
Antibiotics	105	0.94	0.78-1.15
NSAIDs	84	1.29	1.04-1.60
Opioids	60	2.80	2.18-3.59
Minor analgesics	242	0.86	0.75-0.98
Anticonvulsants	16	1.55	0.94-2.56
Sedatives, hypnotics	7	1.73	0.69-3.56#
Antidepressants	188	3.84	3.33-4.43
Drugs for rhinitis	47	0.89	0.66-1.18
Antiasthmatics	158	1.44	1.23-1.69
Cough medicines	11	0.59	0.33-1.06
Antihistamines	187	0.97	0.84-1.13

#observed over expected number with exact Poisson 95% confidence interval.

Table 23.5. Some maternal diagnoses associated with the use of antihypertensives

Diagnosis	Drug use in early pregnancy			Drug use later in pregnancy		
	Number	OR/RR	95% CI	Number	OR/RR	95% CI
Pre-existing diabetes	266	4.31	3.83-4.85	220	3.10	2.72-3.54
Gestational diabetes	89	1.78	1.44-2.20	107	1.98	1.63-2.40
Preeclampsia	684	4.07	3.76-4.41	-	-	-
Hyperemesis gravidarum	93	1.81	1.47-2.22	115	1.98	1.64-2.38
Placenta previa	94	1.58	1.28-1.95	116	1.77	1.47-2.13
Abruptio placentae	118	1.92	1.60-2.32	141	2.06	1.74-2.44
Antepartum bleeding	102	1.52	1.24-1.86	119	1.66	1.38-2.00
Intrapartum bleeding	148	1.49	1.23-1.71	179	1.56	1.34-1.82
Postpartum bleeding	279	1.25	1.11-1.42	289	1.26	1.12-1.42
Delivery induction	937	3.05	2.82-3.29	1251	4.44	4.15-4.75
Caesarean section	1216	2.14	1.99-2.29	1319	2.24	2.09-2.39

OUTCOME AFTER MATERNAL USE OF ANTIHYPERTENSIVES

Infant Sex

After early use of antihypertensives, 1850 of the infants born were male and 1856 female which gives a sex ratio of 1.00 (95% CI 0.93-1.06). This sex ratio is thus marginally below the normal sex ratio of 1.06. After later use, there were 1943 male and 1883 female infants, sex ratio 1.03 (95% CI 0.97-1.10).

Multiple Births

After early use of antihypertensives, there were 58 twin deliveries and two triplet deliveries. The odds ratio for twinning was 0.92 (95% CI 0.71-1.20). After later use, there were 78 twin deliveries with an OR of 1.23 (95% CI 0.98-1.54).

Table 23.6. Infant mortality after maternal use of antihypertensives

Variable studied	Drug use in early pregnancy			Drug use later in pregnancy		
	Number	OR/RR	95% CI	Number	OR/RR	95% CI
Stillbirth	35	2.30	1.66-2.39	32	2.07	1.47-2.93
Early neonatal death	9	1.42	0.65-2.70#	12	1.86	0.96-3.15#

There is thus a marked increase in the stillbirth rate and a suggested but not statistically significant increase in the early neonatal death rate.

Table 23.7. Pregnancy duration and infant birth weight at maternal use of antihypertensives

Variable studied	Drug use in early pregnancy			Drug use later in pregnancy		
	Number	OR/RR	95% CI	Number	OR/RR	95% CI
<37 weeks	522	3.15	2.88-3.44	592	3.59	3.30-3.90
<2500g	409	3.76	3.40-4.14	526	5.14	4.72-5.60
≥4500g	100	0.58	0.47-0.70	80	0.42	0.34-0.52
SGA	244	3.29	2.89-3.73	300	4.27	3.83-4.77
LGA	218	0.83	0.72-0.95	202	0.70	0.60-0.81

There is thus a marked increase in the rate of preterm birth and intrauterine growth retardation both after early and later exposure to antihypertensive drugs.

Table 23.8. Neonatal diagnoses after maternal use of antihypertensives

Diagnosis	Drug use in early pregnancy			Drug use later in pregnancy		
	Number	OR	95% CI	Number	OR	95% CI
Hypoglycaemia	390	2.70	2.44-3.00	421	2.92	2.65-3.23
Respiratory diagnoses	353	1.83	1.64-2.04	403	2.13	1.92-2.36
Low Apgar score	138	1.75	1.47-2.08	147	1.92	1.63-2.26
CNS diagnoses	48	1.74	1.31-2.32	51	1.74	1.32-2.29
Jaundice	339	2.22	1.98-2.48	419	2.64	2.36-2.92

All five neonatal diagnoses studied thus occurred in excess.

There was thus an excess of congenital malformations which seems specifically due to cardiovascular defects. Among other malformations, only cystic kidneys occurred more often than expected but this is based on only five cases: Two of these were coded as polycystic kidneys of infantile type, one as unspecified sponge kidney, and two as cystic dysplasia. Among the four neural tube defects, one was anencephaly and three spina bifida.

The strong association between hypertension and diabetes could explain the effect on cardiac defects. The analysis was therefore repeated after exclusion of women with any type of diabetes diagnosis. The over-all odds ratio declined only little: OR = 1.89 (95% CI 1.44-2.48).

Table 23.9. Congenital malformations in infants whose mothers had used antihypertensives in early pregnancy

Congenital malformation	Number	OR	95% CI
All malformation	225	1.25	1.07-1.45
Relatively severe malformation	166	1.32	1.11-1.58
Chromosome anomalies	5	0.49	0.19-1.27#
Without chromosome anomalies			
Any cardiovascular defect	75	1.96	1.51-2.53
VSD and/or ASD	40	1.71	1.19-2.47
Unspecified cardiac defect	8	2.46	1.20-5.05#
Without cardiovascular defect	92	1.09	0.86-1.38
Any CNS malformation	7	1.50	0.60-3.09#
Neural tube defects	4	2.70	0.74-6.92#
Ear malformations	7	0.81	0.33-1.67#
Orofacial clefts	5	0.70	0.23-1.64#
Hypospadias	14	1.06	0.55-2.04
Cystic kidneys	5	3.22	1.05-7.52#
Pes equinovarus	9	1.61	0.74-3.05#
Hip (sub)luxation, unstable hip	18	0.76	0.46-1.26
Poly/syndactyly	10	1.42	0.68-2.61#

#observed over expected number with exact Poisson 95% confidence interval.

In order to search for specific relationships between infant cardiac defects and groups of antihypertensive use, exposure for each group was studied after exclusion of maternal diabetes. Due to low numbers, ACE inhibitors and angiotensin II inhibitors were added together.

Table 23.10. Cardiac defects in infants exposed to different types of antihypertensives in early pregnancy

Antihypertensive drug group	Number of cardiac defects	Number of infants	OR	95% CI
Centrally acting agents	6	126	4.06	1.49-8.83#
Beta-blocking agents	51	3030	1.67	1.23-2.28
Calcium channel blockers	11	320	3.54	1.77-6.33#
ACE-inhibitors and angiotensine II inhibitors	8	181	4.35	1.88-8.56#

#observed over expected number with exact Poisson 95% confidence interval.

All eight infants with cardiovascular defects in the last group were exposed to ACE-inhibitors.

The much lower OR for beta blocking agents could be explained by the use of these drugs at other conditions than hypertension, e.g., arrhythmia and as migraine prophylaxis. If this group was studied after restriction to women who had a delivery diagnosis of chronic hypertension, the OR increased to 2.17 (95% CI 1.27-3.42), based on 18 cardiovascular defects among 841 exposed infants.

There is thus a significantly increased risk for an infant cardiovascular defect, irrespective of antihypertensive drug group used. The rate of cardiovascular defects does not vary significantly between drug groups ($\chi 2$=5.0 for 3 d.f., p=0.17) if the rate for beta blockers in the presence of a diagnosis of chronic hypertension is used.

Summary

Early pregnancy treatment for maternal chronic hypertension is associated with a number of pregnancy and neonatal complications including an increased risk for infant congenital cardiovascular malformations. There seems to be little drug specificity which speaks in favour of an effect of underlying maternal pathology but it is also possible that there is a drug group specific effect, for instance via hypotension in the foetal circulation.

References

[1] Rey E, Couturier A (1994) The prognosis of pregnancy in women with chronic hypertension. *Am J Obst Gynecol 181*: 410-416.

[2] McCowan LM, Buist RG, North RA, Gamble G. (1996) Perinatal morbidiy in chronic hypertension. *Br J Obstet Gynecol 103*: 123-129.

[3] Sibai BM, Caritis SN, Hauth JC, MacPherson C, VanDorsten JP, Klebanoff M, Landon M, Paul RH, Meis PJ, Modovnik M, Dombrowski MP, Thurnau GR, Moawad AH, Roberts J. (2000) Preterm delivery in women with pregestational diabetes or chronic hypertension relative to women with uncomplicated pregnancies. The National Institute of Child Health and Human Development – Fetal Medicine Units Network. *Am J Obst Gynecol 183*: 1520-1524.

[4] Ray JG, Burrows RF, Burrows E et al (2001) McMaster outcome study of hypertension in pregnancy. *Early Human Develop 64*: 129-143.

[5] Abalos E, Duley L, Steyn DW, Dudley JA, Dyer S, Gideon PS, Hall K, Ray WA. (2007) Antihypertensive drug therapy for mild to moderate hypertension during pregnancy. *Cochrane Database of Systematic Reviews Issue 1*. Art.No.: CD002252, DOI: 10.1002/14651858.CD002252.pub2.

[6] Heinonen OP, Slone D, Shapiro S (1977) *Birth Defects and Drugs in Pregnancy*. Publishing Sciences Group, Inc. Littleton, Mass.

[7] Källén B, Otterblad Olausson P (2003) Maternal drug use in early pregnancy and infant cardiovascular defect. *Reprod Toxicol 17*: 255-261.

[8] Cooper WO, Hernandez-Diaz S, Arbogast P et al (2006) Major congenital malformations after first-trimester exposure to ACE inhibitors. *New Engl J Med 354*: 2443-2451.

[9] Weber-Schoendorfer C, Hannemann D, Mester R, Eléfant E, Cuppers-Maarschalkerweerd B, Arnon J, Vial T, Rodriguez-Pinilla E, Clementi M, Robert-Gnansia E, de Santis M, Malm H, Dolivo A, Schaefer C. The safety of calcium channel blockers during pregnancy: A prospective, multicenter, observational study. *Reprod Toxicol* 2008; 26: 24-30.

Chapter 24

DIURETICS

The main use of diuretics in early pregnancy is associated with hypertension and diuretics are often given together with antihypertensive drugs. At mild hypertension, diuretics may be given alone. It is therefore likely that the effect of diuretic use in early pregnancy should resemble that of antihypertensive use (see Chapter 23). In late pregnancy, diuretics can cross the placenta and affect foetal electrolytics. An association between the use of diuretics and neonatal thrombopenia has been described, notably for thiazides but also for loop diuretics.

Table 24.1. Number of women identified using diuretics

Total	759
Reported use in early pregnancy	502
Got prescription later in pregnancy	390
Both early and later use	133

Type of drug	ATC code	Early use	Later use
Low-ceiling diuretics (thiazides)	C03A,C03B	93	63
Bendroflumethiazide	C03AA01	68	51
Bendroflumethiazide + potassium	C03AB01	3	2
Hydrochlorthiazide	C03AA03	21	8
Chlortalidone	C03BA04	1	0
Undefined	C03AD01	0	2
High-ceiling diuretics (loop diuretics)	C03C	234	201
Furosemide	C03CA01	226	195
Bumetanide	C03CA02	4	4
Torasemide	C03CA04	4	2
Potassium-sparing agents	C03D	103	106
Spironolactone	C03DA01	98	104
Potassium canrenoate	C03DA02	1	0
Amiloride	C03DB01	5	3
Thiazides and potassium-sparing agents	C03E	76	33
Amiloride+hydrochlorthiazide	C03EA01	76	33
Unspecified	C03	7	4

Diuretics used during early pregnancy are generally regarded as safe but few large studies exist. One study found no association between maternal diuretic use and infant malformations, based on 280 exposures [1]. As the major indication for diuretics is hypertension, it is to be expected that similar effects as with antihypertensive drugs should be found (cf. Chapter 23). When used during late pregnancy, thiazides can pass to the foetus and cause disturbances of electrolytes. Cases of thrombocytopenia have also been described after the use of thiazides or loop diuretics during late pregnancy.

Table 24.2. Combinations of diuretics used

Drug groups	Early use	Later use
Low-ceiling diuretics+high-ceiling diuretics	0	1
Low-ceiling diuretics+potassium-sparing agents	0	2
Low-ceiling diuretics+combined diuretics and potassium-sparing agents	3	0
High-ceiling diuretics+potassium-sparing agents	5	6
High-ceiling diuretics+combined diuretics and potassium-sparing agents	2	1
Potassium-sparing agents+combined diuretics and potassium sparing agents	1	1

Table 24.3. Characteristics of women using diuretics

Variable studied	Number	OR	95% CI
Maternal age			
< 25 years	13	0.17	0.10-0.28
25-34 years	290	1.00	reference
±35 years	199	2.38	1.97-2.88
Parity			
1	194	1.40	1.16-1.70
2	149	0.74	0.61-0.90
3	94	0.97	0.77-1.22
≥4	65	0.99	0.75-1.31
Smoking			
Unknown	19		
No	397	1.00	reference
Yes	86	1.70	1.22-2.35
Previous miscarriages			
No	360	1.00	reference
Yes	142	1.16	0.95-1.42
BMI			
Unknown	39	-	-
<19.8	20	0.89	0.56-1.43
19.8-25.9	195	1.00	reference
≥26	248	2.81	2.34-3.37
Unwanted childlessness			
No	428	1.00	reference
Yes	74	1.68	1.31-2.16
Country of birth			
Unknown	1	-	-
Sweden	431	1.00	reference
Other Nordic country	21	1.39	0.89-2.16
Non-Nordic country	49	0.62	0.40-0.84

CHARACTERISTICS OF WOMEN USING DIURETICS

Based on women reporting the drug in early pregnancy (n=502). Each variable is adjusted for all other variables and year of delivery. Comparison with all women who gave birth during the period and with information from the first antenatal care (n=967 742). The odds ratios for maternal age, parity, smoking in early pregnancy, number of previous miscarriages, BMI, subfertility, and country of birth are adjusted for all other variables (Table 24.3).

Some further maternal characteristics were analyzed, adjusting for year of delivery, maternal age, parity, smoking, and BMI (Table 24.4).

Table 24.4. Some further characteristics of women using diuretics

Variable studied	Number	OR	95% CI
Education (1996-2001, 241 women with drugs, 506238 in population)			
Unknown	1		
<12 years	27	0.90	0.58-1.39
12 years	139	1.00	reference
≥13 years	74	0.67	0.50-0.90
Family situation			
Unknown	9	-	
Co-habiting	459	1.00	reference
Living alone	17	1.14	0.69-1.87
Other family situation	17	1.47	0.89-2.42
Work outside home			
Unknown	57	-	
Full time	224	1.00	reference
Part time	140	1.29	1.04-1.59
None	81	0.96	0.73-1.26

Table 24.5. Concomitant drug use (early pregnancy)

Drug group	Number	OR/RR	95% CI
Drugs for stomach ulcer and reflux	15	2.01	1.83-4.96#
Drugs for inflammatory bowel disease	9	5.63	2.57-10.7#
Insulin	36	17.0	13.2-21.8
Multivitamins	28	0.93	0.67-1.39
Folic acid	29	1.17	0.79-1.73
Antihypertensives	159	71.8	63.7-80.8
Progestogens	4	1.48	0.40-3.79#
Systemic corticosteroids	25	13.2	8.52-19.4#
Thyroid drugs	28	3.16	2.10-4.57
Antibiotics	20	1.26	0.81-1.98
NSAIDs	17	1.71	0.99-2.74#
Opioids	11	3.41	1.70-6.09#
Minor analgesics	42	1.04	0.76-1.43
Sedatives, hypnotics	9	2.85	1.30-5.41#
Antidepressants	29	3.49	2.33-4.01#
Drugs for rhinitis	16	2.18	1.25-3.07#
Antiasthmatics	34	2.17	1.54-3.07
Antihistamines	24	0.92	0.55-1.45

observed over expected number with exact Poisson 95% confidence interval.

The maternal characteristics resemble relatively much those found for antihypertensives (Chapter 23) which is reasonable but as numbers are lower, confidence intervals are wider.

Also the pattern of concomitant drug use resembles that shown for antihypertensives (Chapter 23). The association with systemic corticosteroids is stronger, however, and the association with drugs for rhinitis was not seen for antihypertensives.

Table 24.6. Some maternal diagnoses associated with the use of diuretics

Diagnosis	Drug use in early pregnancy			Drug use later in pregnancy		
	Number	OR/RR	95% CI	Number	OR/RR	95% CI
Pre-existing diabetes	54	5.26	4.09-6.77	31	3.47	2.36-4.93
Chronic hypertension	140	19.1	16.3-22.3	93	16.0	13.2-19.4
Gestational diabetes	12	1.43	0.81-2.53#	13	2.08	1.11-3.56#
Preeclampsia	99	3.67	2.98-4.53	72	3.34	2.61-4.27
Hyperemesis gravidarum	15	1.75	0.98-2.89#	13	1.97	1.05-3.36#
Placenta previa	15	2.07	1.16-3.41#	13	1.79	0.95-3.06#
Abruptio placentae	12	1.20	0.67-2.12	14	1.80	0.98-3.02#
Antepartum bleeding	16	1.49	0.91-2.45	14	1.66	0.91-2.79#
Intrapartum bleeding	20	1.28	0.82-2.00	21	1.72	1.12-2.66
Postpartum bleeding	40	1.28	0.93-1.38	38	1.60	1.14-2.23
Delivery induction	132	2.98	2.43-3.64	109	3.08	2.47-3.85
Caesarean section	197	2.46	2.06-2.93	140	2.13	1.74-2.61

#observed over expected number with exact Poisson 95% confidence interval.

Pregnancy complications thus occur at an increased rate similar to what is seen after antihypertensives (cf. Chapter 23) and delivery inductions and caesarean sections are more common than expected. The effect on delivery induction after later use of diuretics is weaker than that seen after antihypertensives.

OUTCOME AFTER MATERNAL USE OF DIURETICS

Infant Sex

After early use of diuretics, there were 277 male and 234 female infants born, sex ratio 1.18 (95% CI 1.00-1.41) and after later use there were 187 male and 214 female infants born, sex ratio 0.87 (95% CI 0.72-1.06). The latter sex ratio is thus marginally low – the normal sex ratio is 1.06.

Multiple Births

After early exposure to diuretics, there were four twin deliveries (RR =1.78, 95% CI 0.48-4.55) and two triplet deliveries. After later exposure there were 11 twin deliveries (RR = 1.73, 95% CI 0.86-3.09). Neither risk increase was thus statistically significant.

Table 24.7. Infant mortality after maternal use of diuretics

Variable studied	Drug use in early pregnancy			Drug use later in pregnancy		
	Number	RR	95% CI	Number	RR	95% CI
Stillbirth	4	1.78	0.48-4.55	2	1.16	0.14-4.19
Early neonatal death	2	2.01	0.24-7.27	1	-	-

#observed over expected number with exact Poisson 95% confidence interval.

The small size of the material makes estimates very uncertain.

Table 24.8. Pregnancy duration and infant birth weight at maternal use of diuretics

Variable studied	Drug use in early pregnancy			Drug use later in pregnancy		
	Number	OR/RR	95% CI	Number	OR/RR	95% CI
<37 weeks	108	4.98	4.09-6.06	69	3.91	3.06-4.99
<2500g	72	4.57	3.62-5.76	51	4.27	3.23-5.63
≥4500g	27	1.07	0.73-1.58	22	1.14	0.74-1.76
SGA	33	2.88	2.04-4.06	26	2.88	1.96-4.24
LGA	42	1.12	0.81-1.53	39	1.46	1.04-2.06

There is thus a similar effect on preterm birth, low birth weight, and SGA as after antihypertensives (Chapter 23). In contrast to those drugs, a significantly increased risk for LGA is seen after later use of diuretics.

Table 24.9. Neonatal diagnoses after maternal use of diuretics

Diagnosis	Drug use in early pregnancy			Drug use later in pregnancy		
	Number	OR/RR	95% CI	Number	OR/RR	95% CI
Hypoglycaemia	57	2.65	2.03-3.46	32	1.80	1.27-2.57
Respiratory diagnoses	73	2.77	2.18-3.53	54	2.71	2.05-3.58
Low Apgar score	23	2.02	1.33-3.07	13	1.51	0.86-2.63
CNS diagnoses	13	3.37	1.99-5.71#	8	2.45	1.06-4.82#
Jaundice	64	2.96	2.29-3.83	45	2.69	1.98-3.66
Thrombocytopenia	16	3.13	1.50-5.07#	6	1.81	0.67-3.95#

#observed over expected number with exact Poisson 95% confidence interval.

All the studied diagnoses show excess risks of 2-4 times after early exposure and 1.5-3 times after later exposure.

Among the 16 infants with thrombocytopenia after early exposure, 11 had been exposed to high-ceiling diuretics (loop diuretics), two to potassium-saving diuretics, and three to thiazide diuretics. Among the six infants with thromocytopenia after later exposure, 5 were exposed to high-ceiling diuretics.

The risk estimates resemble those after antihypertensive drug exposure (cf. Chapter 23) but confidence intervals are wide. A formally significant increase in orofacial clefts is seen which was not noted after antihypertensive drugs but it is based on only four cases, two with cleft lip/palate and two with isolated cleft palate. One of the cleft lip/palate infants also had craniosynostosis, one of the cleft palate infants had microcephaly and the other had a syndrome diagnosis with anomalies in the facial appearance.

Table 24.10. Congenital malformations in infants whose mothers had used diuretics in early pregnancy

Congenital malformation	Number	OR/RR	95% CI
All malformation	34	1.56	1.05-2.33
Relatively severe malformation	25	1.53	0.96-2.46
Chromosome anomalies	0	0.00	0.00-2.20#
Without chromosome anomalies			
Any cardiovascular defect	7	1.41	0.57-2.90#
VSD and/or ASD	4	1.46	0.40-3.74#
Orofacial cleft	4	4.41	1.20-11-3#
Hypospadias	3	2.23	0.46-6.51#

#observed over expected number with exact Poisson 95% confidence interval.

The odds ratio for any malformation was slightly lower when the woman had not reported the use of an antihypertensive (OR = 1.46, 95% CI 0.89-2.39) than when she had done so (OR = 1.80, 95% CI 0.92-3.55). This difference may be random and neither odds ratio is by itself statistically significant. Use of diuretics without antihypertensives may indicate mild hypertension.

SUMMARY

The effects noted after maternal use of diuretics resemble much those seen after the use of antihypertensives and there is also a strong association between the two types of drugs. As discussed in Chapter 23, these effects may be due to underlying pathology. The expected association between late use of diuretics and infant thrombocytopenia was not statistically significant due to small numbers but it was seen after early use (many of these women continued using the drugs also later in pregnancy). Both after early and later use, high-ceiling diuretics (loop diuretics) dominated among mothers of infants with thrombocytopenia.

REFERENCES

[1] Heinonen OP, Slone D, Shapiro S. *Birth Defects and Drugs in Pregnancy.* Publishing Sciences Group Inc., Littletone, MA.1977.

Chapter 25

SERUM LIPID REDUCING AGENTS

Among serum lipid agents, only resines are regarded as safe during pregnancy. In case of a planned pregnancy, it is recommended to stop the use of serum lipid reducing agents, but if pregnancy occurs during treatment there is no definitely shown risk for teratogenesis and there is no reason to discuss a pregnancy termination because of usage of these drugs. Further large-scale data are needed to evaluate possible specific teratogenic risks, e.g., the tentative association between statins and holoprosencephaly.

Different groups of lipid lowering agents are used. Statins are inhibitors of 3-hydroxy-3-methylglutaryl coenzyme A (HMG CoA) and reduce the biosynthesis of cholesterol. Fibrates activate a PPAR-receptor and results in the reduction of triglycerides and increase of HDL in the blood. Resines act locally in the gut by binding to bile acids and indirectly affect LDL-cholesterol in the blood. Nicotinic acid inhibits lipase which transforms triglycerides to free fatty acids.

Among lipid reducing agents, most interest has been given statins, partly because they show teratogenic properties in animal experiments [1] and therefore are regarded as potentially unsafe during human pregnancy. Two studies have searched for unusual patterns of malformations among malformed infants, reported as adverse drug reports [2-3]. In one of the studies [2], 22 cases of structural defects were identified and among them were four severe midline CNS defects (one with holoprosencepahly) and five limb reduction defects. In the second study [3], also 22 malformed infants after maternal use of statins were summarized. In this study the two patterns described in the previous paper could not be found. A post-marketing surveillance of lovastatin and simvastatin [1] identified 131 reports of exposure during the first trimester of pregnancy. Nine infants with congenital malformations were identified, five after lovastatin and four after simvastatin exposure. There was one case of VATER association, one infant with holoprosencephaly, and one with spina bifida. The other six infants had cleft lip/palate, a cardiac defect, polydactyly, hypospadias, club foot, and trisomy 18, respectively. In a new report of this kind [4], 154 liveborn infants were identified, now with five malformations to which was added one foetal death with a malformation. All occurred after simvastatin exposure. A small TIS study [5] identified 46 exposed infants with one of them malformed: a cervical soft tissue mass which was evaluated as a minor anomaly. Another study [6] identified 64 infants exposed to statins in the first trimester and 14 exposed to fibrate or nicotinic acid. There were three infants with malformations in both groups. All three malformed infants in the statin group had heart malformations. Among the fibrate/nicotinic acid exposed malformed infants, one had a cardiac defect, one an unspecified musculoskeletal defect, and one tuberous sclerosis with an eye malformation (all three exposed to fenofibrate).

Little is known about fibrate use during pregnancy and such use is not recommended. Resines are not absorbed and are therefore regarded as harmless. An early study found an increased risk of congenital malformations after high doses of nicotinic acid [7] but this has never been confirmed.

Table 25.1. Number of women identified using serum lipid reducing drugs

Total	249
Reported use in early pregnancy	176
Got prescription later in pregnancy	118
Both early and later use	45

Type of drug	ATC code	Early use	Later use
HMG CoA reductase inhibitors (statins)	C10AA	76	13
Simvastatin	C10AA01	39	4
Pravastatin	C10AA03	10	1
Fluvastatin	C10AA04	4	0
Atorvastatin	C10AA05	23	8
Fibrates	C10AB	8	11
Clofibrate	C10AB01	1	0
Bezafibrate	C10AB02	1	0
Gemfibrozil	C10AB04	4	0
Fenofibrate	C10AB05	2	1
Bile acid sequestrans (resines)	C10AC	90	103
Colestyramine	C10AC01	68	93
Colestipol	C10AC02	23	21
Nicotinic acid derivates	C10AD	1	3
Niceritrol	C10AD01	0	1
Nicotinic acid	C10AD02	1	2
Unspecified	C10A	3	0

One woman used both an HMG CoA reductase inhibitor and a fibrate in early pregnancy and one in both early and late pregnancy used both a resine and nicotinic acid derivate.

Characteristics of Women Using Lipid Reducing Drugs

Based on women reporting the drug in early pregnancy (n=176). Each variable is adjusted for all other variables and year of delivery. Comparison with all women who gave birth during the period and with information from the first antenatal care (n=967 742). The odds ratios for maternal age, parity, smoking in early pregnancy, number of previous miscarriages, BMI, subfertility, and country of birth are adjusted for all other variables (Table 25.2).

Table 25.2. Characteristics of women using lipid reducing drugs in early pregnancy

Variable studied	Number	OR	95% CI
Maternal age			
<25 years	19	0.72	0.44-1.20
25-34 years	101	1.00	reference
≥35 years	56	2.07	1.45-2.97
Parity			
1	74	1.29	0.92-1.81
≥2	102	1.00	reference
Smoking			
Unknown	5	-	-
No	136	1.00	reference
Yes	35	2.48	1.42-4.33
Previous miscarriage			
No	138	1.00	reference
Yes	38	0.87	0.59-1.23
BMI			
Unknown	13	-	-
<19.8	11	1.12	0.59-2.11
19.8-25.9	80	1.00	reference
≥26	72	2.08	1.51-2.86
Unwanted childlessness			
No	158	1.00	reference
Yes	18	1.22	0.72-2.04

Some further maternal characteristics were analyzed, adjusting for year of delivery, maternal age, parity, smoking, and BMI but numbers were low. No significant deviations from expected values were seen for maternal education, family situation or work situation. Women born in non-Nordic countries were under-represented (n=8, OR = 0.26, 95% CI 0.14-0.51).

Table 25.3. Concomitant drug use (early pregnancy)

Drug group	Number	OR/RR	95% CI
Drugs for stomach ulcer and reflux	11	5.56	2.77-9.94#
Drugs for inflammatory bowel disease	12	23.5	12.2-41.1#
Insulin	11	18.3	9.15-32.6#
Multivitamins	12	1.35	0.70-2.36#
Folic acid	13	1.41	0.75-2.41#
Antihypertensives	15	14.9	8,31-24.5#
Thyroid drugs	6	1.99	0.73-4.78#
Antibiotics	5	0.93	0.30-2.16#
NSAIDs	3	0.78	0.16-2.39#
Minor analgesics	10	0.63	0.33-1.18#
Sedatives, hypnotics	5	3.91	1.27-9.12#
Antidepressants	10	2.82	1.35-5.20#
Drugs for rhinitis	5	3.91	1.27-9.12#
Antiasthmatics	10	1.77	0.95-3.25#
Antihistamines	9	0.94	0.43-1.79

#observed over expected number with exact Poisson 95% confidence interval.

There is a strong association with the use of insulin and antihypertensives but also with drugs for inflammatory bowel disease and stomach ulcer and reflux, psychoactive drugs, and drugs for rhinitis.

Table 25.4. Some maternal diagnoses associated with the use of lipid reducing drugs

Diagnosis	Drug use in early pregnancy			Drug use later in pregnancy		
	Number	OR/RR	95% CI	Number	OR/RR	95% CI
Pre-existing diabetes	21	6.98	4.32-10.7#	7	4.00	1.61-8.24#
Chronic hypertension	10	3.38	1.62-6.21#	8	4.30	1.86-8.47#
Gestational diabetes	1	0.47	0.01-2.63#	5	4.00	1.30-9.33#
Preeclampsia	20	2.04	1.25-3.15#	9	1.48	0.68-2.80#
Hyperemesis gravidarum	1	0.44	0.01-2.47#	6	4.29	1.57-9.33#
Placenta previa	1	0.37	0.01-2.06#	5	3.18	1.03-7.43#
Abruptio placentae	3	1.05	0.22-3.07#	6	3.26	1.20-2.10#
Antepartum bleeding	2	0.64	0.08-2.32#	6	3.33	1.22-7.26#
Intrapartum bleeding	3	0.58	0.12-1.70#	5	2.16	0.70-5.05#
Postpartum bleeding	10	0.95	0.50-1.81	12	1.77	0.91-3.09#
Delivery induction	28	1.45	0.96-2.19	28	2.33	1.54-3.52
Caesarean section	47	1.59	1.13-2.24	28	1.45	0.94-2.23

#observed over expected number with exact Poisson 95% confidence interval.

Due to low numbers, confidence intervals are large and few conditions reach statistical significance. There is a strong association with preexisting diabetes and – after later use – with gestational diabetes and also with chronic hypertension. After early use, the risk for preeclampsia is increased and later use is associated with a number of pregnancy complications. Both delivery induction and caesarean section occured in an increased frequency.

Outcome after Maternal Use of Lipid Reducing Drugs

Infant Sex

Among infants born after maternal use of lipid lowering drugs in early pregnancy, there were 97 males and 80 females, sex ratio = 1.21 (95% CI 0.90-1.64). After maternal use of such drugs later in pregnancy, there were 61 males and 59 females, sex ratio 1.03 (95% CI 0.72-1.49). The normal sex ratio of 1.06 is thus contained within both confidence intervals.

Multiple Births

After early use of lipid lowering drugs, there was one twin delivery, after later use two.

Infant Mortality

Only one death occurred: after late exposure for colestyramine. Death occurred on the 3rd day of life and was an unexpected sudden death.

Table 25.5. Pregnancy duration and infant birth weight at maternal use of lipid reducing drugs

Variable studied	Drug use in early pregnancy			Drug use later in pregnancy		
	Number	OR/RR	95% CI	Number	OR/RR	95% CI
<37 weeks	25	2.66	1.72-3.93#	14	2.40	1.31-4.02#
<2500g	9	1.48	0.68-2.81#	11	2.81	1.40-5.02#
≥4500g	6	0.80	0.29-1.74#	1	0.19	0.02-1.09#
SGA	3	0.73	0.15-2.14#	4	1.50	0.41-3.85#
LGA	12	1.06	0.58-1.92	7	0.93	0.38-1.92#

#observed over expected number with exact Poisson 95% confidence interval.

Both after early and later exposure to lipid reducing drugs, an increased risk for preterm birth was seen, after later exposure also an increased risk for low birth weight. Intrauterine growth did not seem to be affected.

Table 25.6. Neonatal diagnoses after maternal use of serum lipid reducing drugs

Diagnosis	Drug use in early pregnancy			Drug use later in pregnancy		
	Number	OR/RR	95% CI	Number	OR/RR	95% CI
Hypoglycaemia	23	3.22	2.04-4.83#	7	1.55	0.62-3.19#
Respiratory diagnoses	16	1.65	0.94-2.68#	3	0.51	0.11-1.49#
Low Apgar score	5	1.21	0.39-2.82#	0	0.00	0.00-1.65#
CNS diagnoses	2	1.41	0.17-5.09#	0	-	-
Jaundice	14	1.91	1.12-3.27	12	2.40	1.24-4.20#

#observed over expected number with exact Poisson 95% confidence interval.

Only hypoglycaemia and jaundice occurred in significantly increased frequencies.

Table 25.7. Congenital malformations in infants whose mothers had used lipid reducing drugs in early pregnancy

Congenital malformation	Number	RR	95% CI
All malformation	12	1.40	0.72-2.44
Relatively severe malformation	10	1.67	0.80-3.06
Chromosome anomalies	2	3.62	0.44-13.1
Without chromosome anomalies			
Any cardiovascular defect	5	2.73	0.89-6.38

There was thus no statistically significant excess of malformed infants. The infant malformation diagnoses and maternal drug usage was as follows:

Table 25.8. List of infants with congenital malformations after maternal use of serum lipid reducing drugs

Congenital malformation	Lipid reducing drug	Other drug
Relative severe malformations		
Ventricular septum defect	clofibrate	salmeterol, budesonide, cromoglicic acid
Ventricular and atrium septum defect	simvastatin	enalapril
Unspecified cardiac defect	simvastatin	
Unspecified cardiac defect	colestipol	folic acid, iron, mesalazine, loperamide
Unspecified cardiac defect	atorvastatin	insulin
Pes equinovarus	colestyramine	iron
Polydactyly	pravastatin	prolactine
Syndactyly	niceritrol	
Down syndrome	colestyramine	
Down syndrome	colestyramine	loperamide
Mild and variable conditions		
Undescended testicle	simvastatin	
Hip (sub)luxation, unstable hip	unspecified	folic acid

In this limited material no statistically significant sign of teratogenicity was seen

Summary

Only little information is available on the use during pregnancy of lipid lowering agents. There is a strong co-morbidity with diabetes, chronic hypertension, and inflammatory bowel disease, also demonstrated by concomitant drug use. Pregnancy complications occur in excess and this is true also for preterm birth. In this limited material, no certain effects on congenital malformation risk was seen and the observed heart defects were mild or uncertain.

References

[1] Manson JM, Freyssinges C, Ducrocq MB, Stephenson WP. Postmarketing surveillance of lovastatin and simvastatin exposure during pregnancy. *Reprod Toxicol* 1996; 10: 439-446.

[2] Edison RJ, Muenke M. Mechanistic and epidemiologic considerations in the evaluation of adverse birth outcomes following gestational exposure to statins. *Amer J Med Genet* 2004; 131A: 287-298.

[3] Petersen EE, Mitchell AA, Carey JC, Werler MW, Louik C, Rasmussen SA, and the National Birth Defects Prevention Study. Maternal exposure to statins and risk for birth defects: A case-series approach. *Amer J Med Genet* 2008: 146A: 2701-2705.

[4] Pollack PS, Shields KE, Burnett DM, Osborne MJ, Cunningham ML, Stepanavage ME. Pregnancy outcomes after maternal exposure to simvastatin and lovastatin. *Birth Def Res (Part A)* 2007; 73: 888-896.

[5] Taguchi N, Rubin ET, Hosokawa A, Choi J, Ying AY, Moretti ME, Koren G, Ito S. Prenatal exposure to HMG-CoA reductase inhibitors: Effects on foetal and neonatal outcomes. *Reprod Toxicol* 2008; 26: 175-177.
[6] Ofori B, Rey E, Bérard A. Risk of congenital anomalies in pregnant users of statin drugs. *Brit J Clin Pharmacol* 2007; 64: 496-509.
[7] Nelson MM, Forfar JO. Associations between drugs administered during pregnancy and congenital abnormalities of the foetus. *Br Med J* 1971;1:523-7.

Chapter 26

DERMATOLOGICAL DRUGS

Some systemically used drugs for skin disease, notably retinoids like isotretinoin, etretinate and acitretin, are strong teratogens and must be avoided during pregnancy. If early pregnancy exposure has occurred, a termination of the pregnancy should be discussed. Topical use of tretinoin or adapalene could carry a risk and should be avoided, but if exposure has occurred there is hardly reason to discuss a pregnancy termination. There seems to be no certain teratogenic or other harmful effect of the topical use of corticosteroids. Most topical dematological drugs can be used without risk during pregnancy.

Most dermatological drugs are used topically and only few of such drugs have been discussed from the point of view of teratogenicity.

Acne treatment: Some case reports of malformed infants after topical use of tretinoin exist [1-2], but two studies, both limited in size, found no evidence of teratogenicity [3-4]. One study, concentrating on minor malformations [5] found no effect of maternal topical use of tretinoin. Systemic treatment is possible with isotretinoin which is a well documented human teratogen [6] with a relatively high risk of severe congenital malformations, mainly as a result of an inhibition of cranial neural list development. In a Canadian population study, 90 women became pregnant during isotretinoin treatment, 76 of them terminated their pregnancy, and nine had a live birth with one infant malformed [7].

Psoriasis treatment: Two retinoids are used for systemic treatment of psoriasis: etretinate and acitretin. Etretinate is a classical human teratogen [8]. Acitretin is metabolized to etretinate and some case reports on typical etretinate malformations after acitretin exist [9-10]. A recent review on the safety of dermatological drugs used at psoriasis is available [11].

Topical treatment with corticosteroids: As some corticosteroids can be absorbed at topical treatment, notably of inflamed skin, the question has been raised if such treatment could share the effects of systemic corticosteroid treatment and notably the risk increase in orofacial clefts. One small case-control study found a high risk increase for orofacial clefts after maternal use of topical corticosteroids [12]. Other studies have not supported the finding [13,14].

Other treatments: Another topically used drug which has been suspected of teratogenicity is minoxidil where case reports of congenital malformations are available [15-16]. Minoxidil is absorbed through the skin.

Table 26.1. Number of women identified using dermatological drugs

Total	7925
Reported use in early pregnancy	4266
Got prescription later in pregnancy	4038
Both early and later use	379

Type of drug	ATC code	Early use	Later use
Antibiotic antifungals (topical)	D01AA	37	46
Antifungal imidazole derivates (topical)	D01AC	1307	2320
Other antifungals (topical)	D01AE	72	32
Antifungals (systemic)	D01BA	14	1
Emollients and protectives	D02	109	71
Antipruritics (topical)	D04	4	7
Antipsoriatics (topical)	D05A	115	32
Antipsoriatics (systemic)	D05B	2	0
Antibiotics (topical)	D06A	36	41
Chemotherapeutics (topical)	D06B	210	68
Corticosteroids (topical)	D07	2151	1192
Antiseptics, disinfectants (topical)	D08	13	10
Medicated dressings	D09	8	11
Antiacne preparations (topical)	D10A	347	312
Antiacne drug (systemic)	D10B	11	0
Antihidrotics	D11AA	1	0
Medicated shampoos	D11AC	7	2
Other dermatologics	D11AX	14	1
Unspecified	D	9	0

A majority of these drugs are used topically. Among them, corticosteroids will be discussed separately. Few of the drugs were used systemically in early pregnancy.

Table 26.2. Systemically used drugs for dermatological treatment

	ATC code	Early use	Later use
Systemic antifungals			
Griseofulvin	D01BA01	1	0
Terbinafine	D01BA02	13	1
Systemic antipsoriatics			
Etretinate	D01BB01	1	0
Acitretin	D01BB02	1	0
Systemic antiacne drugs			
Isotretinoin	D10BA01	11	0
Weak corticoids (Group I)	D07-A	588	285
Hydrocortisone	D07AA01	509	223
Hydrocortisone with antibiotics	D07CA01	78	61
Hydrocortisone with urea	D07XA01	4	1
Moderately potent corticoids (Group II)	D07A-B	524	370
Clobetasone	D07AB01	125	156
Hydrocortisone butyrate	D07AB02	297	177
Fluprednedine	D07AB07	12	2
Desonide	D07AB08	1	0
Triamcinolone	D07AB09	1	0
Triamcinolone with antiseptics	D07BB03	51	19
Triamcinolone with antibiotics	D07CB01	22	19

Table 26.2. Systemically used drugs for dermatological treatment

	ATC code	Early use	Later use
Triamcinolone with nystatin or antiseptic	D07XB02	1	0
Alcomethsone	D07AB10	10	2
Flumetasone with antibiotics	D07XB01	4	5
Fluprednidene with antibiotics	D07CB02	2	0
Flumetasone vith antiseptics	D07BB01	1	0
Potent corticoids (Group III)	D07-C	1098	563
Betamethasone	D07AC01	584	283
Betamethasone with antiseptics	D07BC01	6	1
Betamethasone with antibiotics	D07CC01	1	2
Betamethasone with salicylic acid	D07XC01	61	15
Desoximetasone	D07AC03	58	80
Fluocinolone	D07AC04	9	3
Mometasone	D07AC12	381	178
Fluticasone	D07AC17	35	21
Very potent corticoids (Group IV)	D07-D	203	87
Clobetasol	D07AD01	203	87
Unspecified	D07	30	4

Characteristics of Women using Dermatological Drugs

Based on women reporting corticosteroids topically in early pregnancy (n=2 151) or using dermatological drugs other than topical corticosteroids (n=2 114, one unknown maternal age). Each variable is adjusted for all other variables and year of delivery. Comparison with all women who gave birth during the period and with information from the first antenatal care (n=967 742). The odds ratios for maternal age, parity, smoking in early pregnancy, number of previous miscarriages, BMI, subfertility, and country of birth are adjusted for all other variables and are shown in Figure 26.1.

Some further maternal characteristics were analyzed, adjusting for year of delivery, maternal age, parity, smoking, and BMI (Table 26.3).

The maternal age distribution is unusual for both groups with a maximum at 25-34 years. The two groups of women have similar characteristics even though some differences exist (e.g., the risk for non-Nordic women).

The association between the use of corticosteroids topically and atopic conditions is obvious. The same association, although weaker, is seen for other dermatological drugs. For both groups there is an excess use of antibiotics and also of antihistamines used for NVP.

There is a lower than expected risk for preexisting diabetes and chronic hypertension. Most pregnancy complications occur with normal frequency, some even in a lower than expected frequency.

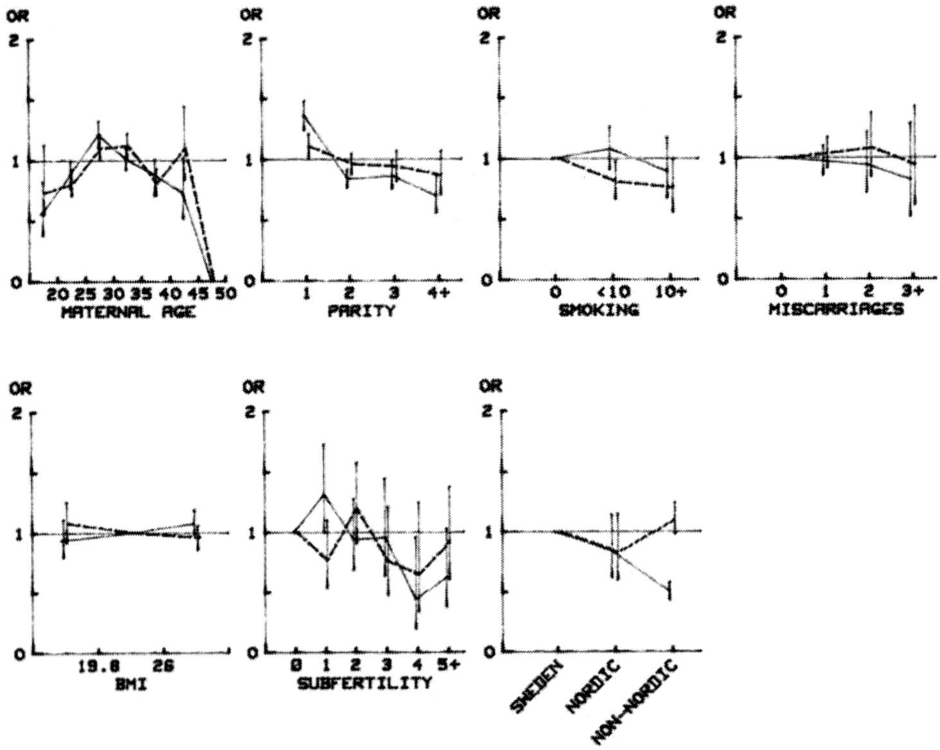

Figure 26.1. Odds ratios for seven maternal characteristics. Unbroken lines refer to topical corticosteroids, dashed graphs to other dermatological drugs. The odds ratios (OR) for each variable are adjusted for the other variables and year of delivery. Vertical lines mark 95% confidence intervals. For maternal age and parity, each class is compared with all other classes.

Table 26.3. Some further characteristics of women using dermatological drugs in early pregnancy

Variable studied	Topical corticosteroids			Other dermatological drugs		
	Number	OR	95% CI	Number	OR	95% CI
Education (1996-2001, 1015 women with topical corticoids, 967 with other dermatological drugs, 506238 in population)						
Unknown	17	-	-	29	-	-
<12 years	80	0.67	0.52-0.85	87	0.86	0.69-1.12
12 years	547	1.00	reference	462	1.00	reference
13 years	60	1.03	0.78-1.35	53	1.03	0.78-1.38
≥14 years	311	1.02	0.88-1.19	336	1.25	1.08-1.45
Family situation						
Unknown	42	-	-	30	-	-
Co-habiting	2026	1.00	reference	1955	1.00	reference
Living alone	40	0.80	0.57-1.10	52	1.17	0.88-1.56
Other family situation	43	0.79	0.57-1.10	69	1.34	1.03-1.75
Work outside home						
Unknown	267	-	-	269	-	-
Full time	1065	1.00	reference	981	1.00	reference
Part time	556	1.20	1.07-1.34	485	1.00	0.89-1.14
None	263	0.77	0.66-0.90	371	1.15	1.01-1.32

Table 26.4. Concomitant drug use (early pregnancy)

Drug group	Topical corticosteroids			Other dermatological drugs		
	Number	OR/RR	95% CI	Number	OR/RR	95% CI
Drugs for stomach ulcer and reflux	24	1.34	0.89-2.00	19	1.04	0.66-1.64
Drugs for inflammatory bowel disease	6	1.04	0.38-2.27#	6	1.08	0.40-2.36#
Insulin	1	0.14	0.01-0.77#	4	0.57	0.16-1.45
Multivitamins	125	1.03	0.85-1.25	174	1.26	1.07-1.48
Folic acid	99	0.97	0.78-1.19	112	0.95	0.79-1.16
Antihypertensives	8	1.04	0.45-2.06#	8	0.98	0.42-1.94#
Oral contraceptives	3	0.43	0.09-1.27#	7	1.17	0.47-2.42#
Progestogens	8	0.89	0.39-1.76#	8	0.93	0.40-1.84#
Gonadotropins	6	1.19	0.44-2.59#	1	0.22	0.01-1.21#
Systemic corticosteroids	72	8.64	6.67-10.9#	20	2.53	1.55-3.91#
Thyroid drugs	21	0.81	0.53-1.24	26	0.98	0.66-1.44
Antibiotics	141	2.28	1.93-2.69	276	4.79	4.26-5.38
NSAIDs	42	1.06	0.78-1.44	42	1.18	0.87-1.61
Opioids	10	0.96	0.51-1.79	21	2.02	1.32-3.09
Minor analgesics	169	1.02	0.87-1.19	264	1.85	1.63-2.10
Neuroleptics	7	1.02	0.41-2.11#	9	1.24	0.57-2.36#
Sedatives, hypnotics	8	1.10	0.47-2.16#	7	0.91	0.37-1.88#
Antidepressants	30	1.14	0.79-1.63	22	0.91	0.60-1.39
Drugs for rhinitis	102	3.49	2.81-4.21	61	2.10	1.63-2.70
Antiasthmatics	219	3.50	3.07-4.00	76	1.23	0.98-1.55
Cough medicines	20	1.87	1.20-2.90	21	2.06	1.31-3.14
Antihistamines	319	2.81	2.51-3.15	173	1.48	1.27-1.73
For NVP	126	1.24	1.04-1.48	133	1.36	1.14-1.62
For allergy	216	5.74	5.06-6.51	60	1.54	1.19-1.99

#observed over expected number with exact Poisson 95% confidence interval.

OUTCOME AFTER MATERNAL USE OF DERMATOLOGICAL DRUGS

Infant Sex

Among infants born after maternal use of topical corticosteroids there were 1 166 males and 1 019 females, sex ratio 1.14 (95% CI 1.05-1.24) and after later use there were 615 males and 593 females, sex ratio 1.04 (95% CI 0.93-1.16). Among infants born after maternal use of other dermatological drugs there were 1 090 males and 1 046 females, sex ratio 1.04 (95% CI 0.96-1.13) and after later use 1 454 males and 1 423 females (two with unknown sex), sex ratio 1.02 (95% CI 0.95-1.10). The normal sex ratio of 1.06 was thus contained in all confidence intervals.

Multiple Births

After early use of topical corticosteroids, there were 34 twin deliveries and one triplet delivery. The odds ratio for twinning was 1.09 (95% CI 0.97-1.53). After later use there were 16 twin deliveries, OR = 0.95 (95% CI 0.58-1.56).

Table 26.5. Some maternal diagnoses associated with the use of dermatological drugs

Diagnosis	Drug use in early pregnancy			Drug use later in pregnancy		
	Number	OR	95% CI	Number	OR	95% CI
Topical corticosteroids						
Pre-existing diabetes	13	0.46	0.27-0.79	10	0.62	0.33-1.15
Chronic hypertension	14	0.57	0.34-0.96	10	0.69	0.37-1.28
Gestational diabetes	12	0.62	0.35-1.10	6	0.56	0.25-1.24
Preeclampsia	102	0.98	0.80-1.20	70	1.23	0.97-1.53
Hyperemesis gravidarum	17	0.80	0.44-1.29	10	0.80	0.43-1.48
Placenta previa	18	0.77	0.48-1.22	8	0.59	0.29-1.16
Abruptio placentae	20	0.76	0.49-1.19	11	0.72	0.40-1.29
Antepartum bleeding	20	0.70	0.45-1.08	13	0.83	0.48-1.44
Intrapartum bleeding	38	0.83	0.60-1.15	26	0.96	0.65-1.41
Postpartum bleeding	119	0.97	0.81-1.17	70	1.07	0.84-1.36
Delivery induction	239	1.02	0.89-1.17	164	1.26	1.07-1.49
Caesarean section	360	1.04	0.93-1.17	204	1.03	0.89-1.20
Other dermatological drugs						
Pre-existing diabetes	13	0.48	0.28-0.82	35	0.91	0.65-1.27
Chronic hypertension	16	0.65	0.40-1.07	29	0.86	0.59-1.24
Gestational diabetes	10	0.54	0.29-1.00	25	0.96	0.65-1.43
Preeclampsia	92	0.96	0.78-1.19	126	0.97	0.81-1.16
Hyperemesis gravidarum	10	0.48	0.26-0.87	29	0.97	0.67-1.41
Placenta previa	12	0.52	0.30-0.90	34	1.04	0.74-1.46
Abruptio placentae	10	0.70	0.44-1.11	37	1.01	0.73-1.40
Antepartum bleeding	19	0.66	0.42-1.04	43	1.11	0.82-1.51
Intrapartum bleeding	33	0.73	0.52-1.03	52	0.85	0.64-1.12
Postpartum bleeding	103	0.87	0.72-1.07	165	1.09	0.93-1.28
Delivery induction	239	1.06	0.92-1.21	322	1.06	0.94-1.20
Caesarean section	318	0.93	0.82-1.05	420	0.97	0.87-1.07

After early use of other dermatological drugs, there were 30 twin deliveries (OR = 0.97, 95% CI 0.68-1.40) and after later use 32 twin deliveries (OR = 0.76, 95% CI 0.53-1.09).

Table 26.6. Infant mortality after maternal use of dermatological drugs

Variable studied	Drug use in early pregnancy			Drug use later in pregnancy		
	Number	RR	95% CI	Number	RR	95% CI
Topical corticosteroids						
Stillbirth	7	0.94	0.38-1.95	2	0.48	0.06-1.75
Early neonatal death	6	1.97	0.72-4.29	3	1.76	0.36-5.15
Other dermatological drugs						
Stillbirth	4	0.58	0.16-1.50	10	1.12	0.54-2.06
Early neonatal death	5	1.43	0.46-3.34	5	1.13	0.37-2.63

Even though some risk estimates are high, none reaches statistical significance.

Table 26.7. Pregnancy duration and infant birth weight at maternal use of dermatologic drugs

Variable studied	Drug use in early pregnancy			Drug use later in pregnancy		
	Number	OR	95% CI	Number	OR	95% CI
Topical corticosteroids						
<37 weeks	106	1.03	0.84-1.25	56	0.97	0.74-1.26
<2500g	55	0.83	0.63-1.08	32	0.87	0.61-1.24
≥4500g	80	0.94	0.75-1.18	39	0.82	0.60-1.13
SGA	45	0.94	0.70-1.27	31	1.21	0.84-1.75
LGA	122	1.04	0.86-1.26	63	0.94	0.72-1.22
Other dermatological drugs						
<37 weeks	97	0.96	0.78-1.18	128	0.95	0.79-1.13
<2500g	69	1.09	0.85-1.39	78	0.92	0.73-1.16
≥4500g	88	1.03	0.83-1.28	127	1.05	0.81-1.37
SGA	58	1.32	1.02-1.73	59	1.05	0.81-1.37
LGA	117	0.94	0.77-1.13	174	0.95	0.81-1.11

There is only one apparently deviating value: SGA after other dermatological drugs in early pregnancy.

Table 26.8. Neonatal diagnoses after maternal use of dermatological drugs

Diagnosis	Drug use in early pregnancy			Drug use later in pregnancy		
	Number	OR/RR	95% CI	Number	OR/RR	95% CI
Topical corticosteroids						
Hypoglycaemia	76	0.96	0.76-1.21	41	0.94	0.68-1.28
Respiratory diagnoses	107	0.98	0.80-1.19	45	0.78	0.38-1.05
Low Apgar score	31	0.74	0.52-1.05	21	0.95	0.61-1.47
CNS diagnoses	14	1.00	0.59-1.68	8	0.96	0.41-1.89#
Jaundice	86	0.95	0.76-1.18	44	0.85	0.63-1.15
Other dermatological drugs						
Hypoglycaemia	67	0.88	0.69-1.13	93	0.94	0.76-1.16
Respiratory diagnoses	113	1.10	0.91-1.33	108	0.80	0.66-0.97
Low Apgar score	41	1.04	0.76-1.42	50	1.00	0.76-1.33
CNS diagnoses	13	0.98	0.57-1.70	18	0.91	0.57-1.46
Jaundice	85	0.97	0.78-1.21	108	0.96	0.79-1.17

#observed over expected number with exact Poisson 95% confidence interval.

No deviations in the neonatal outcome were seen.

Topical Corticosteroids

There were four cases of orofacial cleft which agrees with the expected number. Among them two were stillborn. The mother of one had used betamethasone, the second mother had also used betamethasone but also mometasone and hydrocortisone with antibiotics and also cetirizine. Among the remaining two mothers, one had used hydrocortisone butyrate and the other had used fluticasone and paracetamol.

Table 26.9. Congenital malformations in infants whose mothers had used dermatological drugs in early pregnancy

Congenital malformation	Topical corticosteroids			Other dermatological drugs		
	Number	OR/RR	95% CI	Number	OR/RR	95% CI
All malformation	91	0.87	0.71-1.08	89	0.90	0.73-1.12
Relatively severe malformation	57	0.81	0.62-1.06	51	0.76	0.58-1.01
Chromosome anomalies	5	1.47	0.48-3.43#	3	0.70	0.14-2.05#
Without chromosome anomalies						
Ear malformations	3	0.60	0.05-2.24#	4	0.91	0.25-2.32#
Any cardiovascular defect	22	0.92	0.60-1.41	22	0.99	0.65-1.51
VSD and/or ASD	10	0.78	0.42-1.45	14	1.16	0.69-1.97
Orofacial clefts	4	1.00	0.37-2.69#	3	0.78	0.16-2.29#
Hypospadias	4	0.64	0.18-1.65#	3	0.51	0.15-1.50#
Pes equinovarus	4	1.31	0.37-2.64#	1	0.34	0.01-1.91#
Poly/syndactyly	5	1.13	0.37-2.64#	4	0.95	0.26-2.43#
Hip (sub)luxation, unstable hip	16	1.10	0.67-1.81	18	1.33	0.83-2.11

#observed over expected number with exact Poisson 95% confidence interval.

The odds ratio for any relatively severe congenital malformation for potent corticosteroids (n=1112) was 0.94 (95% CI 0.67-1.32) and for very potent corticosteroids (n=205) 0.97 (95% CI 0.43-2.19).

There was thus no signs of a teratogenic effect of topical use of corticosteroids but the number of clefts observed is so low that the upper confidence limit does not exclude a 2.7 times increased odds ratio.

Other Dermatological Drugs

Most of the other dermatological drugs are used topically and with few exceptions, no teratogenic effect can be expected. One such drug is minoxidil but only seven exposures were reported. No exposure for finasterid was registered and only seven exposures for tacrolimus. None of the 14 infants had a malformation diagnosis.

Another group of a certain interest is topical anti-acne drugs which are vitamin A derivates: tretinoin and adapalen. There were only 30 exposures for tretinoin with one infant with a congenital malformation, polydactyly. There was no exposure to adapalen. Among other drugs used for acne can be mentioned topical clindamycin. Among 217 exposed infants, nine were malformed (OR= 0.97, 95% CI 0.49-1.91). One of these infants had Potter sequence with bilateral kidney agenesis, anal atresia, and genital malformations.

Among systemically used drugs, 13 infants were exposed to the antimycotic drug terbenafine – none had a malformation diagnosis. Eleven mothers reported the use of isotretinoin – none of the infants was malformed.

Summary

Basically no ill effects were noted from maternal use of dermatologic drugs but the most well known or suspected teratogens were only represented by few exposures. The absence of a malformation among the eleven infants exposed to isotretinoin is astonishing due to the strong teratogenic effect of this drug. Swedish women who get prescriptions for this drug (which is only obtainable on a special licence) are strictly instructed to avoid pregnancy. It is likely that women who anyway got pregnant using isotretinoin to a large extent had induced abortions but some may have stopped the drug as soon as they realized they were pregnant and then continued their pregnancy. In this limited material, no signs of teratogenicity from topical use of tretinoin were seen.

REFERENCES

[1] Camera G, Pregliasco P. Ear malformation in baby born to mother using tretinoin cream. *Lanceet* 1992; 339: 687.

[2] Lipson AH, Collins F, Webster WS. Multiple congenital defects associated with maternal use of topical tretinoin. *Lancet* 1993; 341: 1352-1353.

[3] Jick SS, Terris BZ, Jick H. First trimester topical tretinoin and congenital disorders. *Lancet* 1993; 341: 1181-1182.

[4] Shapiro L Pastuszak A, Curto G, Koren G. Safety of first-trimester exposure to topical tretinoin: prospective cohort study. *Lancet* 1997;350: 1143-1144.

[5] Loureiro K, Kao KK, Jones KL, Alvarado S, Chavez C, Dick L, Felix R, Johnson D, Chambers CD. Minor malformations characteristic of the retinoic acid embryopathy and other birth outcomes in children of women exposed to topical tretinoin during early pregnancy. *Amer J Med Gener* 2005; 136A: 117-121.

[6] Lammer EJ, Chen DT, Hoar RM, Agnish ND, Benke PJ, Braun JT, Curry CJ, Fernhoff PM, Grix Jr AW, Lott IT, Richard JM, Sun SS. Retinoic acid embryopathy. *New Engl J Med* 1985; 313: 837-841.

[7] Bérard A, Azoulay L, Koren G, Perreault S, Oraichi D. Isotretinoin, pregnancies, abortions and birth defects: a population-based perspective. *Br J Clin Pharmacol* 2007; 63: 196-205.

[8] Geiger JM, Baudin M, Saurat JH. Teratogenic risk with etretinate and acitretin treatment. *Dermatology* 1994; 189: 109-116.

[9] de DieSmulders CEM, Surkenboom MCJM, Veraart J, van Karwijk C, Sastrowijoto P, van der Linden E. Severe limb defects and craniofacial anomalies in a fetus conceived during acitretin therapy. *Teratology* 1995; 52: 215-219.

[10] Barbero P, Lotersztein V, Bronberg R, Perez M, Alba L. Acitrein embryopathy: A case report. *Birth Def Res (Part A)* 2004; 70: 831-833.

[11] Lam J, Poliftka JE, Dohil MA. Safety of dermatologic drugs used in pregnant patients with psoriasis and other inflammatory skin diseases. *J Am Acad Dermatol* 2008; 59: 295-315.

[12] Edwards MJ, Agho KA, Attia J, Diaz P, Hayes T, Illingworth A, Roddick LG. Case-control study of cleft lip or palate after maternal use of topical corticosteroids during pregnancy. *Amer J Med Genet* 2003; 120A: 459-463.

[13] Carmichael SI, Shaw GM, Ma C, Werler MM, Rasmussen SA, Lammer EJ, for the National Birth Defects Prevention Study. Maternal corticosteroid use and orofacial clefts. *Amer J Obst Gynecol* 2007; 197: 585.e1-585.e7.

[14] Mygind H, Thulstrup AM, Pedersen L, Larsen H. Risk of intrauterine growth retardation, malformations and other birth outcomes in children after topical use of corticosteroids in pregnancy. *Acta Obst Gynecol Scand* 2002; 81: 234-239.

[15] Kaler SG, Patrinos ME, Lambert GH, Myers TF, Karlman R, Anderson CL. Hypertrichosis and congenital anomalies associated with maternal use of minoxidil. *Pediatrics* 1987; 79: 434-436.
[16] Smorlesi C, Caldarella A, Caramelli L, Di Lotto S, Moroni F. Topically applied minoxidil may casue fetal malformation: a case report. *Birth Def Res (Part A)* 2003; 67: 997-1001.

Chapter 27

GYNAECOLOGICAL DRUGS

Use of vaginal anti-infectives or antiseptics appears not to be associated with any ill effects on the pregnancy or neonatal outcome, including congenital malformations. Little is known about possible negative effects of the use of prostaglandins in early pregnancy – such use should be avoided but if exposure has occurred there is hardly any reason to discuss a termination of the pregnancy. The same is true for the use of methylergometrine.

Table 27.1. Number of women identified using

Total	1193
Reported use in early pregnancy	516
Got prescription later in pregnancy	702
Both early and later use	25

Type of drug	ATC code	Early use	Later use
Antiinfectives and antiseptics used vaginally	G01A	487	694
Clindamycin	G01AA10	31	32
Combination of sulfonamides	G01AE10	12	4
Metronidazole	G01AF01	121	133
Clotrimazole	G01AF02	204	291
Miconazole	G01AF04	1	5
Terconazol	G01AG02	2	2
Policresulen	G01AX03	13	20
Unspecified	G01	4	2
Ergot alkaloids	G02AB	16	3
Methylergometrine	G02AB01	16	3
Prostaglandins	G02AD	6	1
Dinoprost	G02AD01	1	0
Dinoprostone	G02AD02	2	1
Gemeprost	G02AD03	1	0
Unspecified	G02AD	2	0

This group of drugs is heterogeneous and one subgroup (prolactin inhibitors) will be discussed in Chapter 28. Among the remaining drugs, the majority are made up of anti-infective and antiseptics used vaginally. The possible risks involved with vaginal treatment of infections were raised in an early study [1] but a number of studies including at least two meta-analyses [2,3] found no association between prenatal use of metronidazole and birth defects. Case-control studies found a possible association between vaginal use of combined metronidazole and miconazole treatment with poly-syndactyly [4] and with hydrocephaly [5]. Studies on clotrimazole showed no association with congenital malformaions [6] but an indicated protective effect on preterm birth [7]. Systemic treatment with metronidazole seemed to carry no increased risk for congenital malformations [8-10].

The main part of this chapter will deal with anti-infectives and antiseptics used vaginally.

Table 27.2. Characteristics of women using antiinfectives or antiseptics vaginally

Variable studied	Number	OR	95% CI
Maternal age			
<25 years	69	1.02	0.78-1.33
25-34 years	326	1.00	reference
≥35 years	92	0.89	0.70-1.14
Parity			
1	212	0.97	0.80-1.18
≥2	275	1.00	reference
Smoking			
Unknown	18	-	-
No	429	1.00	refrence
Yes	40	1.16	0.67-1.99
Previous miscarriages			
No	369	1.00	reference
Yes	118	1.22	0.99-1.51
BMI			
Unknown	39	-	-
<19.8	35	0.95	0.62-1.35
19.8-25.9	290	1.00	reference
≥26	123	0.95	0.75-1.16
Unwanted childlessness			
No	455	1.00	reference
Yes	32	0.84	0.56-1.26
Country of birth			
Unkown	9	-	-
Sweden	367	1.00	reference
Other Nordic country	7	0.73	0.35-1.53
Non-Nordic country	104	1.38	1.11-1.72

Variable studied	Number	OR	95% CI
Maternal age			
<25 years	69	1.02	0.78-1.33
25-34 years	326	1.00	reference
≥35 years	92	0.89	0.70-1.14
Parity			
1	212	0.97	0.80-1.18
≥2	275	1.00	reference
Smoking			
Unknown	18	-	-

Characteristics of Women using Anti-infectives or Antiseptics Vaginally

Based on women reporting the drug in early pregnancy (n=487). Each variable is adjusted for all other variables and year of delivery. Comparison with all women who gave birth during the period and with information from the first antenatal care (n=967 742). The odds ratios for maternal age, parity, smoking in early pregnancy, number of previous miscarriages, BMI, sub fertility, and country of birth are adjusted for all other variables Table 27.2).

Some further maternal characteristics were analyzed, adjusting for year of delivery, maternal age, parity, smoking, and BMI (Table 27.3).

Table 27.3. Some further characteristics of women using anti-infectives or antiseptics vaginally

Variable studied	Number	OR	95% CI
Education (1996-2001, 42 women with drugs, 526 695 in population)			
Unknown	2	-	-
<12 years	7	2.24	0.86-5.85
12 years	17	1.00	reference
≥13 years	16	1.38	0.71-2.69
Family situation			
Unknown	14	-	
Co-habiting	443	1.00	reference
Living alone	13	1.09	0.54-2.22
Other family situation	17	1.12	0.66-1.90
Work outside home			
Unknown	52	-	
Full time	210	1.00	reference
Part time	110	0.95	0.72-1.25
None	115	1.27	0.96-1.68

The only indicated deviation from expected values refers to the variable being born ouside the Nordic countries.

There is a clear-cut association with systemic antibiotics and also with drugs for rhinitis and cough (perhaps indicating common cold problems) but not with antiasthmatics. There is also an excess use of antihistamines, mainly for NVP.

Table 27.4. Concomittant drug use (early pregnancy), anti-infectives or antiseptics vaginally

Drug group	Number	OR/RR	95% CI
Drugs for stomach ulcer and reflux	9	2.07	0.95-3.93#
Multivitamins	79	1.31	1.01-1-70
Folic acid	51	1.13	0.85-1.51
Thyroid drugs	6	0.84	0.31-1.83#
Antibiotics	87	7.65	6.27-9.34
NSAIDs	9	1.34	0.61-2.54#
Opioids	4	1.19	0.32-3.05#
Minor analgesics	48	1.91	1.41-2.57

Table 27.4. Continued

Drug group	Number	OR/RR	95% CI
Neuroleptics	7	3.74	1.51-7.71#
Antidepressants	5	0.76	0.25-§.78#
Drugs for rhinitis	15	2.35	1.32-3.88#
Antiasthmatics	13	0.99	0.57-1.72
Cough medicines	7	3.63	1.46-7.47#
Antihistamines	38	1.57	1.13-2.18
For NVP	31	1.49	1.04-2.14
For allergy	10	1.20	0.58-2.21#

There were thus no statistically significant deviations in maternal diagnoses studied, neither before nor during pregnancy.

Table 27.5. Some maternal diagnoses after the use of anti-infectives or antiseptics vaginally

Diagnosis	Drug use in early pregnancy			Drug use later in pregnancy		
	Number	OR/RR	95% CI	Number	OR/RR	95% CI
Pre-existing diabetes	8	1.23	0.53-2.42#	11	1.10	0.55-1.97
Chronic hypertension	8	1.39	0.60-2.73#	12	1.36	0.70-2.38#
Gestational diabetes	8	1.88	0.81-3.70#	10	1.47	0.71-2.71#
Preeclampsia	23	1.07	0.70-1.64	35	1.13	0.80-1.60
Hyperemesis gravidarum	10	2.04	0.98-3.75#	13	1.67	0.89-2.86
Placenta previa	10	1.80	0.86-3.30#	11	1.27	0.63-2.27#
Abruptio placentae	9	1.50	0.69-2.85#	12	1.30	0.67-2.27#
Antepartum bleeding	9	1.40	0.64-2.65#	13	1.35	0.72-2.32#
Intrapartum bleeding	15	1.36	0.80-2.31	19	1.18	0.74-1.86
Postpartum bleeding	35	1.28	0.90-1.81	48	1.27	0.94-1.70
Delivery induction	63	1.14	0.87-1.50	87	1.15	0.92-1.45
Caesarean section	79	0.97	0.75-1.24	122	1.09	0.89-1.33

#observed over expected number with exact Poisson 95% confidence interval.

Outcome after Maternal use of Anti-infectives or Antiseptics Vaginally

Infant Sex

After use of these drugs in early pregnancy, 242 male and 250 female infants were born, a sex ratio of 0.97 (95% CI 0.81-1.16) and after later exposure there were 348 male and 358 female infants, sex ratio 0.97 (95% CI 0.84-1.13). Both sex ratios are thus lower than the normal sex ratio of 1.06 but statistical significance is not reached.

Multiple Births

After early exposure to these drugs, there were five twin deliveries (RR = 0.77, 95% CI 0.25-1.80) and after later exposure 12 twin deliveries (OR = 1.27, 95% CI 0.72-2.26). Twinning rates thus appeared normal.

Table 27.6. Infant mortality after maternal use of antiinfectives or antiseptics vaginally

Variable studied	Drug use in early pregnancy			Drug use later in pregnancy		
	Number	RR	95% CI	Number	RR	95% CI
Stillbirth	2	1.40	0.17-5.02	3	1.62	0.33-4.75
Early neonatal death	1	-	-	1	-	-

No significantly increased mortality is seen but confidence intervals are wide.

Table 27.7. Pregnancy duration and infant birth weight at maternal use of anti-infectives or antiseptics vaginally

Variable studied	Drug use in early pregnancy			Drug use later in pregnancy		
	Number	OR	95% CI	Number	OR	95% CI
<37 weeks	23	0.99	0.65-1.51	40	1.26	0.91-1.75
<2500g	14	0.94	0.54-1.62	28	1.42	0.97-2.08
≥4500g	22	1.16	0.75-1.79	29	1.04	0.71-1.52
SGA	9	0.91	0.41-1.72	16	1.19	0.72-1.97
LGA	38	1.35	0.96-1.89	39	0.90	0.65-1.26

No significant deviations are thus seen in these variables.

When clomitrazole was studied specifically, there were eight preterm births among 199, RR = 0.87, 95% CI 0.37-1.71.

Table 27.8. Neonatal diagnoses after maternal use of anti-infectives or antiseptics vaginally

Diagnosis	Drug use in early pregnancy			Drug use later in pregnancy		
	Number	OR/RR	95% CI	Number	OR/RR	95% CI
Hypoglycaemia	11	0.63	0.35-1.14	26	1.11	0.74-1.64
Respiratory diagnoses	24	1.07	0.71-1.62	20	0.63	0.40-0.98
Low Apgar score	13	1.46	0.85-2.54	8	0.66	0.33-1.32#
CNS diagnoses	3	0.84	0.17-2.45#	3	0.62	0.13-1.82#
Jaundice	24	1.18	0.78-1.79	26	0.90	0.60-1.33

#observed over expected number with exact Poisson 95% confidence interval.

No neonatal diagnoses thus occurred statistically more often than expected.

Table 27.9. Congenital malformations in infants whose mothers had used anti-infectives or antiseptics vaginally

Congenital malformation	Number	OR	95% CI
All malformation	20	0.94	0.60-1.48
Relatively severe malformation	15	1.06	0.63-1.78
Chromosome anomalies	1	1.19	0.03-6.63#
Without chromosome anomalies			
Any cardiovascular defect	6	1.17	0.63-1.78#
Hypospadias	2	1.36	0.18-5.31#

#observed over expected number with exact Poisson 95% confidence interval.

There was one infant with poly- or syndactyly (and also a ventricular septum defect) and none with hydrocephaly.

Among 16 infants exposed to methylergometrine, two were malformed: one had Down syndrome (which can hardly be due to drugs taken during pregnancy); the other had a ventricular septum defect. Among 13 infants exposed to prostaglandins, one had a diagnosis of unstable hip.

No certain signs of teratogenic effects were thus seen.

Summary

There were no signs of ill effects after vaginal treatments with anti-infectives or antiseptics. Even though the size of the material is limited, there was little support for the idea that use of clotrimazole would reduce the risk for preterm birth, nor for an association between metronidazole use and poly- or syndactyly or hydrocephaly.

References

[1] Rosa FW, Baum C, Shaw M. Pregnancy outcomes after first-trimester vaginities drug therapy. *Obster Gynecol* 1987; 69: 751-755.

[2] Burtin P, Taddio A, Ariburnu O, Einarson TR, Koren G. Safety of metronidazole in pregnancy: a meta-analysis. *Am J Obst Gynecol* 1995; 172: 525-529.

[3] Caro-Patón T, Carvajal A, de Diego IM, Martín-Arias LH, Requejo AA, Rodriguez Pinilla E. Is metronidazole teratogenic? A meta-analysis. *Br J Clin Pharmacol* 1997; 44: 179-182.

[4] Kazy Z, Puhó E, Czeizel AE. The possible association between the combination of vaginal metronidazole and miconazole treatment and poly-syndactyly. Poplation-based case-control teratologic study. *Reprod Toxicol* 2005; 20: 89-94.

[5] Kazy Z, Puhó E, Czeizel AE. Teratogenic potential of vaginal metronidazole treatment during pregnancy. *Europ J Obst Gynecol* 2005; 123: 174-178.

[6] Czeizel AE, Tóth M, Rockenbauer M. No teratogenic effect after clotrimazole therapy during pregnancy. *Epidemiology* 1999; 10: 437-440.

[7] Czeizel AE, Fladung B, Vargha P. Preterm birth reduction after clotrimazole treatment duriing pregnancy. *Eur J Obst Gynecol* 2004; 116: 157-163.

[8] Czeizel AE, Rockenbauer M. A population-based case-control teratologic study of oral metronidazole treatment during pregnancy. *Br J Obstet Gynecol* 1998; 105: 322-327.

[9] Sørensen HT, Larsen H, Jensen ES, Thulstrup AM, Schønheyder HC, Nielsen GL, Czeizel A and the EUROMAP Study Group. Safety of metronidazole during pregnancy: a cohort study of risk of congenital abnormalities, preterm delivery and low birth weight in 124 women. *J Antimicrobial Chemother* 1999; 44: 854-855.

[10] Diav-Citrin O, Schechtman S, Gotteiner T, Arnon J, Ornoy A. Pregnancy outcome after gestational exposure to metronidazole: a prospective cohort study. *Teratology* 2001; 63: 186-192.

Chapter 28

PROLACTINE INHIBITORS AND DOPAMINE AGONISTS

Infertility treatment with prolactine inhibitors appears to carry no increased risk of pregnancy or neonatal complications and no increased risk of congenital malformations has been observed, at least not for bromocriptine or cabergoline treatments. Less data are available for quinagolide but no evidence for an increased malformation risk exists. Little is known of the use of dopamine agonists for parkinsonism in pregnant women but it is unlikely that the drugs should have a negative effect on the embryo in this situation.

This group of drugs has as main indications hyperprolactinaemia, infertility, and parkinsonism. In Sweden, bromocriptine and cabergoline are used for both infertility and parkinsonism, quinagolide only for infertility, and pramipexole and apomorfin only for parkinsonism. Infertility treatment with prolactine inhibitors obviously takes place before pregnancy but often continues until pregnancy has been verified when it should be stopped.

Bromocriptine therapy of infertility is regarded as safe [1,2]. One study of cabergoline treatment in early pregnancy [3] identified 148 liveborn infants, two of which were malformed (one with megaureter, one with scapocephaly) to which can be added three induced abortions because of identified malformations: one Down syndrome, one limb-body wall complex, and one hydrocephaly. Another study [4] of 49 live births found one malformed infant (trisomy 18) to which can be added one induced abortion due to a congenital malformation (nature not known).

Table 28.1. Number of women identified usingprolactine inhibitors or dopamine agonists

Total	877
Reported use in early pregnancy	765
Got prescription later in pregnancy	119
Both early and later use	35

Type of drug	ATC code	Early use	Later use
Bromocriptine	G02CB01/N04BC01	560	85
Cabergoline	G02CB03/N04BC06	60	13
Quinagolide	G02CB04	143	19
Pramipexole	N04BC05	3	3
Apomorphine	N04BC07	1	0

Characteristics of Women using Prolactine Inhibitors or Dopamine Agonists

Based on women reporting the drug in early pregnancy (n=765). Each variable is adjusted for all other variables and year of delivery. Comparison with all women who gav birth during the period and with information from the first antenatal care (n=967 742). The odds ratios for maternal age, parity, smoking in early pregnancy, number of previous miscarriages, BMI, subfertility, and country of birth are adjusted for all other variables (Table 28.2).

Table 28.2. Characteristics of women using prolactine inhibitors or dopamine agonists

Variable studied	Number	OR	95% CI
Maternal age			
<25 years	43	0.31	0.23-0.41
25-34 years	536	1.00	reference
≥35 years	186	1.67	1.41-1.99
Parity			
1	437	2.26	1.95-2.61
2+	328	1.00	reference
Smoking			
Unknown	11	-	-
No	717	1.00	reference
Yes	35	0.37	0.20-0.70
Previous miscarriages			
No	589	1.00	reference
Yes	176	1.20	1.01-1.42
BMI			
Unknown	67	-	-
<19.8	54	0.94	0.71-1.25
19.8-25.9	456	1.00	reference
≥26	186	1.06	0.89-1.27
Unwanted childlessness			
N0	517	1.00	reference
Yes	248	4.44	3.80-5.19

Some further maternal characteristics were analyzed, adjusting for year of delivery, maternal age, parity, smoking, and BMI (Table 28.3).

Table 28.3. Some further characteristics of women using prolactine inhibitors or dopamine agonists in early pregnancy

Variable studied	Number	OR	95% CI
Education (1996-2001, 274 women with drugs, 526 695 in population)			
Unknown	1	-	-
<12 years	12	0.57	0.31-1.07
12 years	123	1.00	reference
≥13 years	138	1.26	0.98-1.63
Family situation			
Unknown	7	-	
Co-habiting	735	1.00	reference
Living alone	11	0.64	0.33-1.23
Other family situation	12	0.93	0.51-1.70
Work outside home			
Unknown	79	-	
Full time	444	1.00	reference
Part time	160	0.98	0.79-1.21
None	82	0.82	0.62-1.06

The relatively small number of women in this group makes confidence intervals wide.

High age, first parity, previous miscarriages and subfertility are definite risk factors as can be expected. These women smoke less than expected.

Table 28.4.Concomittant drug use (early pregnancy)

Drug group	Number	OR/RR	95% CI
Drugs for stomach ulcer and reflux	4	0.62	0.39-3.79#
Insulin	4	1.55	0.42-3.97#
Multivitamins	28	0.86	0.59-1.27
Folic acid	31	0.98	0.68-1.40
Oral contraceptives	5	2.59	0.84-6.05#
Progestogens	10	2.00	0.96-3.68#
Gonadotrophines	21	8.86	5.49-13.5#
Systemic corticosteroids	4	1.31	0.30-3.36#
Thyroid drugs	34	3.37	2.43-4.68
Antibiotics	22	0.99	0.65-1.52
NSAIDs	15	1.00	0.60-1.66
Opioids	4	1.31	0.36-3.36#
Minor analgesics	39	0.60	0.44-0.83
Sedatives, hypnotics	5	1.56	0.51-3.65#
Antidepressants	13	1.35	0.72-2.31#
Drugs for rhinitis	6	0.50	0.23-1.10#
Antiasthmatics	10	0.42	0.23-0.77
Cough medicines	4	1.01	0.28-2.59#
Antihistamines	30	0.67	0.47-0.97

#observed over expected number with exact Poisson 95% confidence interval.

As expected there is a clear-cut association with gonadotropins. The second drug group which is clearly associated is thyroid drugs.

After later exposures, most diagnoses were not represented by any case. There were seven instances of preeclampsia (RR = 1.11, 95% CI 0.45-2.30) and four of postpartum bleeding (RR = 0.70, 95% CI 0.23-1.63). Delivery induction occurred in 10 cases (OR = 0.69, 95% CI 0.36-1.32) and caesarean section in 29 cases (OR = 1.32, 95% CI 0.85-1.99).

Table 28.5. Some maternal diagnoses associated with the use of prolactine inhibitors or dopamine agonists. This Table is restricted to early pregnancy use

Diagnosis	Number	OR/RR	95% CI
Pre-existing diabetes	11	1.03	0.56-1.89
Chronic hypertension	8	0.81	0.35-1.60#
Gestational diabetes	5	0.67	0.22-1.56#
Preeclampsia	45	1.11	0.82-1.51
Hyperemesis gravidarum	7	0.88	0.35-1.80#
Placenta previa	7	0.73	0.29-1.51#
Abruptio placentae	8	0.78	0.38-1.60
Antepartum bleeding	10	0.89	0.47-1.68
Intrapartum bleeding	21	1.17	0.75-1.82
Postpartum bleeding	49	1.05	0.78-1.40
Delivery induction	111	1.33	1.08-1.63
Caesarean section	148	1.07	0.89-1.28

#observed over expected number with exact Poisson 95% confidence interval.

There were thus no certain effect on pregnancy morbidity.

Outcome after Maternal use of Prolactine Inhibitors or Dopamine Agonists

Infant Sex

After early eposure, the sex ratio was exactly normal: 1.06 (95% CI 0.92-1.22) based on 407 male and 384 female infants. After later exposure there were 58 male and 63 female infants born, sex ratio = 0.92, 95% CI 0.64-1.32).

Multiple Births

There was an excess of twin deliveries (n=22) after early exposure: OR = 1.67 (95% CI 1.09-2.57). There were two triplet deliveries. After later exposure there were only two twin deliveries: RR = 1.04 (95% CI 0.13-3.74). The excess in twinning is explained by the association with treatments for subfertility.

Infant Mortality

There were three stillbirths after early exposure (RR = 1.09, 95% CI 0.21-3.02) and one after later exposure. One infant died before the age of 7 days after early exposure.

After later exposure, there were 11 preterm births, RR = 1.74 (95% CI 0.87-3.10).

The only neonatal diagnosis with a risk estimate which approached statistical significance was CNS diagnoses but this risk increase may well be random.

Table 28.6. Pregnancy duration and infant birth weight at maternal use of prolactine inhibitors or dopamine agonists.This Table is restricted to early pregnancy use

Variable studied	Number	OR/RR	95% CI
<37 weeks	43	1.14	0.84-1.55
<2500g	31	1.24	0.86-1.79
≥4500g	25	0.85	0.57-1.27
SGA	16	0.89	0.54-1.46
LGA	37	0.94	0.67-1.32

Table 28.7. Neonatal diagnoses after maternal use of prolactine inhibitors or dopamine agonists

Diagnosis	Drug use in early pregnancy			Drug use later in pregnancy		
	Number	OR/RR	95% CI	Number	OR/RR	95% CI
Hypoglycaemia	39	1.29	0.94-1.78	8	1.50	0.65-2.96#
Respiratory diagnoses	40	0.96	0.65-1.24	6	0.97	0.36-2.11#
Low Apgar score	18	1.06	0.66-1.70	3	1.20	0.25-3.59#
CNS diagnoses	8	1.41	0.61-2.79	4	3.60	0.98-9.23#
Jaundice	38	1.11	0.80-1.55	9	1.58	0.79-3.16#

Table 28.8. Congenital malformations in infants whose mothers had used prolactine inhibitors or dopamine agonists in early pregnancy

Congenital malformation	Number	OR	95% CI
All malformation	37	0.93	0.67-1.30
Relatively severe malformation	22	0.83	0.54-1.27
Chromosome anomalies	0	0.00	0.00-2.04#
Without chromosome anomalies			
Any cardiovascular defect	10	1.14	0.55-2.10#
VSD and/or ASD	7	1.56	0.63-3.21#
Hypospadias	3	1.22	0.25-3.58#

Among other relatively severe malformations can be mentioned the following ones: ectopic anus, urethra atresia/stenosis, craniostenosis, phocomelic limb reduction, neurofibromatosis.

There were thus no signs of an increased risk of congenital malformations after early exposure or treatment before conception, the majority of which were for infertility.. Sixty of these treatments consisted of *cabergoline*, three infants were malformed (RR = 1.10, 95% CI 0.23-3.31): one had craniostenosis, one hypospadias, and one unstable hip. *Quinagolide* had been used by mothers of 147 infants. Six of these had a congenital malformation diagnosis (RR = 0.93, 95% CI 0.34-2.02). Among them there was only one relatively severe: a ventricular septum defect.

There was a later exposure for prolactine inhibitors or dopamine agonists in 121 infants. Most likely these were exposed because of maternal parkinsonism and probably the majority had been exposed also early in pregnancy (even if only recorded in 35 instances). There were seven infants with congenital malformations (RR 1.32, 95% CI 0.53-2.72). Three of them were mild and variable conditions, one had hypospadias and the remaining three all had a ventricular septum defect (RR = 3.49, 95% CI 0.72-10.2). This may thus be random.

Summary

There are no signs of ill effect of the use of prolactine inhibitors for infertility - most of if of course before conception. It cannot be evaluated how many women continued into pregnancy with these drugs. Only few exposures occurred as therapy for parkinsonism and it is difficult to separate those from the infertility treatments.

References

[1] Weil C. The safety of bromocriptine in hyperprolactinaemic female infertility: a literature review. *Curr Med Res Opin* 1986; 10: 172-195.

[2] Krupp P, Monka C. Bromocriptine in pregnancy; safety aspects. *Klin Wochenschr* 1987; 65: 823-827.

[3] Robert E, Musatti L, Piscitelli G, Ferrari CI. Pregnancy outcome after treatment with the ergot derivative, cabergoline. *Reprod Toxicol* 1996; 10: 333-337.

[4] Ricci E, Parazzini F, Motta T, Ferrari CI, Colao A, Clavenna A, Rocchi F, Gangi E, Paracchi S, Landi ML, Beck-Peccoz P, Bonati M. Pregnancy outcome after cabergoline treatment in early weeks of gestation. *Reprod Toxicol* 2002; 16: 791-793.

Chapter 29

ORAL CONTRACEPTIVES

Oral contraceptives should obviously not be used during pregnancy but some exposed pregnancies will occur after contraceptive failure. The pregnancy outcome seems to be normal after such exposure and no increased risk of congenital malformations is seen. There is no reason to discuss a termination of pregnancy because of an exposure to oral contraceptives.

Table 29.1. Number of women identified using oral contraceptives

Reported use in early pregnancy	3028

Type of drug	ATC code	Number
Progestogen + estrogen, fixed preparation	G03AA	961
Lynesterol + ethinylestradiol	G03AA03	40
Norethisterone + ethinylestradiol	G03AA05	11
Levonorgestrel + ethinylestradiol	G03AA07	380
Desogestrel + ethinylestradiol	G03AA09	492
Drospirenon + ethinylestradiol	G03AA12	14
Unspecified	G03AA00	25
Progestogen+estradiol, sequential preparation	G03AB	944
Levonorgestrel + ethinylestradiol	G03AB03	660
Norethisterone + ethinylestradiol	G03AB04	284
Progestogens	G03AC	1113
Norethisterone	G03AC01	200
Lynestrenol	G03AC02	322
Levonorgestrel	G03AC03	498
Medoxyprogesterone	G03AC06	4
Etonogestrel	G03AC08	1
Desogestrel	G03AC09	86
Unspecified	G03AC	7
Unspecified oral contraceptive	G03A	21

Inadvertent use of oral contraceptives in early pregnancy may occur, for instance after diarrhoea, but some drugs like anticonvulsants and certain antibiotics also interact with oral contraceptives. The question of foetal exposure for oral contraceptive could be harmful has been discussed in some studies, most of them relatively early. In some of them [1-3], a slight increase in malformation risk was seen, in one of the studies only among smoking mothers [2]. A special interest was shown malformations in the urinary tract [4] and hypospadias because of the possibility that hormones as components of the oral contraceptives could affect masculinisation of the genital organs but this could not be supported in one international study [5]. An increased risk of Down syndrome was suggested in pregnancies occurring after stopping oral contraceptives [6] but further studies could not confirm the result [7-8]. A recent small TIS study [9] found no ill effects of oral contraceptives exposure in the periconceptional period but the power of the study was very low.

Obviously, oral contraceptive exposures are only relevant in early pregnancy.

Characteristics of Women using Oral Contraceptives in Early Pregnancy

Based on women reporting the drug in early pregnancy (n=7913, one missing maternal age). Each variable is adjusted for all other variables and year of delivery. Comparison with all women who gave birth during the period and with information from the first antenatal care (n=967 742). The odds ratios for maternal age, parity, smoking in early pregnancy, number of previous miscarriages, BMI, subfertility, and country of birth are adjusted for all other variables and are shown in Figure 29.1.

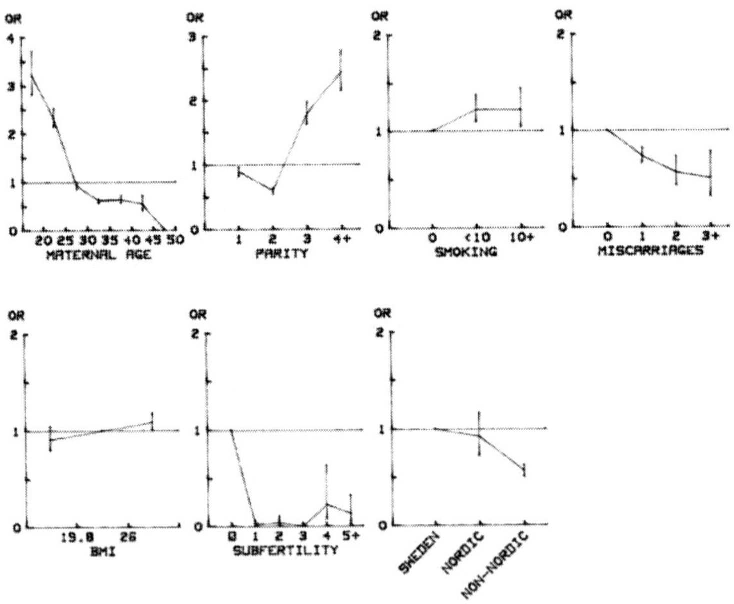

Figure 29.1. Odds ratios for seven maternal characteristics. The odds ratios (OR) for each variable are adjusted for the other variables and year of delivery. Vertical lines mark 95% confidence intervals. For maternal age and parity, each class is compared with all other classes.

Some further maternal characteristics were analyzed, adjusting for year of delivery, maternal age, parity, smoking, and BMI (Table 29.2).

Table 29.2. Some further characteristics of women using oral contraceptives in early pregnancy

Variable studied	Number	OR	95% CI
Education (1996-2001, 1693 women with drugs, 526 695 in population)			
Unknown	26	-	-
<12 years	295	0.88	0.77-1.02
12 years	980	1.00	reference
13-14 years	67	0.82	0.64-1.06
>14 years	271	0.72	0.62-0.83
Family situation			
Unknown	78	-	
Co-habiting	2466	1.00	reference
Living alone	241	2.64	2.31-3.02
Other family situation	243	2.28	1.97-2.64
Work outside home			
Unknown		-	
Full time		1.00	reference
Part time		1.04	0.94-1.15
None		1.01	0.01-1.13

There is thus a marked excess of low maternal age and high parity and a moderate excess of smokers and women with a high BMI. These women have a lower rate of previous miscarriages and practically no signs of subfertility. Women born outside the Nordic country are underrepresented.

Table 29.3.Concomittant drug use (early pregnancy)

Drug group	Number	OR/RR	95% CI
Drugs for stomach ulcer and reflux	49	2.01	1.52-2.66
Drugs for inflammatory bowel disease	5	0.78	0.25-1.81#
Insulin	7	0.73	0.29-1.50
Multivitamins	63	0.77	0.60-0.99
Folic acid	84	0.70	0.55-0.90
Systemic corticosteroids	7	0.67	0.32-1.40
Thyroid drugs	20	0.63	0.40-0.97
Antibiotics	152	1.37	1.15-1.63
NSAIDs	123	2.03	1.69-2.42
Opioids	49	3.17	2.41-4.15
Minor analgesics	342	1.61	0.93-2.79
Anticonvulsants	13	1.59	0.85-2.72#
Neuroleptics	9	0.86	0.45-1.65
Sedatives, hypnotics	4	0.46	0.12-1.17#
Antidepressants	65	1.71	1.34-2.18
Drugs for rhinitis	43	1.19	0.88-1.60
Antiasthmatics	103	0.97	0.80-1.19
Cough medicines	17	1.19	0.74-1.91
Antihistamines	170	0.92	0.78-1.07

#observed over expected number with exact Poisson 95% confidence interval.

As expected there is an excess use of antibiotics and anticonvulsants but also with drugs for stomach ulcer and gastro-oesophageal reflux, NSAID drugs, and antidepressants.

Table 29.4. Some maternal diagnoses associated with the use of oral contraceptives in early pregnancy

Diagnosis	Number	OR/RR	95% CI
Pre-existing diabetes	27	0.71	0.48-1.03
Chronic hypertension	31	0.95	0.67-1.37
Gestational diabetes	18	0.67	0.42-1.07
Preeclampsia	149	1.10	0.93-1.30
Hyperemesis gravidarum	20	0.68	0.44-1.05
Placenta previa	23	0.69	0.46-1.06
Abruptio placentae	27	0.74	0.50-1.08
Antepartum bleeding	29	0.73	0.51-1.06
Intrapartum bleeding	47	0.84	0.63-1.12
Postpartum bleeding	179	1.11	0.95-1.29
Delivery induction	347	1.08	0.96-1.21
Caesarean section	440	1.02	0.92-1.13

#observed over expected number with exact Poisson 95% confidence interval.

No certain deviations from expected values were thus seen.

Outcome after Maternal use of Oral Contraceptives in Early Pregnancy

Infant Sex

After maternal use of oral contraceptives in early pregnancy, there were 1 602 male and 1 455 female infants born (two with unknown sex). Sex ratio was 1.10 (95% CI 1.03-1.18), thus not significantly different from the normal sex ratio of 1.06.

Multiple Births

There were 32 twin deliveries after maternal use of oral contraceptives in early pregnancy, OR 0.79 (95% CI 0.56-1.13).

Table 29.5. Infant mortality after maternal use of oral contraceptives in early pregnancy

Variable studied	Number	RR	5% CI
Stillbirth	12	1.16	0.66-2.06
Early neonatal death	4	0.88	0.24-2.24

No increase in perinatal death risk was thus seen.

Table 29.6. Pregnancy duration and infant birth weight at maternal use of oral contraceptives in early pregnancy

Variable studied	Number	OR/RR	95% CI
<37 weeks	167	1.09	0.93-1.28
<2500g	122	1.25	1.04-1.50
≥4500g	119	0.97	0.81-1.17
SGA	78	1.13	0.90-1.42
LGA	164	0.93	0.79-1.09

There is thus an excess of low birth infants but not of preterm births or SGA.

Table 29.7. Neonatal diagnoses after maternal use of oral contraceptives in early pregnancy

Diagnosis	Number	OR/RR	95% CI
Hypoglycaemia	97	0.90	0.73-1.10
Respiratory diagnoses	171	1.16	0.99-1.35
Low Apgar score	59	1.00	0.77-1.30
CNS diagnoses	24	1.38	0.92-2.06
Jaundice	106	0.85	0.70-1.04

No certain excess of infants with any of these diagnoses was seen.

Table 29.8. Congenital malformations in infants whose mothers had used oral contraceptives in early pregnancy

Congenital malformation	Number	OR	95% CI
All malformation	150	1.05	0.89-1.25
Relatively severe malformation	107	1.09	0.90-1.33
Chromosome anomalies	4	0.75	0.21-1.93#
Without chromosome anomalies			
Any CNS defect	3	0.80	0.16-2.33#
Ear malformations	12	1.61	0.83-2.81#
Any cardiovascular defect	35	1.11	0.79-1.55
VSD and/or ASD	16	0.97	0.59-1.60
Orofacial clefts	7	1.24	0.50-2.55#
Hypospadias	6	0.68	0.25-1.48#
Poly/syndactyly	3	0.49	0.10-1.43#
Pes equinovarus	8	1.80	0.78-3.54#
Hip (sub)luxation, instable hip	14	0.88	0.52-1.46

#observed over expected number with exact Poisson 95% confidence interval.

Table 29.9. Relatively severe malformations in infants whose mothers used oral contraceptives in early pregnancy according to contraceptive type

Oral contraceptive group	No. of infants	No. of malformed infants	OR	95% CI
Progestogen+estrogen, fixed preparation	974	42	1.36	0.99-1.85
Progestogen+estrogen, sequential preparation	951	30	0.90	0.67-1.39
Progestogens	1124	35	0.99	0.70-1.39

There was thus no significant overrisk for a congenital malformation even though the upper confidence limits may approach 3-4 for specific conditions.

There was no difference between the three main groups of oral contraceptives with respect to the risk of a relatively severe malformation, even though the OR estimate is higher (and near statistical significance) for the progestogen+estrogen, fixed group. The $\chi 2$ for a comparison of the four groups (without any adjustments) is 2.73, p=0.26.

The highest RR for a specific malformation type was 3.03 (95% CI 0.98-7.07) for orofacial clefts and progestogen+estrogen, fixed preparation, based on five cases (1.7 expected).

Summary

By and large pregnancy outcome after (inadvertent) use of oral contraceptives in early pregnancy was normal. A moderate excess of low birth weight infants does not agree with the absence of an effect both on preterm birth and SGA and is probably random in spite of formal statistical significance. In this material there are no indications of an increased risk for congenital malformations but an association with a rare condition cannot be excluded.

References

[1] Janerich D T, Piper JM, Glebatis DM. Oral contraceptives and birth defects. *Amer J Epidemiol* 1980; 112: 73-79.

[2] Harlap S, Shiono PH, Ramcharan S. Congenital abnormalities in the offspring of women who used oral and other contraceptives around the time of conception. *Int J Fertility* 1985; 30: 39-47.

[3] Pardthaisong T, Gray RH. In utero exposure to steroid contraceptives and outcome of pregnancy. *Amer J Epidemiol* 1991; 134: 795-803.

[4] Li D-K. Daling JR, Mueller BA, Hickok DE, Fantel AG, Weiss NS. Oral contraceptive use after conception in relation to the risk of congenital urinary tract anomalies. *Teratology* 1995; 51: 30.36.

[5] Källén B, Mastroiacovo P, Lancaster PAL, Mutchinick O, Kringelbach M, Martínez-Frías ML, Robert E, Castilla EE. Oral contraceptives in the etiology of isolated hypospadias. *Contraception* 1991; 44: 173-182.

[6] Lejeune J, Prieur M. Contracéptives oroux et trisomie 21. *Ann Génet* 1979; 22: 61-66.

[7] Ericson A, Källén B, Lindsten J. Lack of correlation between contraceptive pills and Down´s syndrome. *Acta Obst Gynecol Scand* 1983; 62:511-514.

[8] Källén B. Maternal use of oral contraceptives and Down syndrome. *Contraception* 1989: 39: 503-506.

[9] Ahn HK, Choi JS, Han JY, Kim MH, Chung JH, Ryu HM, Kim MY, Yang JH, Koong MK, Nava-Ocampo AA, Koren G. Pregnancy outcome after exposure to oral contraceptives during the periconceptional period. *Human Exp Toxicol* 2008; 27: 307-313.

Chapter 30

SEX HORMONES OTHER THAN ORAL CONTRACEPTIVES

Use of progestogens in Sweden is mainly associated with infertility treatment. Clear-cut effects on pregnancy complications and neonatal problems are seen but these are with all probability due to the underlying subfertility and not to progestogen treatment. There seems to be no increased risk for a congenital malformation – the apparent association with pylorostenosis is probably random. Exposure for androgens and anti-androgens are extremely rare but should be avoided as these drugs may affect sex differentiation.

Sex hormones other than oral contraceptives have been used for various purposes and an association with such treatment and various outcomes has been described. Most well known is perhaps the association between maternal use of diethylstilbestrol, an estrogen, with clear cell adenocarcinoma of the vagina and cervix of female infants and with other genital tract anomalies also in male offspring [1]. Much discussion has also concerned the possible association between maternal use of gestagens and infant malformations, including cardiac defects and hypospadias [2-5]. Use of androgen drugs can masculinise a female foetus and use of antiandrogenic drugs can feminise a male foetus, resulting in for instance hypospadias.

Progestogens are in Sweden mainly used in connexion with infertility treatment, e.g., IVF. In other countries, progestogens have often been used at early pregnancy complications like threatened abortion. This will easily result in serious confounding. An international study of this subject found little evidence for a causal association between gestagen treatment and hypospadias [6]. A case-control study of hydroxyprogesterone treatment found a slightly increased risk of any type of congenital malformation but the use of the drug was strongly confounded by threatened abortion (present in about 90% of the exposed cases or controls) [7].

Combined estrogen and progestogen drugs like raloxifen are primarily used at post climacteric problems and exposure during pregnancy should be rare. Cyproterone, mainly used in combination with estrogens for severe acne, should not be used during pregnancy but inadvertent exposure will occur. Danazol has the main indication in endometriosis, mifepristone together with prostaglandin in medical abortion.

Table 30.1. Number of women identified using sex hormones other than oral contraceptives

Total	4679
Reported use in early pregnancy	4185
Got prescription later in pregnancy	786
Both early and later use	292

Type of drug	ATC code	Early use	Later use
Androgens	G03B	2	0
Testosterone	G03BA03	1	0
Unspecified	G03B	1	0
Estrogens	G03C	408	154
Estradiol	G03CA03	395	147
Estriol	G03CA04	6	6
Conjugated estrogens	G03CA57	1	0
Dienestrol	G03CB01	2	1
Unspecified	G03C	4	0
Progestogens	G03D	4449	789
Medroxyprogesterone	G03DA02 or L02AB02	550	84
Progesterone	G03DA04	2928	564
Dydrogesterone	G03DB01	212	63
Norethisterone	G03DC02	348	29
Lynestrenol	G03DC03	7	0
Tibolone	G03DC05	1	3
Unspecified progestogens	G03D	403	46
Progestogen and estrogen	G03F	47	6
Norgestrel+estrogen	G03FB01	7	2
Norethisterone+estrogen	G03FB05	36	4
Medroxyprogesterone+estrogen	G03FB06	4	0
Antiandrogens	G03H	13	7
Cyproterone	G03HA01	2	0
Cyproterone+estrogen	G03HB01	11	7
Other sex hormones	G03X	17	9
Danazol	G03XA01	2	2
Mifepristone	G03XB01	8	1
Raloxifen	G03XC01	7	6

Among these women, 359 had used more than one sex hormone preparation: 356 a combination of one progestogen and one estrogen and 3 women who reported the use of a combination of such drugs with progestogen (2 cases) or estrogen and progestogen (1 case) to which can be added 47 women (see above) who had used fixed combinations of progestogens and estrogen.

The vast majority of exposures thus concerned progestogens, possibly together with estrogens.

Characteristics of Women using Progestogen Drugs

Based on women reporting progestogen drugs (possibly together with estrogens) in early pregnancy (n=4055, one missing maternal age). Each variable is adjusted for all other variables and year of delivery. Comparison with all women who gave birth during the period and with information from the first antenatal care (n=967 742). The odds ratios for maternal age, parity, smoking in early pregnancy, number of previous miscarriages, BMI, subfertility, and country of birth are adjusted for all other variables and are shown in Figure 30.1.

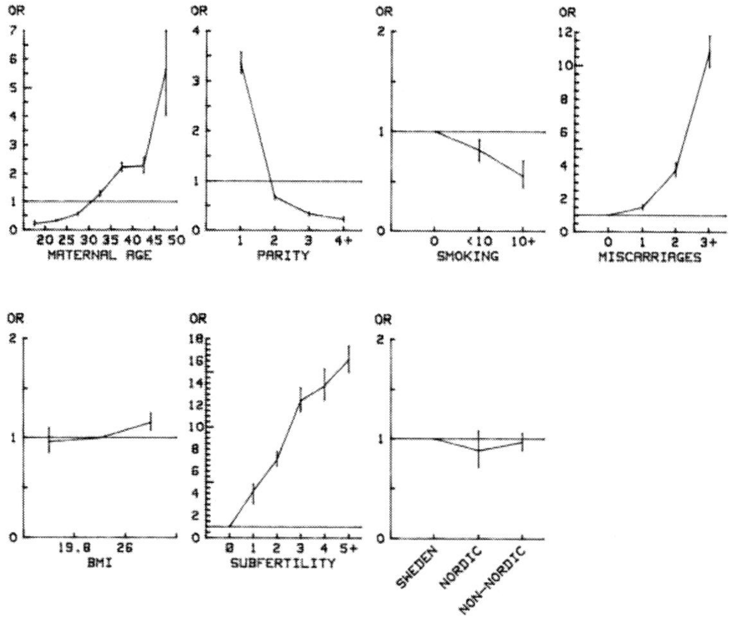

Figure 30.1. Odds ratios for seven maternal characteristics. The odds ratios (OR) for each variable are adjusted for the other variables and year of delivery. Vertical lines mark 95% confidence intervals. For maternal age and parity, each class is compared with all other classes.

Table 30.2. Some further maternal characteristics associated with the use or progestogen drugs

Variable studied	Number	OR	95% CI
Education (1996-2001, 2224 women with drugs, 526 695 in population)			
Unknown	39	-	-
<12 years	172	1.01	0.86-1.20
12 years	1066	1.00	Reference
13-14 years	150	0.97	0.82-1.16
≥14 years	797	0.89	0.81-0.98
Family situation			
Unknown	67	-	
Co-habiting	3904	1.00	Reference
Living alone	41	0.40	0.29-0.55
Other family situation	43	0.52	0.38-0.72
Work outside home			
Unknown	416	-	
Full time	2381	1.00	Reference
Part time	775	0.98	0.89-1.07
None	483	0.86	0.77-0.96

Some further maternal characteristics were analyzed, adjusting for year of delivery, maternal age, parity, smoking, and BMI (Table 30.2).

The most prominent characteristics are obviously associated with subfertility: the increasing use with increasing age, the excess of first parities, previous miscarriages, and duration of subfertility, estimated as years of unwanted childlessness.

Table 30.3. Concomitant drug use (early pregnancy)

Drug group	Number	OR/RR	95% CI
Drugs for stomach ulcer and reflux	35	0.86	0.62-1.21
Drugs for inflammatory bowel disease	12	0.93	0.52-1.65
Insulin	8	0.51	0.26-1.01
Multivitamins	160	0.81	0.69-0.96
Folic acid	511	3.21	2.94-3.52
Antihypertensive	13	0.69	0.40-1.18
Oral contraceptives	5	0.51	0.21-1.20
Gonadotrophines	252	19.6	17.7-21.7
Systemic corticosteroids	28	1.59	1.10-2.31
Thyroid drugs	58	0.88	0.68-1.15
Antibiotics	116	0.88	0.73-1.06
NSAIDs	42	0.47	0.35-0.63
Opioids	22	1.08	0.71-1.65
Minor analgesics	296	0.82	0.73-0.93
Drugs for migraine	9	0.57	0.30-1.08
Anticonvulsants	9	0.71	0.37-1.37
Neuoleptics	9	0.66	0.34-1.25
Sedatives, hypnotics	14	0.64	0.38-1.08
Antidepressants	35	0.60	0.43-0.83
Drugs for rhinitis	61	0.86	0.67-1.10
Antiasthmatics	88	0.64	0.52-0.79
Cough medicines	24	0.97	0.65-1.45
Antihistamines	195	0.80	0.70-0.93

There is a strong association with the use of folic acid (which is often given in connexion with IVF), gonadotrophines, and (weaker) with corticosteroids. For most other drugs, less use is reported than expected.

Table 30.4. Some maternal diagnoses associated with the use of progestogen drugs

Diagnosis	Drug use in early pregnancy			Drug use later in pregnancy		
	Number	OR/RR	95% CI	Number	OR/RR	95% CI
Pre-existing diabetes	60	1.03	0.79-1.33	17	1.40	0.86-2.28
Chronic hypertension	70	1.23	0.97-1.56	15	1.19	0.71-2.01
Gestational diabetes	58	1.46	1.07-1.82	13	1.53	0.82-2.83#
Preeclampsia	318	1.38	1.27-1.55	66	1.52	1.17-1.97
Hyperemesis gravidarum	57	1.30	1.00-1.70	15	1.60	0.89-2.63#
Placenta previa	83	1.60	1.28-1.99	20	1.81	1.16-2.83
Abruptio placentae	82	1.49	1.20-1.86	16	1.41	0.85-2.34
Antepartum bleeding	94	1.51	1.23-1.86	16	1.31	0.79-2.17
Intrapartum bleeding	157	1.53	1.31-1.80	38	1.62	1.13-2.26
Postpartum bleeding	303	1.21	1.07-1.36	68	1.53	1.19-1.97
Delivery induction	618	1.43	1.31-1.56	147	1.79	1.48-2.16
Caesarean section	1168	1.63	1.52-1.74	226	1.52	1.29-1.79

#observed over expected number with exact Poisson 95% confidence interval.

There is thus an increased risk for all studied pregnancy complications. No adjustment for subfertility was made and these effects are probably secondary to subfertility, a main indication for use of progestogens. Similar effects are seen after IVF procedures [8].

OUTCOME AFTER MATERNAL USE OF PROGESTOGENS

Infant Sex

After maternal use of progestogen drugs in early pregnancy, there were 2257 male and 2235 female infants born (two infants had unknown sex). The sex ratio was 1.01 (95% CI 0.95-1.07). After later exposure, there were 389 male and 404 female infants, sex ratio 0.96 (95% CI 0.84-1.11). Both sex ratios were thus low but the normal sex ratio (1.06) was contained in both confidence intervals.

Multiple Births

There is a marked excess of multiple births. After early use of progestogens, there were 443 twin and three triplet deliveries: the OR for twinning was 6.65 (95%CI 6.07-7.26). After later exposure, there were 52 twin deliveries and one triplet delivery: the OR for twinning was 4.08 (95% CI 3.10-5.38). These effects are reasonably due to simultaneous use of ovarian stimulation and IVF.

Table 30.5. Pregnancy duration and infant birth weight at maternal use of progestogen drugs

Variable studied	Drug use in early pregnancy			Drug use later in pregnancy		
	Number	OR/RR	95% CI	Number	OR/RR	95% CI
<37 weeks	300	1.58	1.40-1.78	56	1.58	1.20-2.08
<2500g	199	1.53	1.33-1.77	31	1.29	0.89-1.85
≥4500g	143	1.04	0.88-1.24	23	0.87	0.57-1.33
SGA	107	1.06	0.87-1.29	19	1.04	0.65-1.66
LGA	300	1.17	1.01-1.36	38	1.07	0.76-1.50

After early use, there is an excess of preterm birth and low birth weight and a slight increase of LGA while after later use only an increased risk for preterm birth is seen – a possible consequence of therapy of threatened preterm birth with progestogens.

Table 30.6. Infant mortality after maternal use of progestogen drugs

Variable studied	Drug use in early pregnancy			Drug use later in pregnancy		
	Number	OR/RR	95% CI	Number	OR/RR	95% CI
Stillbirth	23	1.24	0.82-1.87	2	0.60	0.07-2.18#
Early neonatal death	12	1.62	0.84-2.83#	3	1.32	0.48-6.77#

#observed over expected number with exact Poisson 95% confidence interval.

No statistically significant excess in mortality is thus seen.

Table 30.7. Neonatal diagnoses after maternal use of progestogen drugs

Diagnosis	Drug use in early pregnancy			Drug use later in pregnancy		
	Number	OR/RR	95% CI	Number	OR/RR	95% CI
Hypoglycaemia	300	1.62	1.44-1.82	56	1.49	1.13-1.96
Respiratory diagnoses	447	1.72	1.56-1.90	64	1.39	1.07-1.81
Low Apgar score	161	1.53	1.31-1.79	19	1.04	0.65-1.65
CNS diagnoses	39	1.21	0.88-1.66	7	1.03	0.41-2.11#
Jaundice	340	1.78	1.59-1.99	69	1.98	1.54-2.54

#observed over expected number with exact Poisson 95% confidence interval.

There is thus an excess morbidity among the newborn infants, notably after early exposure which is strongly related to subfertility.

Table 30.8. Congenital malformations in infants whose mothers had used progestogens (possible with estrogens) in early pregnancy

Congenital malformation	Number	OR	95% CI
All malformations	243	1.08	0.95-1.24
Relatively severe malformations	175	1.15	0.98-1.34
Chromosome anomalies	9	0.78	0.41-1.51
Without chromosome anomalies			
Any CNS malformation	3	0.55	0.11-1.60#
Eye malformations	7	1.50	0.60-3.08#
Ear malformations	6	0.56	0.26-1.24
Orofacial clefts	5	0.63	0.20-1.47#
Any cardiovascular defect	59	1.19	0.92-1.55
VSD and/or ASD	33	1.28	0.90-1.80
Pylorostenosis	8	2.63	1.14-5.19#
Oesophageal atresia	3	1.94	0.40-5.66#
Small gut atresia	3	3.13	0.64-9.13#
Anal atresia	3	1.55	0.32-4.54#
Hypospadias	12	0.82	0.46-1.49
Pes equinovarus	7	1.10	0.44-2.26#
Poly/syndactyly	11	1.28	0.64-2.29#
Hip (sub)luxation, instable hip	27	0.85	0.58-1.25

#observed over expected number with exact Poisson 95% confidence interval.

There is one condition which shows an excess, pylorostenosis, but the OR estimates for oesophageal, small gut, and anal atresia are also high although not statistically significant. There were seven infants with one of the latter three conditions (four expected). Fifteen infants had one or more of the four alimentary atresia with an RR = 2.10 (95% CI 1.18-3.47). In spite of the apparent statistical significance this excess may be random. Pylorostenosis usually develops relatively late in development while notably oesophageal and anal atresia develop early.

After exposures to other hormones than progestogens, numbers are limited (Table 30.9).

There is thus a significant excess of infants with VSD and/or ASD after estrogen exposure while no statistically significant excess of such malformations was seen after progestogen exposure. This finding, however, is based on only eight cases and even if formally statistically significant may be random.

Table 30.9. Congenital malformations in infants whose mothers used other sex hormones than progestogens

Hormone group	No. of infants	No. malformed	OR/RR	95% CI
Any malformation				
Androgen drug	2	0	0.00	-
Any estrogen drug[a]	470	29	1.26	0.86-1.85
Only estrogen drug	114	7	1.28	0.51-2.63#
Antiandrogen drug	13	0	0.00	-
Antigonadotrophine/progesterone drug	18	0	0.00	
Relatively severe malformation				
Any estrogen drug[a]	470	24	1.51	1.00-2.28
Cardiovacular malformation				
Any estrogen drug[a]	470	10	1.69	0.81-3.12#
VSD and/or ASD				
Any estrogen drug[a]	470	8	2.44	1.05-4.81#

[a]Includes estrogens given together with progestogens.

Among the seven malformed infants, exposed only to estrogens, there were five exposed to estradiol: one infant with anencephaly, two with pylorostenosis, one with polydactyly, one with spina bifida occulta and one with an unspecified skin malformation. One infant with Meckel diverticle was exposed to estriol, and one infant with a ventricular septum defect was exposed to an unspecified estrogen.

SUMMARY

The use of sex hormones included in this Chapter is strongly associated with subfertility and infertility treatment. Many of the excess morbidity during pregnancy and neonatally are probably due to underlying subfertility, as discussed in detail in studies on IVF [9]. There is no clear-cut effect on malformation rate, notably after exposure to progestogens. The only exception is a significantly increased risk for pylorostenosis (also indicated after estrogen exposure although then based on only two cases). A causal association seems unlikely as pylorostenosis is thought to arise late in pregnancy, perhaps even postnatally.

REFERENCES

[1] Mittendorf R. Teratogen update: carcinogenesis and teratogenesis associated with exposure to dietylstilbestrol (DES) in utero. *Teratology* 1995; 51: 435-445.

[2] Heinonen OP, Slone D, Monson RR, Hook EB, Shapiro S. Cardiovascular birth defects and anteenatal exposure to female sex hormones. *New Engl J Med* 1977; 296: 67-70.

[3] Aarskog D. Maternal progestins as a possible cause of hypospadias. *New Engl J Med* 1979; 300: 75-78.

[4] Calzolari E, ContieroMR, Roncatari E, Mattiuz PL, Volpato S. Aetiological factors in hypospadias. *J Med Genet* 1986; 23: 333-337.

[5] Harris EL. Genetic epidemiology of hypospadias. *Epidemiol Rev* 1990;12: 29.40.

[6] Källén B, Martínez-Frías ML, Castilla EE, Robert E, Lancaster PAL, Kringelbach M, Mutchinick OM, Mastroiacovo P. Hormone therapy during pregnancy and isolated hypospadias: an international case-control study. *Int J Risk Safety Med* 1992; 3: 183-198.

[7] Dudás I, Gidai J, Czeizel AE. Population-based case-control teratogenic study of hydroxyprogesterone treatment during pregnancy. *Cong Anomal* 2006; 46: 194-198.

[8] Källén B, Finnström O, Nygren KG, Otterblad Olausson P, Wennerholm U-B. In vitro fertilization in Sweden: obstetric charactristics, maternal morbidity and mortality. *BJOG* 2005; 112: 1529-1535.

[9] Källén B, Finnström O, Nygren KG, Otterblad Olausson P. In vitro fertilization (IVF) in Sweden: Risk for congenital malformations after different IVF methods. *Birth Def Res (Part A)* 2005; 73: 162-169.

Chapter 31

Ovulation Stimulants

An increased risk for pregnancy and delivery complications and also for neonatal morbidity and congenital malformations is seen after ovulation stimulation and no major difference seems to exist between gonadotropin and clomifene therapy. Notably the increased risk for congenital malformations seems to be due to underlying infertility and not to the treatments.

The possible risks with the use of ovarian stimulation and notably with clomifene have been much discussed. Early studies [1-4] found no general increase in malformation risk after ovarian stimulation but a concern was raised over a possible association between use of clomifene and neural tube defects and especially anencephaly. Some reviews, however, found no ground for this association [5]. In a previous study based on the Swedish Medical Birth Register [6], a statistically significant increase in malformation rate was found after ovarian stimulation but it disappeared when adjustment was made for years of involuntary childlessness. A recent review [7] underlined the association between infertility and an increased risk for congenital malformations. Another review [8] indicated the possibility that clomifene treatment may be associated with an increased risk for neural tube defects and severe hypospadias in the offspring.

In the Medical Birth Register, information on ovulation stimulation can be obtained from two sources: reports from the pregnant woman that such drugs had been used, and a mark made by the midwife in the record, if the pregnancy was the result of an ovarian stimulation. The first source is incomplete because the pregnant woman is asked about drugs used during pregnancy and ovarian stimulants are used before pregnancy and therefore usually not reported. Only this source can be used if the nature of the stimulation is to be studied. The midwife mark is not always made when an ovarian stimulation has occurred and records for more than half of the women who had reported use of such drugs lacked a mark. For characteristics of women with ovarian stimulation and the general outcome of pregnancy and delivery, all cases were used irrespective of source, but for the analysis of specific ovarian stimulant use, of concomitant drug use, and outcomes after specific drugs, only women who had reported ovarian stimulation could be analyzed.

See also Chapter 33 on gonadotrophine-releasing drugs and gonadotrophine agonists.

Table 31.1. Number of women identified reporting ovulation stimulants

Totally identified cases of ovarian stimulation	13 873
Use reported by woman in early pregnancy	2 178
Midwife mark for ovulation stimulation	12 550
Both sources of information	855

Type of drug	ATC code	Number
Gonadotrophines	G03GA	973
Chorionic gonadotropin	G03GA01	816
Chorionic gonadotrophn alfa	G03GA08	2
Human menopausal gonadotropin	G03GA02	27
Urofollitropin	G03GA04	49
Follitropin alfa	G03GA05	105
Follitropin beta	G03GA06	92
Unspecified	G03GA	6
Ovulation stimulants, synthetic	G03GB	1260
Clomifene	G03GB02	1260

The use of both gonadotropin and clomifene was reported by 55 women.

Characteristics of Women using Ovarian Stimulants

Based on women reporting the drug in early pregnancy (n=13 861, 12 missing maternal age). Each variable is adjusted for all other variables and year of delivery. Comparison with all women who gave birth during the period and with information from the first antenatal care (n=967 742). The odds ratios for maternal age, parity, smoking in early pregnancy, number of previous miscarriages, BMI, subfertility, and country of birth are adjusted for all other variables and are shown in Figure 31.1. OR for subfertility was calculated with 1 year as a reference. The reason is that all women who did not report years of unwanted childlessness after gonadotropin use must have had subfertility while in the background data the majority of such women had no subfertility why any comparisons based on that group will be biased.

Some further maternal characteristics were analyzed, adjusting for year of delivery, maternal age, parity, smoking, and BMI (Table 31.2).

Women undergoing ovarian stimulation thus show many specific characteristics: high age, low parity, previous miscarriages, high BMI, subfertility measured as years of unwanted childlessness. They smoke less than expected and women born outside the Nordic countries are under-represented.

There is a strong association with the use of progestogens and folic acid while many other drugs are used less often than expected.

Both pre-existing pathology and pregnancy complications thus occur in an increased frequency.

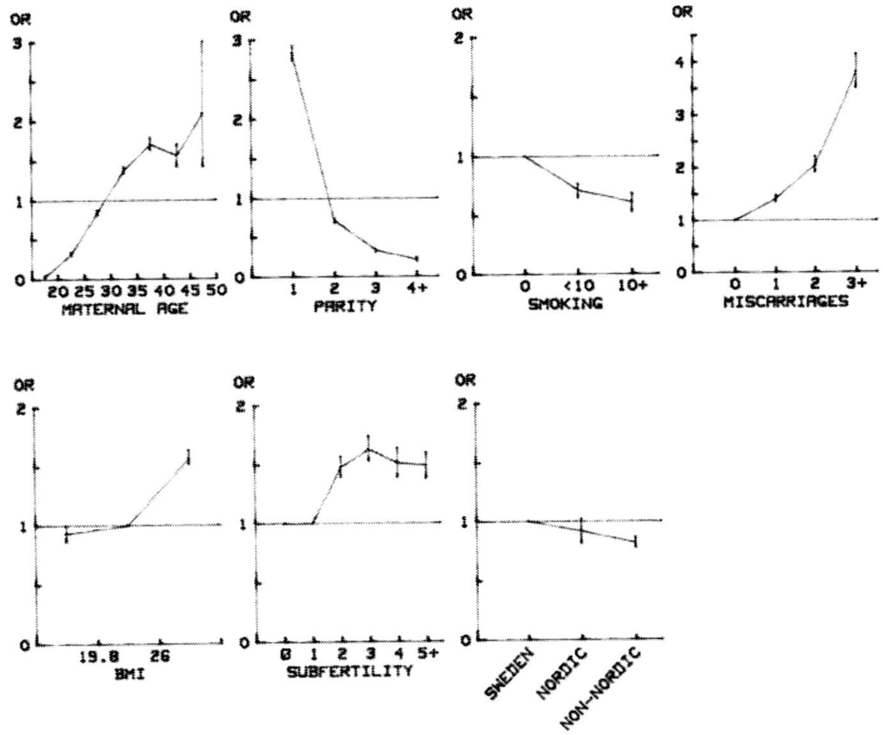

Figure 31.1. Odds ratios for seven maternal characteristics. The odds ratios (OR) for each variable are adjusted for the other variables and year of delivery. Vertical lines mark 95% confidence intervals. For maternal age and parity, each class is compared with all other classes.

Table 31.2. Some further characteristics of women using ovarian stimulants

Variable studied	Number	OR	95% CI
Education (1996-2001, 7 009 women with drugs, 526 695 in population)			
Unknown	111		
<12 years	524	0.99	0.90-1.09
12 years	3660	1.00	reference
13-14 years	394	0.78	0.70-0.87
≥14 years	2320	0.81	0.77-0.85
Family situation			
Unknown	154	-	
Co-habiting	13411	1.00	reference
Living alone	69	0.21	0.17-0.27
Other family situation	69	0.25	0.19-0.31
Work outside home			
Unknown	1269	-	
Full time	8137	1.00	reference
Part time	2947	1.02	0.97-1.07
None	1350	0.69	0.65-0.73

Table 31.3. Concomitant drug use (early pregnancy)

Drug group	Number	OR/RR	95% CI
Drugs for stomach ulcer and reflux	19	1.01	0.64-1.59
Drugs for inflammatory bowel disease	5	0.80	0.26-1.87#
Insulin	9	1.16	0.53-2.20#
Multivitamins	52	0.68	0.52-0.90
Folic acid	107	1.42	1.17-1.73
Antihypertensives	11	1.12	0.56-2.00#
Progestogens	237	19.0	17.2-21.1
Systemic corticosteroids	11	1.18	0.59-2.10#
Thyroid drugs	28	0.93	0.64-1.35
Antibiotics	56	0.78	0.60-1.02
NSAIDs	25	0.57	0.39-0.84
Opioids	10	1.01	0.48-1.86#
Minor analgesics	111	0.57	0.48-0.69
Anticonvulsants	5	0.67	0.22-1.56#
Sedatives, hypnotics	11	1.18	0.59-2.11#
Antidepressants	22	0.85	0.56-1.28
Drugs for rhinitis	21	0.56	0.38-0.88
Antiasthmatics	58	0.80	0.62-1.03
Antihistamines	89	0.68	0.55-0.84

#observed over expected number with exact Poisson 95% confidence interval.

Table 31.4. Some maternal diagnoses associated with the use of ovarian stimulants

Diagnosis	Number	OR/RR	95% CI
Pre-existing diabetes	296	1.56	1.39-1.76
Chronic hypertension	283	1.53	1.41-1.80
Gestational diabetes	240	1.75	1.53-1.99
Preeclampsia	1062	1.39	1.30-1.48
Hyperemesis gravidarum	243	1.73	1.52-1.96
Placenta previa	294	1.81	1.60-2.03
Abruptio placentae	311	1.81	1.62-2.03
Antepartum bleeding	3.22	1.58	1.41-1.77
Intrapartum bleeding	503	1.59	1.45-1.74
Postpartum bleeding	974	1.10	1.03-1.18
Delivery induction	2030	1.34	1.28-1.41
Caesarean section	3379	1.39	1.34-1.45

Outcome after Maternal use of Ovarian Stimulants

Infant Sex

Among infants born, sex was unknown in three, 7 823 were male and 7 335 female, sex ratio 1.04, 95% CI 1.01-1.07 which thus contains the normal sex ratio of 1.06.

Multiple Births

There were 1 032 twin deliveries and 50 triplet deliveries. The odds ratio for twining was 5.05 (95% CI 4.75-5.36). The about 7% twinning rate is to some extent due to a high twinning rate after IVF, usually made after ovulation stimulation.

Table 31.5. Infant mortality after maternal use of ovarian stimulants

Variable studied	Number	OR	95% CI
Stillbirth	67	1.14	0.89-1.45
Early neonatal death	53	2.30	1.75-3.02

#observed over expected number with exact Poisson 95% confidence interval.

There is an increased risk for perinatal death, significant only for early neonatal death.

Table 31.6. Pregnancy duration and infant birth weight at maternal use of ovarian stimulants

Variable studied	Number	OR	95% CI
<37 weeks	918	1.37	1.28-1.47
<2500g	681	1.57	1.45-1.70
≥4500g	500	0.99	0.90-1.08
SGA	458	1.39	1.26-1.53
LGA	674	1.04	0.96-1.13

There is thus an increased risk for preterm birth and intrauterine growth retardation.

Table 31.7. Neonatal diagnoses after maternal use of ovarian stimulants

Diagnosis	Number	OR/RR	95% CI
Hypoglycaemia	1042	1.75	1.65-1.87
Respiratory diagnoses	1309	1.55	1.46-1.64
Low Apgar score	571	1.63	1.50-1.78
CNS diagnoses	173	1.54	1.32-1.80
Jaundice	1203	1.85	1.74-1.96

All studied neonatal diagnoses thus occur at an increased rate.

When the ovarian stimulant used was known, a separate analysis for gonadotropins and for clomifene could be made (Table 31.9).

There is thus an increased risk for congenital malformations in infants born after maternal treatment with ovarian stimulants. The most remarkably increased risk refers to CNS malformations and especially neural tube defects but an increased risk can be seen also for hypospadias and for pes equinovarus. The OR for anal atresia is close to statistical significance with a lower confidence limit of 0.99. There is no major difference between gonadotropins and clomifene with respect to neural tube defects but there are only three cases in each group. Other OR estimates may differ between the two groups but confidence intervals are wide. The total rate of all malformations or relatively severe malformations is significantly increased after gonadotropins but not increased after clomifene, but these two ORs may estimate one and the same common OR (1.37 for relatively severe malformations).

Table 31.8. Congenital malformations in infants whose mothers had used ovarian stimulants

Congenital malformation	All cases known			With known drug		
	Number	OR	95% CI	Number	OR	95% CI
All malformations	841	1.14	1.06-1.23	143	1.25	1.06-1.48
Relatively severe malformations	596	1.20	1.10-1.30	106	1.37	1.13-1.67
Chromosome anomalies	27	0.85	0.57-1.25	7	1.44	0.58-2.97#
Without chromosome anomalies						
Any CNS malformation	33	1.72	1.22-2.43	8	2.42	1.04-4.76#
Neural tube defects	12	1.96	1.01-3.43#	6	5.45	2.00-11.9#
Eye malformations	14	0.93	0.55-1.57	3	1.12	0.23-3.28#
Ear malformations	51	1.41	1.07-1.87	5	0.86	0.28-2.00#
Orofacial cleft	32	1.14	0.80-1.63	4	0.94	0.20-2.42#
Any cardiovascular defect	189	1.15	0.99-1.33	37	1.46	1.05-2.02
VSD and/or ASD	88	1.00	0.80-1.24	22	1.69	1.11-2.58
Oesophageal atresia	8	1.60	0.69-3.15#	1	-	
Small gut atresia	6	1.58	0.58-3.45#	1	-	
Anal atresia	12	1.91	0.99-3.34#	3	3.13	0.64-9.13#
Pylorostenosis	14	1.34	0.79-2.27	1	-	
Body wall defect	3	0.79	0.16-2.32#	0	-	
Diaphragmatic hernia	4	0.95	0.26-2.73#	1	-	
Hypospadias	63	1.43	1.12-1.84	9	1.30	0.60-2.48#
Kidney a/dysgenesis	7	1.78	0.72-3.67#	0	-	
Cystic kidney	8	1.34	0.58-2.65#	0	-	
Pes equinovarus	35	1.66	1.18-2.32	9	2.83	1.29-5.37#
Hip (sub)luxation, instable hip	104	0.97	0.79-1.18	14	0.85	0.50-1.44
Poly/syndactyly	33	1.11	0.78-1.57	6	1.33	0.49-2.90#
Limb reduction defect	13	1.43	0.76-2.44#	1	-	
Craniostenosis	16	1.68	0.96-2.73	2	-	

#observed over expected number with exact Poisson 95% confidence interval.

Table 31.9. Congenital malformations in infants whose mothers used gonadotrophines or clomifene

Congenital malformation	Gonadotropins			Clomifene		
	Number	OR	95% CI	Number	OR	95% CI
All malformations	79	1.52	1.21-1.91	68	1.05	0.82-1.34
Relatively severe malformations	63	1.78	1.38-2.30	45	1.03	0.76-1.38
All CNS malformations	5	3.25	1.05-7.58#	3	1.59	0.33-4.64#
Neural tube defects	3	6.25	1.29-18.3#	3	4.48	0.92-13.1#
Any cardiovascular defect	21	1.79	1.16-2.76	37	1.46	1.05-2.02
VSD and/or ASD	11	1.77	0.88-3.16#	12	1.67	0.86-2.91#
Hypospadias	4	1.27	0.34-3.24#	5	1.28	0.42-2.99#
Pes equinovarus	7	4.93	1.98-10.2#	3	1.63	0.34-4.76#
Hip (sub)luxation, instable hip	6	0.79	0.29-1.32#	8	0.87	0.38-1.72#
Poly/syndactyly	4	1.98	0.54-5.07#	2	0.77	0.09-2.77#

#observed over expected number with exact Poisson 95% confidence interval.

The risk for a congenital malformation may be seriously confounded by the underlying condition which results in ovarian stimulation treatment: subfertility. As pointed out above, this factor is difficult to adjust for, because in the group "no years of unwanted childlessness" may be hidden in a group with missing information. Therefore, analysis adjusting for stated period of unwanted childlessness was restricted to those who said one year or more. For the above-demonstrated excess risks, the results of an adjustment of this sort are given below.

Among all combinations studied, thus only one reached statistical significance: pes equinovarus after gonadotropins. Also this may be random, however, as many tests were made. The declines in OR for all malformations and for relatively severe malformations show that the major determinant is the underlying subfertility status. Similar findings were made in an analysis of congenital defects after IVF treatment [9].

Table 31.10. Congenital malformations showing excess risk in Table 31.9. Risk estimates are now adjusted for the length of known unwanted childlessness as a measure of subfertility

Congenital malformation	Group	Number	OR/RR	95% CI
All malformations	All cases known	661	1.08	0.94-1.13
	With known drug	68	1.00	0.78-1.42
	Gonadotropins	39	1.19	0.85-1.67
Relatively severe malformations	All cases known	460	1.04	0.93-1.15
	With known drug	48	1.06	0.78-1.42
	Gonadotropins	30	1.37	0.93-2.80
All CNS malformations	All cases known	23	1.21	0.77-1.92
Neural tube defects	All cases known	6	1.01	0.51-2.20#
All cardiovascular malformations	With known drug	16	1.10	0.66-1.84
	Gonadotropins	8	1.07	0.46-2.10#
	Clomifene	9	1.20	0.55-2.27#
Pes equinovarus	All cases known	30	1.31	0.87-1.98
	Gonadotropins	5	3.92	1.63-9.47#

#observed over expected number with exact Poisson 95% confidence interval.

SUMMARY

Pregnancies occurring after ovulation stimulation are characterized by an increased risk for a number of different pregnancy and neonatal complications, including an increased risk for congenital malformations. There is no certain difference between gonadotropin and clomifene treatment. The effect on malformation rate seems to disappear when adjustment for the infertility status is made and is probably not due to drug treatment but to the underlying infertility condition. There is a marked increased risk for CNS malformations including neural tube defects both after treatment with gonadotropin and with clomifene but also this effect seems to disappear when adjustment for subfertility is made. The situation resembles much that observed after IVF treatments.

REFERENCES

[1] Hack M, Brish M, Serr DM, Insler V, Salomy M, Lunenfeld B. Outcome of pregnancy after induced ovulation. Follow-up of pregnancies and children born after clomiphene therapy. *JAMA* 1970; 220: 1329-1333.

[2] Ash H, Greenblatt RB. Update on the safety and efficiency of clomiphene citrate as a therapeutic agent. *J Reprod Med* 1976; 17: 175-180.

[3] Ahlgren M, Källén B, Rannevik G. Outcome of pregnancy after clomiphene therapy. *Acta Obst Gynecol Scand* 1976; 55: 371-375.

[4] MacGregor AH, Schardein JL. Congenital anomalies and hormones during pregnancy. A critical revies. *Teratology* 1980; 7: 199-202.

[5] Greenland S, Ackerman DL.Clomiphene citrate and neural tube defects: A pooled analysis of controlled epidemiological studies and recommendations for future studies. *Fertil Steril* 1995; 64: 936-941.

[6] Källén B, Otterblad Olausson P, Nygren KG. Neonatal outcome in pregnancies from ovarian stimulation. *Obstet Gynecol* 2002; 100: 414-419.

[7] Farhi J, Fisch B. Risk of major congenital malformations associated with infertility and its treatment by extent of iatrogenic intervention. *Pediatr Endocrinol Rev* 2007; 4:352-357.

[8] Elizur SE, Tulandi T. Drugs in infertility and fetal safety. *Fertil Steril* 2008; 89: 1595-1602.

[9] Källén B, Finnstrom O, Nygren KG, Otterblad Olausson P. In vitro fertilization (IVF) in Sweden: Risk for congenital malformations after different IVF methods. *Birth Def Res (Part A)* 2005; 73: 162-169.

Chapter 32

UROLOGICALS

Little can be said about possible risks associated with antispasmodics during pregnancy but available data do not indicate an increased risk for congenital malformations. Exposure in early pregnancy therefore does not motivate a discussion of a termination of the pregnancy.

The majority of these drugs, used during pregnancy, are anticholinergics and are used as urinary antispasmodics. Little is known about their use during pregnancy. The preparation of magnesium hydroxide (Emgesan®) categorized during this heading is used for recurrent kidney stones. Alfa-adrenoreceptor antagonists are used at prostatic hypertrophy and the use by pregnant women is unexpected.

Table 32.1. Number of women identified using urologicals

Total	273
Reported use in early pregnancy	111
Got prescription later in pregnancy	186
Both early and later use	24

Type of drug	ATC code	Early use	Later use
Urinary concrement solvent	G04BC	4	0
Urinary antispasmodics	G04BD	48	21
Emepronium	G04BD01	15	11
Oxybutynin	G04BD04	8	1
Tolterodin	G04BD07	24	9
Solifenacin	G04BD08	1	0
Other urologics	G04BX	56	163
Magnesium hydroxide	G04BX01	56	163
Alfa-adreno receptor antagonist	G04CA	2	0
Alfuzosin	G04CA01	2	0
Unspecified	G04	2	0

CHARACTERISTICS OF WOMEN USING UROLOGICAL DRUGS

Based on women reporting the drug in early pregnancy (n=111). Each variable is adjusted for all other variables and year of delivery. Comparison with all women who gave birth during the period and with information from the first antenatal care (n=967 742). The odds ratios for maternal age, parity, smoking in early pregnancy, number of previous miscarriages, BMI, subfertility, and country of birth are adjusted for all other variables (Table 32.2).

Table 32.2.Characteristics of women using urological drugs

Variable studied	Number	OR	95% CI
Maternal age			
<25 years	14	0.92	0.47-1.78
25-34 years	59	1.00	reference
≥35 years	38	2.16	1.40-3.33
Parity			
1	46	1.13	0.75-1.69
≥2	65	1.00	reference
Smoking			
Unknown	7	-	-
No	85	1.00	reference
Yes	19	1.68	0.63-4.51
Previous miscarriages			
No	86	1.00	reference
Any	25	0.96	0.61-1.52
BMI			
Unknown	9	-	-
<19.8	12	1.60	0.86-2.98
19.8-25.9	64	1.00	reference
≥26	26	0.83	0.52-1.33

Some further maternal characteristics were analyzed, adjusting for year of delivery, maternal age, parity, smoking, and BMI (Table 32.3).

Table 32.3. Some further characteristics of women using urological drugs

Variable studied	Number	OR	95% CI
Education (1996-2001, 33 women with drugs, 506 268 in population)			
Unknown	4	-	-
<12 years	5	1.55	0.50-4.80
12 years	13	1.00	reference
≥13 years	11	1.11	0.47-2.63
Family situation			
Unknown	3	-	
Co-habiting	94	1.00	reference
Living alone	3	0.97	0.31-3.06
Other family situation	10	3.06	1.49-6.27
Work outside home			
Unknown	14	-	-
Full time	39	1.00	reference
Part time	30	1.65	0.92-2.95
None	27	2.04	1.12-3.73

The low number of exposed cases makes it possible only to analyse relatively common events.

Table 32.4. Concomitant drug use (early pregnancy)

Drug group	Number	OR/RR	95% CI
Multivitamins	11	0.53	0.30-0.95
Folic acid	11	0.87	0.69-1.10
Antibiotics	8	1.26	0.54-2.48#
Opioids	4	4.30	1.17-11.0#
Minor analgesics	9	1.10	0.50-2.08#
Antidepressants	7	4.07	1.64-8.39#
Antiasthmatics	7	1.78	0.72-3.67#
Antihistamines	6	0.84	0.31-1.83#

#observed over expected number with exact Poisson 95% confidence interval.

The only excess of concomitant drug use was opioids and antidepressants, both represented with only few exposures.

Table 32.5. Some maternal diagnoses associated with the urologics

Diagnosis	Drug use in early pregnancy			Drug use later in pregnancy		
	Number	OR/RR	95% CI	Number	OR/RR	95% CI
Preeclampsia	6	1.15	0.42-2.50#	10	1.13	0.54-2.09#
Antepartum bleeding	0	0.00	-	6	2.04	0.75-4.44#
Intrapartum bleeding	3	0.47	0.09-1.36#	4	0.82	0.22-2.11#
Postpartum bleeding	0			6	0.78	0.39-1.56#
Delivery induction	18	1.64	0.96-2.80	28	1.42	0.95-2.13
Caesarean section	27	1.49	0.94-2.36	36	1.16	0.80-1.68

#observed over expected number with exact Poisson 95% confidence interval.

Even though some odds ratios were increased, none reached statistical significance.

Outcome after Maternal use of Urologics

Infant Sex

Among infants born after early use of urologics, 60 were male and 51 female, sex ratio 1.18, 95% CI 0.81-1.73. After later use, 92 were male and 94 female, sex ratio 0.98, 95% CI 0.73-1.31.The confidence intervals contain the normal sex ratio (1.06).

Multiple Births

There were three twin deliveries after early use of urologics, RR = 1.69 (95% CI 0.35-4.93) and two after later use, RR = 0.67, 95% CI 0.08-2.42.

Two infants were stillborn after maternal early use of urologics (RR = 4.60, 95% CI 0.56-16.6) and one after later use. The excess stillbirth risk is based on only few cases and has a wide confidence interval.

Table 32.6. Pregnancy duration and infant birth weight at maternal use of urologics

Variable studied	Drug use in early pregnancy			Drug use later in pregnancy		
	Number	OR/RR	95% CI	Number	OR/RR	95% CI
<37 weeks	13	2.45	1.30-4.19#	19	2.13	1.28-3.32#
<2500g	6	1.66	0.61-3.61#	11	1.99	0.99-3.55#
≥4500g	7	1.55	0.62-3.20#	10	1.15	0.55-2.11#
SGA	2	0.72	0.09-2.60#	4	1.13	0.31-2.89#
LGA	8	1.19	0.52-2.34#	16	1.18	0.70-1.99

#observed over expected number with exact Poisson 95% confidence interval.

There is thus a significant increase in preterm births but no indications of intrauterine growth retardation.

Table 32.7. Neonatal diagnoses after maternal use of urologics

Diagnosis	Drug use in early pregnancy			Drug use later in pregnancy		
	Number	RR	95% CI	Number	RR	95% CI
Hypoglycaemia	1	0.25	0.01-1.41	12	1.80	0.93-3.15
Respiratory diagnoses	10	1.77	0.85-2.26	19	2.22	1.34-3.47
Low Apgar score	0	-	-	8	2.61	1.13-5.13
CNS diagnoses	0	-	-	2	1.71	0.21-6.17
Jaundice	7	1.51	0.61-3.10	18	2.53	1.50-4.00

There is thus an increased risk for neonatal pathology after exposure during late part of the pregnancy.

Among the 111 infants born after early exposure to urologics, seven had a malformation: RR = 1.39 (95% CI 0.56-2.86). Six of these infants were exposed to magnesium hydroxide (a total of 56 infants) with RR = 2.50 (95% CI 0.92-5.44). The risk increase is thus not statistically significant. The seven infants had the following diagnoses:

- Congenital tracheomalacia
- Tongue tie (oxybutinin exposure)
- Hypospadias
- Undescended testicle (2 infants)
- Nevus
- Down syndrome.

SUMMARY

The study material is small but some deviations in delivery outcome is seen which may well be explained by underlying maternal pathology, e.g., recurrent urinary tract infections. No certain teratogenic risk is seen and the recorded malformations are mainly mild conditions.

Chapter 33

HYPOPHYSEAL AND HYPOTHALAMIC HORMONES (EXCEPT GONADOTROPHINES) AND ANALOGUES

Diabetes insipidus is a rare disease in pregnancy. Only limited information exists on the safety of the use of vasopressin or vasopressin analogues. The present data, although restricted in size, do not suggest an increased risk for congenital malformations and if exposure has occurred in early pregnancy, there is no reason to discuss a termination of the pregnancy.

Use of gonadotropin-releasing drugs and gonadotropin agonists are strongly associated with infertility and the effects on pregnancy and neonatal conditions are probably due to the infertility and not to its treatment.

This group of drug is heterogeneous. The majority of exposures are represented by vasopressin analogues at diabetes insipidus and gonadotropin-releasing hormones used at infertility. Somatropin is used at growth disturbances. Gonadotropin agonists are used in association with IVF.

Little is known about diabetes insipidus during pregnancy and its therapy with vasopressin or vasopressin analogues [1,2], but no major effects on pregnancy outcome have been found.

CHARACTERISTICS OF WOMEN USING HYPOPHYSEAL OR HYPOTHALAMIC DRUGS

Based on women reporting the drug in early pregnancy (n=176 for women using vasopressin analogues, n=224 for women using gonadotropin-releasing hormones or gonadotropin agonists). Each variable is adjusted for all other variables and year of delivery. Comparison with all women who gave birth during the period and with information from the first antenatal care (n=967 742). The odds ratios for maternal age, parity, smoking in early pregnancy, number of previous miscarriages, BMI, subfertility, and country of birth are adjusted for all other variables (Table 33.2).

Table 33.1. Number of women identified using using hypophyseal or hypothalamic drugs in early pregnancy

Total	521
Reported use in early pregnancy	429
Got prescription later in pregnancy	126
Both early and later use	34

Type of drug	ATC code	Early use	Later use
ACTH	H01AA	3	1
Corticotropin	H01AA01	1	0
Tetracosactide	H01AA02	2	1
Somatotropin	H01AC01	26	15
Vasopressin and analogues	H01BA	176	54
Desmopressin	H01BA02	73	35
Lypressin	H01BA03	103	19
Oxytocin	H01BB02	5	3
Antigrowth hormone	H01BC	1	0
Ocreotide	H01BC02	1	0
Gonadotrophine-releasing hormones	H01CA	218	51
Gonadorelin	H01CA01	9	32
Nafarelin	H01CA02	122	19
Unspecified	H01CA	87	0
Gonadorophine agonists	H01CC	6	3
Ganirelix	H01CC01	0	1
Cetrorelix	H01CC02	6	2

Some further maternal characteristics were analyzed, adjusting for year of delivery, maternal age, parity, smoking, and BMI (Table 33.3).

The characteristics of women using vasopressin analogues hardly deviate from expected values. The only exception is an increased risk for short education. Women who reported the use of gonadotropin-releasing hormones or gonadotropin agonists show typical characteristics of women with fertility problems: an increased risk of high maternal age and of first parity, low risk of smoking, and a strong association with a more than one year period of unwanted childlessness.

Use of vasopressin analogues was thus associated with drugs for stomach ulcer and systemic corticosteroids and also with thyroid drugs and antihistamines used at NVP. Use of gonadotropin-releasing drugs or gonadotropin agonists were as expected very strongly associated with progestogens and gonadotropins and also with folic acid which is often prescribed at IVF procedures.

The only significant risk increase was for caesarean section after maternal use of gonadotropin-releasing drugs or gonadotropin agonists.

Table 33.2. Characteristics of women using hypophyseal or hypothalamic drugs in early pregnancy

Variable studied	Using vasopressin analogues			Using gonadotropin releaser etc.		
	Number	OR	95% CI	Number	OR	95% CI
Maternal age						
<25 years	34	1.22	0.81-1.83	11	0.17	0.09-0.33
25-34 years	112	1.00	reference	147	1.00	reference
≥35 years	30	1.13	0.75-1.72	68	2.55	1.91-3.99
Parity						
1	86	1.29	0.93-1.78	142	3.45	2.61-4.55
≥2	90	1.00	reference	82	1.00	reference
Smoking						
Unknown	3	-	-	6	-	-
No	154	1.00	reference	206	1.00	reference
Yes	19	1.47	0.60-3.63	12	0.14	0.03-0.77
Previous miscarriages						
No	145	1.00	reference	173	1.00	reference
Yes	31	0.86	0.57-1.29	51	1.17	0.86-1.60
BMI						
Unknown	24	-	-	20	-	-
<19.8	15	1.01	0.58-1.75	17	1.02	0.62-1.70
19.8-25.9	105	1.00	reference	136	1.00	reference
≥26	32	0.78	0.52-1.16	51	1.07	0.78-1.48
Subfertility						
No	159	1.00	reference	6[a]	1.00	reference
Yes	17	1.42	0.85-2.37	150	7.62	3.86-15.1
Country of birth						
Unknown	0	-	-	0	-	-
Sweden	134	1.00	reference	199	1.00	reference
Other Nordic country	4	1.01	0.38-2.72	2	0.34	0.09-1.28
Non-Nordic country	38	1.53	1.05-2.22	18	0.59	0.37-0.95

[a]One year of unwanted childlessness used as reference group (see Chapter 31).

Table 33.3. Further characteristics of women who using hypophyseal or hypothalamic drugs in early pregnancy

Variable studied	Using vasopressin analogues			Using gonadotrophine releaser etc.		
	Number	OR	95% CI	Number	OR	95% CI
Education (1996-2001,12 women with vasopressin drug, 135 with gonadotrophine-releasing drugs etc., 506 695 in population)						
Unknown	9	-	-	0	-	-
<12 years	24	2.12	1.28-3.53	8	0.78	0.36-1.39
12 years	57	1.00	reference	73	1.00	reference
≥13 years	38	1.06	0.69-1.64	54	0.70	0.48-1.00
Family situation						
Unknown	5	-	-	2	-	-
Co-habiting	242	1.00	reference	189	1.00	reference
Living alone	1	0.57	-	10	1.66	0.87-3.16
Other family situation	5	1.07	0.42-2.72	4	1.10	0.41-2.96
Work outside home						
Unknown	27	-	-	39	-	-
Full time	148	1.00	reference	82	1.00	reference
Part time	51	1.11	0.80-1.54	44	1.30	0.86-1.95
None	27	0.77	0.49-1.22	40	1.63	1.06-2.51

Table 33.4. Concomitant drug use (early pregnancy)

Drug group	Number	OR/RR	95% CI
Vasopressin analogues			
Drugs for stomach ulcer and reflux	5	3.70	1.20-8.64#
Multivitamins	5	0.95	0.31-2.21#
Folic acid	6	1.27	0.47-2.77#
Systemic corticosteroids	5	7.69	2.50-18.0#
Thyroid drugs	7	4.07	1.64-8.39#
Antibiotics	3	0.57	0.12-1.67#
Minor analgesics	17	1.48	0.91-2.42
Antiasthmatics	9	1.83	0.84-3.47#
Antihistamines	29	3.22	2.16-4.63#
For NVP	25	3.40	2.20-5.01#
For allergy	5	1.62	0.53-3.78#
Gonadotropin-releasing drugs and gonadotropin agonists			
Multivitamins	3	0.35	0.07-1.03#
Folic acid	21	2.41	1.49-3.69
Progestogens	55	26.1	19.6-33.9#
Gonadotropins	93	78.8	63.6-96.6#
Thyroid drugs	4	1.25	0.34-3.70#
Antibiotics	4	0.57	0.16-1.47#
NSAIDs	7	1.50	0.60-3.08#
Minor analgesics	6	0.30	0.14-0.64
Antiasthmatics	5	0.70	0.23-1.64
Antihistamines	11	0.84	0.47-1.51

#observed over expected number with exact Poisson 95% confidence interval.

Table 33.5. Some maternal diagnoses associated with the use of hypophyseal or hypothalamic hormones

Diagnosis	Drug use in early pregnancy			Drug use later in pregnancy		
	Number	OR/RR	95% CI	Number	OR/RR	95% CI
Vasopressin analogues						
Preeclampsia	12	1.59	0.82-2.78#	1	-	-
Postpartum bleeding	12	1.18	0.66-2.13	4	1.38	0.38-3.54#
Delivery induction	24	1.44	0.94-2.21	6	1.02	0.37-2.21#
Caesarean section	32	1.29	0.88-1.90	9	1.04	0.48-1.98#
Gonadotropin-releasing drugs and gonadotropn agonists						
Preeclampsia	16	1.26	0.76-2.10			
Intrapartum bleeding	10	1.87	0.90-3.44#			
Postpartum bleeding	12	0.82	0.45-1.47			
Delivery induction	31	1.24	0.84-1.83			
Caesarean section	60	1.53	1.15-2.05			

#observed over expected number with exact Poisson 95% confidence interval.

Outcome after Maternal use of Hypophyseal Hormones other than Gonadotrophines

Infant Sex

After maternal early use of vasopressin analogues, 92 infants were males, 91 females, giving a sex ratio of 1.01 (95% CI 0.76-1.35) and after later use there were 25 male and 20 female infants, sex ratio 1.20 (95% CI 0.71-2.10). After maternal use of gonadotropin-releasing drugs or gonadotropin agonists, there were 135 male and 122 female infants, sex ratio 1.11 (95% CI 0.87-1.42). The normal sex ratio (1.06) is thus contained in all confidence intervals.

Multiple Births

After maternal early use of vasopressin analogues, there were seven twin deliveries, RR =2.46 (95% CI 0.99-5.06). After later use, there was only one twin delivery. After maternal use of gonadotropin-releasing drugs or gonadotropin agonists, there are 34 twin deliveries, RR=8.17 (95% CI 5.66-11.4).

No stillbirths or early neonatal deaths were observed.

Table 33.6. Pregnancy duration and infant birth weight at maternal use of hypophyseal or hypothalamic drugs

Variable studied	Drug use in early pregnancy			Drug use later in pregnancy		
	Number	RR	95% CI	Number	RR	95% CI
Vasopressin analogues						
<37 weeks	7	0.84	0.34-1.72	6	2.37	0.81-5.08
<2500g	6	1.11	0.41-2.42	4	2.56	0.70-6.57
≥4500g	0	-	-	3	1.44	0.30-4.19
SGA	4	1.06	0.29-2.70	1	-	-
LGA	7	0.76	0.31-1.57	3	1.07	0.22-3.12
Gonadotropin-releasing drugs and gonadotropin agonists						
<37 weeks	11	1.12	0.56-2.00			
<2500g	3	0.45	0.09-1.33			
≥4500g	6	0.88	0.32-1.92			
SGA	2	0.38	0.05-1.38			
LGA	9	1.06	0.48-2.01			

Numbers are thus low and confidence intervals large but no significant deviations are seen.

There was thus an increased risk for neonatal pathology after late maternal use of vasopressin analogues. After use of gonadotropin-releasing drugs or gonadotropin agonists odds ratios were also high but only for CNS diagnoses was formal statistical significance reached.

Table 33.7. Neonatal diagnoses after maternal use of hypophyseal or hypothalamic drugs

Diagnosis	Drug use in early pregnancy			Drug use later in pregnancy		
	Number	OR/RR	95% CI	Number	OR/RR	95% CI
Vasopressin analogues						
Hypoglycaemia	8	1.31	0.56-2.57#	22	2.24	1.45-3.43
Respiratory diagnoses	10	1.00	0.52-1.90	24	1.71	1.13-2.59
Low Apgar score	2	0.49	0.02-1.27#	12	2.07	1.07-3.61#
CNS diagnoses	1	-	-	0	-	-
Jaundice	17	2.28	1.33-3.65#	5	2.25	0.73-5.26
Gonadotropin-releasing drugs and gonadotropin agonists						
Hypoglycaemia	4	2.04	0.56-5.23#			
Respiratory diagnoses	5	1.90	0.62-4.44#			
CNS diagnoses	6	3.41	1.25-7.42#			
Jaundice	16	1.43	0.86-2.38#			

#observed over expected number with exact Poisson 95% confidence interval.

Table 33.8. Congenital malformations in infants whose mothers used hypophyseal or hypothalamic drugs in early pregnancy

Congenital malformation	Number	OR/RR	95% CI
All malformations	20	0.85	0.54-1.32
Somatropin	1	-	-
Vasopressin analogues	6	0.66	0.24-1.44#
Gonadotropin-releasing drugs and gonadotropin agonists	13	1.05	0.60-1.84
Relatively severe malformation			
Vasopressin and analogues	4	0.65	0.181-66#
Gonadotropin-releasing drugs and gonadotropin agonists	11	1.30	0.652-33#

The infant exposed to somatropin had prominent ears.

Among the four infants with relatively severe malformations after vasopressin analogue exposure, three with desmopressin exposure had the following malformations: Arnold-Chiari syndrome with brain reduction, transposition of great vessels, unspecified cardiac defect. One infant with lypressin exposure had hypospadias.

Among the eleven infants with relatively severe malformations after maternal use of gonadotrophine-releasing drugs, four had been exposed by an undefined such drug and the other for nafarelin. The following relatively severe malformations were noted:

1. Congenital ptosis, unspecified CNS malformation, upper alimentary tract malformation.
2. Branchial sinus, fistula or cleft.
3. Median cleft palate
4. Testis aplasia
5. Penis malformation
6. Congenital vesico-uretero-renal reflux

7. Epidermolysis bullosa, pes equinovarus, hypospadias, unilateral renal agenesis, ectopic testis, deformity of spine and chest.
8. Pes equinovarus
9-10. Down syndrome
11. Trisomy 18

There was thus no observable increase in malformation risk but the presence of two multimalformed infants after gonadotropin-releasing drugs is noticeable.

SUMMARY

Vasopressin analogues used during early pregnancy seem not to be associated with a major risk for teratogenesis but such drugs used during the later part of the pregnancy appear to be associated with an increased neonatal morbidity. This could well be due to the underlying disease, diabetes insipidus. Use of gonadotropin-releasing drugs or gonadotropin agonists was uncommon and no conclusions on possible risk increases could be drawn. Probably similar associations exist as with other drugs used at infertility treatment.

REFERENCES

[1] Källén B, Carlsson SS, Bengtsson BK. Diabetes insipidus and use of desmopressin (Minirin) during pregnancy. *Eur J Endocrinol* 1995; 132: 144-146.

[2] Ray JG. DDAVP use during pregnancy: an analysis of its safety for mother and child. *Obstet Gynecol Surv* 1998; 53: 450-455.

Chapter 34

CORTICOSTEROIDS USED SYSTEMICALLY

Maternal use of corticosteroids in early pregnancy usually indicates severe morbidity, e.g., inflammatory bowel disease or asthma, and this affects pregnancy outcome. There is a slight increase in the risk of a congenital malformation after maternal use of glucocorticoids in early pregnancy which seems independent of concomitant drug use. Even though the literature is not quite conclusive, there seems to be an association between glucocorticoid use and cleft lip/palate but not with cleft palate. The association is not strong and if exposure has occurred in early pregnancy, there is no reason to discuss a termination of the pregnancy.

The possible risks associated with the use of glucocorticoids during pregnancy have been much debated. One reason is their use in experimental teratology, mainly to produce cleft palate in mice. A large number of studies using different methodologies have approached the problem if use of corticosteroids in human pregnancy increases the risk for congenital malformations and notably orofacial clefts. A meta-analysis of case-control studies published before 2000 found an odds ratio of 3.35 for oral clefts [1]. A later international study comparing orofacial clefts with other malformations also found an increased risk for cleft lip/palate but not for cleft palate [2]. A small TIS study [3] found a higher rate of congenital malformations among infants exposed to glucocorticoids than in an unexposed group (4.6 versus 2.6%) but the low numbers made the difference statistically non-significant. The most recent study is a case-control study [4] which found an increased risk for cleft lip/palate but not for isolated cleft palate. In that paper, the earlier literature was summarized. An increased risk of preterm birth and a lower median birth weight was found in a prospective study but analysis was crude [3].

There were thus only 68 women who used a mineral corticosteroid in early pregnancy, among them 52 had also used a glucocorticosteroid. In late pregnancy there were 34 women who had used a mineral corticosteroid and among them 26 had also used a glucocorticosteroid. Except for data on congenital malformations, results will be restricted to glucocorticoids, irrespective of simultaneous use of mineral corticoids.

Table 34.1. Number of women identified using corticosteroids

Total	3481
Reported use in early pregnancy	1579
Got prescription later in pregnancy	583
Both early and later use	4477

Type of drug	ATC code	Early use	Later use
Mineralcorticoids	H02AA	68	34
Fludrocortisone	H02AA02	60	34
Unspecified	H02AA	8	0
Glucocorticoids	H02AB	3425	1565
Betamethasone	H02AB01	825	391
Dexamethasone	H02AB02	31	27
Methylprednisolone	H02AB04	121	23
Prednisolone	H02AB06	1051	782
Prednisone	H02AB07	5	9
Triamcinolone	H02AB08	42	12
Hydrocortisone	H02AB09	1322	326
Cortisone	H02AB10	70	21
Prednylidene	H02AB11	6	0
Deflazacont	H02AB13	0	1
Unspecified	H02A	33	4

Characteristics of Women using Glucocorticoids

Based on women reporting the drug in early pregnancy (n=3425). Each variable is adjusted for all other variables and year of delivery. Comparison with all women who gave birth during the period and with information from the first antenatal care (n=967 742). The odds ratios for maternal age, parity, smoking in early pregnancy, number of previous miscarriages, BMI, subfertility, and country of birth are adjusted for all other variables and are shown in Figure 34.1.

Some further maternal characteristics were analyzed, adjusting for year of delivery, maternal age, parity, smoking, and BMI (Table 34.2).

These women thus showed an age distribution with a maximum in the 30-34 years class, an excess of first parity, and an association with three previous miscarriages or more and with unwanted childlessness. There was a slight excess of women with a high BMI and fewer than expected of women were born outside the Nordic countries.

There is thus a very strong association with drugs for inflammatory bowel disease, thyroid drugs, drugs for asthma and rhinitis, and antihistamines, notably such drugs used for allergy. All this indicates the natures of underlying diseases which were the indication for the use of glucocorticosteroids.

The only significant association between concomitant drug use and the use of mineral corticosteroids was drugs used for thyroid disease (16 found, RR = 18.2, 95% CI 10.4-29.5), indicating co-morbidity between Addison´s disease and thyroiditis.

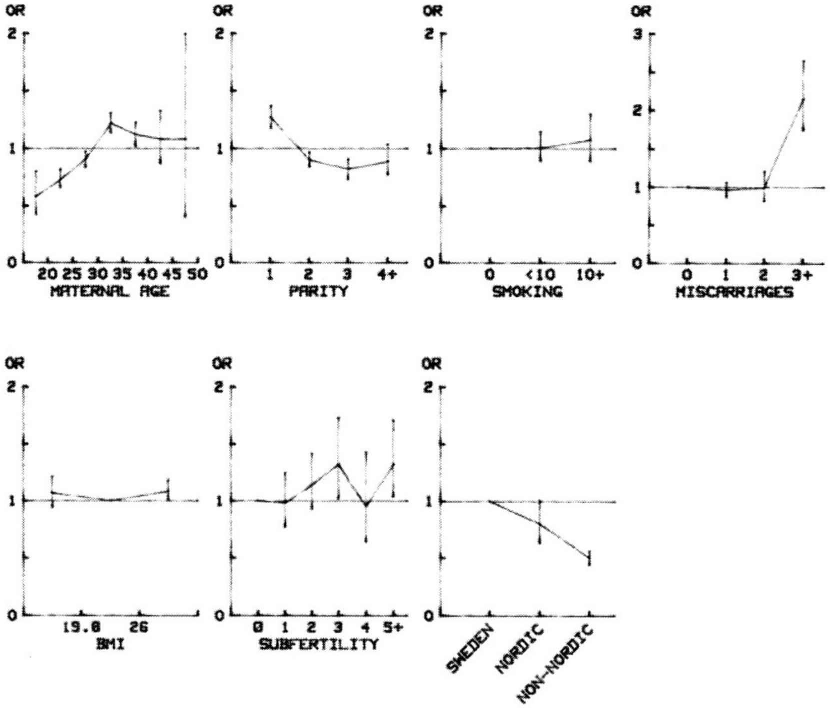

Figure 34.1. Odds ratios for seven maternal characteristics. The odds ratios (OR) for each variable are adjusted for the other variables and year of delivery. Vertical lines mark 95% confidence intervals. For maternal age and parity, each class is compared with all other classes.

Table 34.2. Some further maternal characteristics of women using glucocorticosteroids

Variable studied	Number	OR	95% CI
Education (1996-2001, 1896 women with drugs, 526 695 in population)			
Unknown	21	-	-
<12 years	178	0.86	0.72-1.02
12 years	983	1.00	reference
13-14 years	92	0.83	0.67-1.03
>14 years	622	1.03	0.92-1.15
Family situation			
Unknown	65	-	-
Co-habiting	3180	1.00	reference
Living alone	98	1.16	0.95-1.46
Other family situation	82	1.10	0.86-1.41
Work outside home			
Unknown	462	-	-
Full time	1652	1.00	reference
Part time	794	1.05	0.95.1,15
None	517	0.96	0.86-1.07

Table 34.3. Concomitant drug use (early pregnancy)

Drug group	Number	OR/RR	95% CI
Drugs for stomach ulcer and reflux	84	2.84	2.31-3.50
Drugs for inflammatory bowel disease	235	23.9	20.9-27.2#
Insulin	14	1.08	0.64-1.84
Multivitamins	122	0.65	0.55-0.78
Folic acid	202	1.42	1.23-1.64
Oral contraceptives	7	0.67	0.32-1.40
Progestogens	26	1.57	1.07-2.30
Gonadotrophines	11	1.19	0.59-2.13#
Thyroid drugs	89	2.00	1.62-2.46
Antibiotics	211	1.95	1.70-2.24
NSAIDs	137	2.17	1.84-2.57
Opioids	61	3.53	2.78-4.49
Minor analgesics	292	1.05	0.93-1.18
Anticonvulsants	12	1.22	0.63-2.14#
Sedatives, hypnotics	58	4.40	3.45-5.60
Antidepressants	64	1.54	1.20-1.97
Drugs for rhinitis	156	3.16	2.71-3.69
Antiasthmatics	692	7.84	7.29-8.43
Antihistamines	641	3.72	3.43-4.03
For NVP	284	1.77	1.57-2.00
For allergy	502	8.65	7.98-9.38

#observed over expected number with exact Poisson 95% confidence interval.

Table 34.4. Some maternal diagnoses associated with the use of glucocorticoids

Diagnosis	Drug use in early pregnancy			Drug use later in pregnancy		
	Number	OR	95% CI	Number	OR	95% CI
Pre-existing diabetes	54	1.19	0.91-1.56	38	1.73	1.25-2.39
Chronic hypertension	69	1.67	1.31-2.13	47	2.39	1.79-3.19
Gestational diabetes	37	1.16	0.84-1.62	28	1.90	1.31-2.76
Preeclampsia	216	1.35	1.18-1.56	122	1.69	1.40-2.03
Hyperemesis gravidarum	43	1.24	0.91-1.67	35	2.09	1.50-2.91
Placenta previa	50	1.28	0.97-1.70	37	1.95	1.41-2.70
Abruptio placentae	62	1.42	1.10-1.83	42	2.02	1.50-2.74
Antepartum bleeding	58	1.22	0.94-1.59	37	1.72	1.24-2.38
Intrapartum bleeding	85	1.17	0.94-1.46	58	1.61	1.24-2.09
Postpartum bleeding	178	0.91	0.78-1.06	95	1.10	0.89-1.35
Delivery induction	496	1.47	1.33-1.62	301	2.68	1.83-2.37
Caesarean section	798	1.57	1.45-1.70	422	1.82	1.63-2.04

There is thus an excess of pregnancy morbidity and also an association with pre-existing diabetes and hypertension. The use of glucocorticosteroids in later part of the pregnancy is often due to pregnancy complications, e.g., preeclampsia and HELLP syndrome or threatened preterm birth. Some underlying conditions, like asthma, are also directly associated with many of these pregnancy outcomes.

Outcome after Maternal use of Glucocorticosteroids

Infant Sex

After early use of glucocorticosteroids, there were 1 782 male and 1 708 female infants born, sex ratio 1.04 (95% CI 0.98-1.12). After use later in pregnancy, there were 837 male and 785 female infants, sex ratio 1.07 (95% CI 0.97-1.18). The normal sex ratio of 1.06 is thus included in both confidence intervals.

Multiple Births

After early use of glucocorticosteroids, there were 63 twin deliveries and one triplet delivery. The OR for twinning was 1.21, 95% CI 0.94-1.55. After later use, there were 36 twin deliveries and six triplet deliveries, OR for twinning = 1.53 (95% CI 1.10-2.14).

Table 34.5. Infant mortality after maternal use of glucocorticosteroids

Variable studied	Drug use in early pregnancy			Drug use later in pregnancy		
	Number	OR/RR	95% CI	Number	OR/RR	95% CI
Stillbirth	12	0.93	0.55-1.71	7	1.22	0.49-2.52#
Early neonatal death	7	1.31	0.53-2.69#	5	2.14	0.69-4.99#

#observed over expected number with exact Poisson 95% confidence interval.

No statistically significant risk increase for perinatal mortality is thus seen.

Table 34.6. Pregnancy duration and infant birth weight at maternal use of glucocorticosteroids

Variable studied	Drug use in early pregnancy			Drug use later in pregnancy		
	Number	OR/RR	95% CI	Number	OR/RR	95% CI
<37 weeks	311	1.95	1.73-2.19	186	2.70	2.33-3.13
<2500g	209	2.00	1.74-2.30	133	3.01	2.54-3.58
≥4500g	102	0.73	0.60-0.89	35	0.55	0.09-0.76
SGA	132	1.79	1.50-2.13	63	2.03	1.58-2.61
LGA	173	0.85	0.73-1.00	92	0.99	0.80-1.23

After early use of glucocorticoids there is thus an increased risk for preterm birth and intrauterine growth retardation which is still stronger after later use.

Some types of neonatal pathology were thus increased also after early use of glucocorticosteroids but effects were stronger after later use. The increased risk for adrenal insufficiency is not statistically significant but is an expected effect, notably of glucocorticosteroid use in late pregnancy.

Table 34.7. Neonatal diagnoses after maternal use of glucocorticosteroids

Diagnosis	Drug use in early pregnancy			Drug use later in pregnancy		
	Number	OR/RR	95% CI	Number	OR/RR	95% CI
Hypoglycaemia	172	1.38	1.18-1.61	108	1.92	1.58-2.33
Respiratory diagnoses	212	1.21	1.05-1.39	132	1.80	1.51-2.16
Low Apgar score	73	1.08	0.85-1.36	44	1.57	1.16-2.11
CNS diagnoses	25	1.15	0.77-1.71	16	1.49	0.91-2.43
Jaundice	186	1.32	1.14-1.53	142	2.27	1.91-2.69
Adrenal insufficiency	28	1.16	0.80-1.69	12	1.39	0.72-2.43

Table 34.8. Congenital malformations in infants whose mothers had used glucocorticosteroids in early pregnancy

Congenital malformation	Number	OR	95% CI
All malformations	185	1.10	0.95-1.28
Relatively severe malformations	136	1.19	1.00-1.42
Chromosome anomalies	2	0.27	0.03-0.99#
Without chromosome anomalies			
Any CNS malformation	3	0.68	0.14-1.99#
Eye malformations	4	1.14	0.31-2.91#
Ear malformations	11	1.30	0.65-2.32#
Orofacial clefts	9	1.42	0.65-2.89#
Isolated cleft palate	2	0.74	0.88-3.82#
Cleft lip/palate	7	1.83	0.73-3.77#
Any cardiovascular defect	48	1.27	0.95-1.69
VSD and/or ASD	25	1.28	0.86-1.91
Pylorostenosis	5	2.05	0.67-4.78#
Hypospadias	7	0.71	0.28-1.45#
Severe kidney malformations	3	1.37	0.28-4.00#
Pes qeuinovarus	7	1.44	0.58-2.96#
Hip (sub)luxation, unstable hip	25	1.12	0.76-1.67
Poly/syndactyly	6	0.86	0.32-1.87#
Limb reduction defects	5	2.37	0.77-5.53#
Craniostenosis	4	1.87	0,51-4.79#

#observed over expected number with exact Poisson 95% confidence interval.

There is thus a weak general increase in congenital malformations but no specific type reaches statistical significance. When infants exposed to drugs used for inflammatory bowel disease, thyroid disease, or asthma were removed from the analysis, the OR for relatively severe malformations (99 cases) increased slightly: OR = 1.24 (95% CI 1.01-1.52).

Table 34.9. Odds ratio for relatively severe malformations and specific glucocorticosteroids (with at least 50 exposures)

Glucocorticosteroid	Number of infants	Number malformed	OR/RR	95% CI
Betamethasone	837	29	1.05	0.71-1.53
Methylprednisolone	121	4	1.06	0.86-5.18#
Prednisolone	1075	40	1.15	0.83-1.57
Hydrocortisone	1347	58	1.32	1.01-1.72
Cortisone	71	5	2.02	0.66-4.72#

The proportions of malformed infants do not differ between the five drugs, $\chi 2_{(4\ d.f)}$ = 3.05, p=0.55 and the statistically significant increase for hydrocortisone may well be random.

There were six malformed infants after maternal use of mineral corticosteroids (some of them also used glucocorticosteroids), all regarded as relatively severe RR = 2.58, 95% CI 0.95-5.60. The recorded diagnoses were:

1. Cauda equina malformation and anal atresia (also glucocorticosteroid)
2. Hypospadias (also glucocorticosteroid)
3. Hydronephrosis
4. Craniostenosis
5. Diaphragmatic hernia (also glucocorticosteroid)
6. Mosaic Turner syndrome.

SUMMARY

Systemic corticosteroids are used at a variety of conditions, many of which like asthma have a direct effect on pregnancy and neonatal outcome. There is only a weak indication of a teratogenic effect of glucocorticosteroids. An association with cleft lip/palate is indicated but does not reach statistical significance. The odds ratios for cleft palate and for cleft lip/palate are in the same order of magnitude as those recently described from a retrospective case-control study. There is a suggested increase in adrenal insufficiency notably after late exposure, but statistical significance is not reached.

REFERENCES

[1] Park-Wyllie L, Mazzotta P, Pastuszak A, Moretti ME, Beique L, Hunnisett L, Friesen MH, Jacobson S, Ksapinovic S, Chang D, Diav-Citrin O, Chitayat D, Nulman I, Einarson TR, Koren G. Birth defects after maternal exposure to corticosteroids: prospective cohort study and meta-analysis of epidemiological studies. *Teratology* 2000; 62: 385-392.

[2] Pradat P, Robert-Gnansia E. di Tanna GL, Rosano A, Lisi A, Mastroiacovo P, and ll contributors to the MADRE database. Frist trimester exposure to corticosteroids and oral clefts. *Birth Def Res (Part A)* 2003; 67: 968-970.

[3] Gur C, Diav-Citrin O, Shechtman S,Arnon J, Ornoy A. Pregnancy outcome after first trimester exposure to corticosteroids: a prospective controlled study. *Reprod Toxicol* 2004; 18: 93-101.

[4] Carmichael SL, Shaw GM, Ma C, Werler MM, Rasmussen SA, Lammer EJ for the National Birth Defects Prevention Study. Maternal corticosteroid use and orofacial clefts. *Am J Obst Gynecol* 2007; 197: 585e1-585.e7.

Chapter 35

THYROID DRUGS

Adequate supplementation with thyroxine is important for pregnant women with hypothyreosis. Already early in pregnancy, an increased demand for thyroxine exists which may explain some deviations in pregnancy and neonatal outcomes among women with thyroxine substitution. This may also explain a moderate increase in malformation risk, especially visible for cardiovascular defects and hypospadias. Women using thyroid hormones often have other co-morbidity.

Thyreostatic drugs are known teratogens and should if possible be avoided in early pregnancy. The individual risk after exposure for such drugs is, however, not very large and exposure in early pregnancy is hardly a reason for a discussion of pregnancy termination.

Thyroid hormones are unlikely to damage foetal development. There is, however, an increased demand for thyroid hormones during pregnancy and an increase of thyroid hormones at substitution is regularly needed. Before pregnancy is realized and hormone substitution adjusted, a relative hypothyroidism may theoretically occur but little is known about this problem in spite of the fact that hypothyroidism during pregnancy is a frequent complication. A recent study [1] summarized previous literature on the subject and described pregnancy and neonatal outcome in a cohort of more than 8500 women who were substituted with thyroid hormones in early pregnancy. An increased risk for various pregnancy complications was found, an increased risk for neonatal thyroid disease among the newborns, and a weak increase in malformation risk, especially for congenital cardiovascular defects.

Thyreostatic drugs and notably methimazole have been associated with an increased risk of congenital malformations [2-6]. The typical malformations seen are a combination of choanal atresia, oesophageal atresia, scalp defects, facial anomalies, and psychomotor delay [2].

Table 35.1. Number of women identified using thyroid drugs

Total	13 742
Reported use in early pregnancy	11 922
Got prescription later in pregnancy	8 355
Both early and later use	6 535

Type of drug	ATC code	Early use	Later use
Thyroid hormones	H03A	11 767	8 225
Levothyroxin	H03AA01	11 758	8 224
Liothyronin	H03AA02	47	41
Unspecified	H03A	6	1
Thyreostatics	H03B	268	166
Propylthiouracil	H03BA02	187	137
Thiamazole	H03BB02	102	37
Unspecified	H03B	1	0
Unspecified	H03	1	0

The majority of women who used liothyronin also had levothyroxin, 44 of 47 in early pregnancy and all 41 later in pregnancy. In early pregnancy 62 women and in later pregnancy 35 women reported the use of both levothyroxin and a thyreostatic.

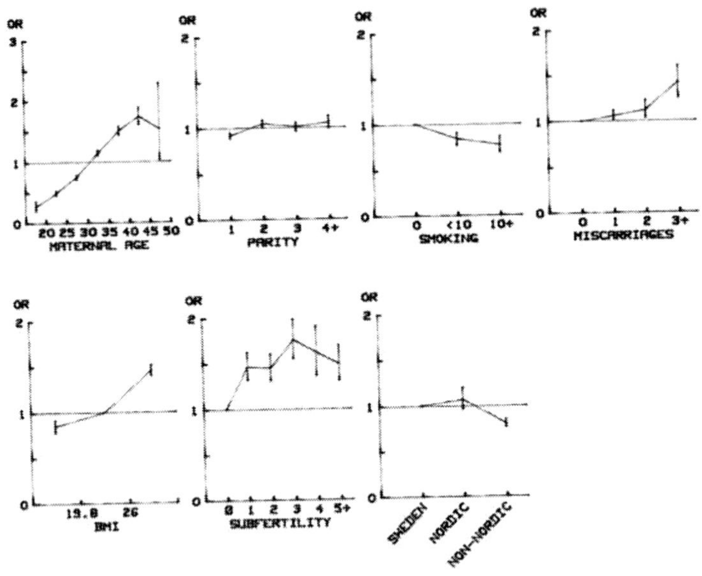

Figure 35.1. Odds ratios for seven maternal characteristics. The odds ratios (OR) for each variable are adjusted for the other variables and year of delivery. Vertical lines mark 95% confidence intervals. For maternal age and parity, each class is compared with all other classes.

Characteristics of Women using Thyroid Drugs

Thyroid Hormones

Based on women reporting the drug in early pregnancy (n=11 966, 1 missing maternal age). Each variable is adjusted for all other variables and year of delivery. Comparison with all women who gave birth during the period and with information from the first antenatal care (n=967 742). The odds ratios for maternal age, parity, smoking in early pregnancy, number of previous miscarriages, BMI, subfertility, and country of birth are adjusted for all other variables and are shown in Figure 35.1.

Some further maternal characteristics were analyzed, adjusting for year of delivery, maternal age, parity, smoking, and BMI (Table 35.2).

Table 35.2. Some further maternal characteristics for women using thyroid hormones

Variable studied	Number	OR	95% CI
Education (1996-2001, 4601 women with drugs, 526 695 in population)			
Unknown	85	-	-
<12 years	459	0.91	0.82-1.01
12 years	2395	1.00	reference
13-14 years	248	0.90	0.79-1.03
>14 years	1412	0.91	0.84-0.97
Family situation			
Unknown	205	-	-
Co-habiting	11087	1.00	reference
Living alone	252	0.98	0.86-1.13
Other family situation	222	0.80	0.69-0.94
Work outside home			
Unknown	1483	-	-
Full time	5479	1.00	reference
Part time	2935	1.02	0.97-1.08
None	1869	0.98	0.92-1.04

Table 35.3. Maternal characteristics of women using thyeostatics in early pregnancy

Variable studied	Number	OR	95% CI
Maternal age			
<25 years	29	0.89	0.59-1.34
25-34 years	169	1.00	reference
≥35 years	70	1.31	0.97-1.76
Parity			
1	92	0.74	0.51-0.97
≥2	176	1.00	reference
Smoking			
Unknown	9	-	-
No	235	1.00	reference
Yes	24	0.55	0.22-1.38
Previous miscarriages			
No	201	1.00	reference
Yes	67	1.14	0.81-1.51
BMI			
Unknown	28	-	-
<19.8	23	1.23	0.80-1.91
19.8-25.9	153	1.00	reference
≥26	84	0.90	0.68-1.21
Country of birth			
Unknown	3	-	-
Sweden	187	1.00	reference
Other Nordic country	6	1.02	0.41-2.29
Non-Nordic country	72	1.90	1.45-2.49

Thyreostatics

Based on women reporting the drug in early pregnancy (n=268). Each variable is adjusted for all other variables and year of delivery. Comparison with all women who gave birth during the period and with information from the first antenatal care (n=967 742). The odds ratios for maternal age, parity, smoking in early pregnancy, number of previous miscarriages, BMI, subfertility, and country of birth are adjusted for all other variables (Table 35.3).

Some further maternal characteristics were analyzed, adjusting for year of delivery, maternal age, parity, smoking, and BMI (Table 35.4).

Table 35.4. Some further maternal characteristics of women using thyreostatics in early pregnancy

Variable studied	Number	OR	95% CI
Education (1996-2001, 126 women with drugs, 526 695 in population)			
Unknown	6	-	-
<12 years	27	2.10	1.34-3.31
12 years	51	1.00	Reference
≥13 years	42	1.17	0.75-1.82
Family situation			
Unknown	5	-	-
Co-habiting	248	1.00	Reference
Living alone	9	1.37	0.68-2.78
Other family situation	6	0.93	0.37-2.36
Work outside home			
Unknown	40	-	-
Full time	96	1.00	Reference
Part time	55	1.01	0.75-1.43
None	77	2.01	1.44-2.81

There is a marked association between maternal age and use of thyroid hormones and the same is indicated for thyreostatics. Low use of both thyroid hormones and thyreostatics is associated with first parity and for thyreostatics the use increases with parity. Both types of drugs are associated with non-smoking and with previous miscarriages. Thyroid hormones but not thyreostatics are associated with a high BMI and with a period of unwanted childlessness. To be born outside the Nordic countries reduces the risk of using thyroid hormones but increases the risk for using thyreostatics. Not to be working outside home is associated with thyreostatics but not with thyroid hormones.

All estimates for thyreostatics are based on relatively low numbers and confidence intervals are therefore wide.

There is thus a strong association between the use of insulin and thyroid hormones or thyreostatics and the same is true for beta-blocking agents (notably for thyreostatics), systemic corticosteroids, and sedatives/hypnotics. There is also an association between the use of thyroid hormones and drugs for inflammatory bowel disease, antidepressants and antiasthmatics.

Table 35.5. Concomitant drug use (early pregnancy)

Drug group	Number	OR	95% CI
Thyroid hormones			
Drugs for stomach ulcer and reflux	128	1.12	0.94-1.34
Drugs for inflammatory bowel disease	51	1.35	1.02-1.78
Insulin	279	6.73	6.03-7.50
Multivitamins	799	0.84	0.78-0.89
Folic acid	804	1.11	1.04-1.20
Beta-blocking agents	117	2.14	1.78-2.57
Oral contraceptives	20	0.61	0.40-0.95
Progestogens	58	0.92	0.71-1.20
Gonadotrophines	28	0.93	0.64-1.35
Systemic corticosteroids	94	2.10	1.72-2.57
Antibiotics	311	0.81	0.72-0.90
NSAIDs	146	0.65	0.55-0.76
Opioids	78	1.11	0.89-1.40
Minor analgesics	545	0.54	0.49-0.58
Anticonvulsants	46	1.26	0.94-1.69
Sedatives, hypnotics	129	2.16	1.82-2.57
Antidepressants	317	1.89	1.69-2.11
Drugs for rhinitis	177	0.94	0.81-1.09
Antiasthmatics	516	1.38	1.26-1.51
Cough medicines	40	0.59	0.43-0.81
Antihistamines	581	0.81	0.75-0.88
Thyreostatics			
Insulin	4	4.35	1.18-11.1#
Multivitamins	12	0.65	0.40-1.07
Folic acid	12	0.84	0.47-1.50
Beta-blocking agents	37	29.1	24.8-40.2#
Systemic corticosteroids	4	3.60	0.98-9.23#
Antibiotics	11	1.24	0.62-2.23#
Minor analgesics	3	0.30	0.14-0.63#
Sedatives, hypnotics	37	30.3	21.4-41.8#
Antihistamines	20	1.34	0.85-2.11

#observed over expected number with exact Poisson 95% confidence interval.

Most pregnancy complications are significantly increased in women who used thyroid hormones in early pregnancy. Rather similar odds ratios were seen after later use but numbers are lower and statistical significance often not reached. Among the relatively few women who used thyreostatics in early or later pregnancy, increased rates of delivery inductions and caesarean sections indicate the presence of pregnancy complications, but the only specific complication which occurs in statistically significant excess is antepartum bleeding.

Outcome after Maternal use of Thyroid Drugs

Infant Sex

After maternal use of thyroid hormones in early pregnancy, there were 6 184 male and 5 807 female infants born (three with unknown sex).The sex ratio was normal, 1.06

(95% CI 1.03-1.10). After later use, there were 4 200 male and 4 150 female infants (two with unknown sex), sex ratio 1.02 (95% CI 0.98-1.06). After maternal use of thyreostatics in early pregnancy there were 144 male and 132 infants born, sex ratio 1.09 (95% CI 0.86-1.38), and after later use 83 male and 88 female infants, sex ratio 0.94 (95% CI 0.70-1.27).

Table 35.6. Some maternal diagnoses associated with the use of thyroid drugs

Diagnosis	Drug use in early pregnancy			Drug use later in pregnancy		
	Number	OR/RR	95% CI	Number	OR/RR	95% CI
Thyroid hormones						
Pre-existing diabetes	479	2.58	2.35-2.82	326	2.40	2.15-2.68
Chronic hypertension	253	1.39	1.22-1.58	185	1.40	1.20-1.62
Gestational diabetes	176	1.27	1.09-1.48	116	1.19	0.99-1.43
Preeclampsia	785	1.35	1.25-1.45	553	1.32	1.21-1.45
Hyperemesis gravidarum	186	1.25	1.07-1.44	130	1.79	1.00-1.43
Placenta previa	205	1.20	1.04-1.38	141	1.14	0.96-1.35
Abruptio placentae	211	1.17	1.02-1.35	144	1.10	0.93-1.30
Antepartum bleeding	235	1.22	1.07-1.40	153	1.14	0.90-1.34
Intrapartum bleeding	367	1.20	1.08-1.33	255	1.10	0.97-1.25
Postpartum bleeding	726	1.05	0.98-1.14	509	1.07	0.98-1.17
Delivery induction	1664	1.27	1.21-1.34	1207	1.28	1.20-1.36
Caesarean section	2588	1.29	1.23-1.35	1849	1.26	1.20-1.33
Thyreostatics						
Pre-existing diabetes	8	2.19	0.94-2.31#	4	1.70	0.46-4.36#
Preeclampsia	15	1.29	0.75-2.23#	7	0.95	0.38-1.96#
Abruptio placentae	6	1.70	0.62-3.70#	2	0.91	0.11-3.30#
Antepartum bleeding	9	2.36	1.08-4.47#	5	2.18	0.77-5.10#
Intrapartum bleeding	10	1.67	0.80-3.80#	7	1.82	0.73-3.76#
Postpartum bleeding	15	1.03	0.61-1.75	10	1.12	0.54-2.05#
Delivery induction	38	1.37	0.96-1.96	31	1.90	1.29-2.82
Caesarean section	61	1.55	1.16-2.08	40	1.66	1.15-2.39

#observed over expected number with exact Poisson 95% confidence interval.

Multiple Births

After maternal use of thyroid hormones in early pregnancy, there were 223 twin deliveries and three triplet deliveries. The odds ratio for twinning was 1.16 (95% CI 1.02-1.33). After later exposure there were 156 twins and two triplet deliveries, OR for twinning was 1.21 (95% CI 1.03-1.42). The increased twinning rate indicates an association with infertility treatment.

After the use of thyreostatics in early pregnancy, there were eight twin deliveries, RR = 1.90 (95% CI 0.82-3.75) and after later use five twin deliveries, RR = 2.05 (95% CI 0.67-4.78).

No increased perinatal mortality risk was thus seen.

Table 35.7. Infant mortality after maternal use of thyroid drugs

Variable studied	Drug use in early pregnancy			Drug use later in pregnancy		
	Number	OR7RR	95% CI	Number	OR/RR	95% CI
Thyroid hormones						
Stillbirth	45	1.06	0.79-1.43	13	0.97	0.52-1.66
Early neonatal death	19	1.04	0.66-1.64	9	0.74	0.34-1.40
Thyreostatics						
Stillbirth	3	3.30	0.68-9.64#	1	-	-
Early neonatal death	0	-	-	0	-	-

#observed over expected number with exact Poisson 95% confidence interval.

Table 35.8. Pregnancy duration and infant birth weight at maternal use of thyroid drugs

Variable studied	Drug use in early pregnancy			Drug use later in pregnancy		
	Number	OR/RR	95% CI	Number	OR/RR	95% CI
Thyroid hormones						
<37 weeks	683	1.24	1.14-1.34	455	1.18	1.07-1.30
<2500g	393	1.13	1.02-1.25	281	1.16	1.02-1.31
≥4500g	541	0.99	0.91-1.08	385	1.02	0.92-1.14
SGA	262	1.17	1.04-1.33	199	1.27	1.10-1.47
LGA	936	1.13	1.05-1.21	663	1.16	1.07-1.26
Thyreostatics						
<37 weeks	17	1.40	0.85-2.31	11	1.38	0.69-2.46#
<2500g	18	2.41	1.48-3.92	8	1.56	0.67-3.07#
≥4500g	9	0.75	0.38-1.45	5	0.76	0.25-1.77#
SGA	10	2.01	0.96-3.70#	3	0.95	0.20-2.78#
LGA	13	0.68	0.39-1.20	10	0.98	0.51-1.89#

#observed over expected number with exact Poisson 95% confidence interval.

There is thus an increased risk for preterm birth, intrauterine growth retardation, and low birth weight after maternal use of thyroid drugs. There is also an increased risk for LGA. All effects remained basically unchanged after exclusion of women with diabetes from the analysis. The OR for LGA, for instance, was then 1.10 (95% CI 1.03-1.18). Similar effects were seen after use of thyreostatics but the only OR which reached statistical significance was for birth weight <2500g.

The only clearly significantly increased risks after use of thyroid hormones were for hypoglycaemia and for jaundice. If women with a diagnosis of diabetes were removed from the analysis, the increased risk for hypoglycaemia disappeared (OR = 0.94, 95% CI 0.85-1.04, after early use and OR = 0.86, 95% CI 0.76-0.98 after later use). The increased risk for jaundice after early exposure decreased but remained significant: OR = 1.10. 95% CI 1.01-1.20.

Removal of women with a diabetes diagnosis from the analysis of hypoglycaemia in infants exposed to thyreostatics reduced the OR to 1.49 (95% CI 0.82-2.51) after early exposure and to 1.88 (95% CI 0.94-3.36) after later exposure. The remaining effects can thus be random.

Table 35.9. Neonatal diagnoses after maternal use of thyroid drugs

Diagnosis	Drug use in early pregnancy			Drug use later in pregnancy		
	Number	OR/RR	95% CI	Number	OR/RR	95% CI
Thyroid hormones						
Hypoglycaemia	623	1.41	1.30-1.53	401	1.29	1.16-1.42
Respiratory diagnoses	635	1.06	0.98-1.15	420	1.05	0.95-1.16
Low Apgar score	248	1.07	0.94-1.21	161	1.06	0.90-1.24
CNS diagnoses	85	1.05	0.85-1.31	54	0.90	0.69-1.18
Jaundice	584	1.20	1.10-1.30	404	1.16	1.05-1.28
Thyreostatics						
Hypoglycaemia	17	1.75	1.02-2.80#	13	2.15	1.14-3.67#
Respiratory diagnoses	15	1.17	0.69-1.98	5	0.65	0.21-1.52#
Low Apgar score	4	0.82	0.22-2.11#	5	1.57	0.51-3.67#
CNS diagnoses	3	1.90	0.39-5.55#	1	-	-
Jaundice	12	1.12	0.62-2.00	14	2.01	1.10-3.38#

#observed over expected number with exact Poisson 95% confidence interval.

Table 35.10. Congenital malformations in infants whose mothers had used thyroid hormones in early pregnancy

Congenital malformation	Number	OR/RR	95% CI
All malformation	624	1.12	1.04-1.22
Relatively severe malformation	452	1.19	1.08-1.19
Chromosome anomalies	39	1.43	1.04-1.98
Among them Down syndrome	27	1.47	1.00-2.16
Without chromosome anomalies			
Any CNS malformation	20	1.52	0.97-2.36
Neural tube defects	5	1.15	0.37-2.68#
Eye malformations	10	0.99	0.53-1.85
Ear malformations	21	0.77	0.49-1.20
Orofacial clefts	24	1.10	0.73-1.66
Median cleft palate	14	1.54	0.84-2.58#
Cleft lip/palate	10	0.72	0.39-1.36#
Any cardiovascular defect	153	1.18	1.00-1.38
VSD and/or ASD	83	1.19	0.95-1.48
Unspecified cardiac defects	13	1.13	0.65-1.98
Pylorostenosis	10	1.21	0.58-2.22#
Oesophageal atresia	5	1.42	0.46-3.32#
Small gut atresia	3	0.99	0.20-2.90#
Anal atresia	9	1.97	0.90-3.75#
Hypospadias	50	1.48	1.12-1.96
Severe kidney malformations	13	1.71	0.91-2.93#
Pes equinovarus	20	1.20	0.87-1.87
Hip (sub)luxation, unstable hip	88	1.18	0.95-1.46
Poly/syndactyly	21	0.86	0.56-1.33
Limb reduction defects	8	1.62	0.70-3.20#
Body wall defects	5	1.96	0.64-4.58#
Diaphragmatic hernia	4	1.42	0.39-3.63#
Craniostenosis	5	0.66	0.22-1.55#

#observed over expected number with exact Poisson 95% confidence interval.

There is thus an increased risk for a chromosome anomaly. In this analysis, adjustment for maternal age was only made using 5-year age classes. The analysis was repeated with one-year age classes. The OR for any chromosome anomaly then decreased to 1.30 (95% CI 0.95-1.79) and for Down syndrome to 1.33 (95% CI 0.95-1.95). Statistical significance was thus lost but the odds ratios were still elevated.

Among neural tube defects, there were two infants with anencephaly and three with spina bifida. There is a seemingly different effect on median cleft palate and cleft lip/palate but this may be random.

The analysis was repeated for relatively severe malformations after exclusion from the analysis of women who had a diagnosis of diabetes or had reported the use of drugs for immunological bowel disease, insulin, beta-blocking agents, systemic corticosteroids, neuroleptics, sedatives, hypnotics, or drugs for asthma. These exclusions reduced the odds ratio estimate slightly and widened the confidence interval (OR = 1.16, 95% CI 1.05-1.28). The same effect was seen on the risk for any cardiovascular defect (OR = 1.14, 95% CI 0.96-1.36) and hypospadias (OR = 1.42, 95% CI 1.05-1.92).

Table 35.11. Congenital malformations in infants born after maternal use of thyreostatics in early pregnancy

Congenital malformation	Number	OR/RR	95% CI
All malformation	17	1.39	0.84-2.30
Relatively severe malformation	14	1.62	0.89-2.73#

#observed over expected number with exact Poisson 95% confidence interval.

A list of the 14 infants with relatively severe malformations and the drugs used is given in Table 35.12.

Table 35.12. Specification of relatively severe congenital malformations and drugs used after maternal use of thyreostatics

Congenital malformation	Thyreostatic	Other drugs
Ventricular septum defect	thiamazole, propylthiouracil	
Atrium septum defect + pulmonary valve stenosis	propylthiouracil	propranolol
Choanal atresia	thiamazole	thyroxine, prednisolone
Oesophageal atresia+ventricular septum defect+aorta malformation	thiamazole	
Ileum atresia	thiamazole	
Pylorostenosis	propylthiouracil	
Meckel diverticle	thiamazole	
Hydronephrosis	thiamazole	iron
Polydactyly	thiamazole	thyroxine, terfenadine
Accessory thum	thiamazole	clomipramine
Accessory finger	thiamazole	thyroxine
Omphalocele	propylthiouracil	iron, cefadroxil
Gastroschisis	thiamazole	thyroxine, terbutaline
Craniostenosis	propylthiouracil	metoprolol, sucralfate

There is thus no statistically significant increase in malformation risk but two of the infants have malformations which have been linked to the use of thyreostatics, choanal atresia and oesophageal atresia.

Summary

Women using thyroxine (most of which have autoimmune thyroiditis) often have other pathology, notably diabetes and immunological bowel disease. There are disturbances in pregnancy and neonatal outcome with an excess of both preterm delivery, SGA and LGA, apparently independent of the co-morbidity with diabetes. There is an increased risk for neonatal jaundice and hypoglycaemia, but the latter is completely explained by co-morbidity with diabetes. There is a moderate increase in the rate of congenital malformations which cannot be explained by co-morbidity with diabetes or use of other drugs. It is seen also for cardiac defects and for hypospadias. There is an indicated excess of chromosome anomalies but this could be random

The number of women using thyreostatics is relatively low and an observed increased risk for congenital malformations may be random. There are, however, two infants with relatively rare malformations which have been linked to the use of thyreostatics.

References

[1] Norstedt Wikner B, Skjöldebrand Sparre L, Stiller C-O, Källén B, Asker C. Maternal use of thyroid hormones in pregnancy and neonatal outcome. *Acta Obst Gynecol* 2008; 87: 617-627.

[2] Milham S, Elledge D. Maternal methimazole and congenital defects in children. *Teratology* 1972;5:125.

[3] Clementi M, Di Gianantonio E, Pelo E, Mammi I, Brasile RT, Tenconi R. Methimazole embryopathy: delineation of the phenotype. *Am J Med Genet* 1999;83:43-6.

[4] DiGianantonio E, Schaefer C, Mastroiacovo P, Cournot MP, Benedicenti F, Reuvers M, Occupati B, Robert E, Bellemin B, Addis A, Arnon J, Clementi M. Adverse effects of prenatal methimazole exposure. *Teratology* 2001;64:262-6.

[5] Ferraris S, Valenzise M, Lerone M, Divizia MT, Rosaia L, Blaid D, Nemelka O, Ferrero GB, Silengo M. Malformations following methimazole exposure in utero: An open issue. *Birth Defects Research Part A* 2003;67:989-92.

[6] Barbero P, Ricagni C, Mercado G, Bronberg R, Torrado M. Choanal atresia associated with prenatal methimazole exposure: three new patients. *Am J Med Genet A* 2004;129:83-6.

Chapter 36

ANTIBIOTICS USED SYSTEMICALLY

A few antibiotics carry a foetal risk when used during pregnancy. Use of tetracycline drugs after the 12th week can cause discolouring of deciduous teeth and aminoglycoside use during late pregnancy can cause ototoxicity. Some categories of antibiotics, e.g., trimethoprim and quinolone derivatives should be avoided in early pregnancy but if exposure has occurred the risk is uncertain and does not motivate a discussion of a termination of pregnancy. The same is true for macrolides (notably erythromycin) and nitrofurantoin which may be associated with a moderately increased risk for cardiovacular defects but these associations are also uncertain. For penicillins and cephalosporins, no harmful effects seem to exist.

Antibiotics are commonly used during pregnancy and are generally regarded as low risk drugs with some exceptions. The analysis of the effects of antibiotics during pregnancy can be confounded by underlying infection [1]. Virus infections may damage a developing embryo and treatment of such infections or secondary bacterial infections with antibiotics can give a false association between antibiotic treatment and foetal damage. This may also be true for urinary tract infections.

Use of tetracycline after week 12 is associated with discolouring and disfiguring of deciduous teeth [2] and use of aminoglycosides, notably streptomycin, dihydrostreptomycin and kanamycin, with inner ear toxicity [3]. Due to its effect on folic acid, use of trimethoprim in early pregnancy has been regarded as a hazard but evidence for it is weak [4]. Most studies on various forms of penicillin have found no signs of teratogenicity [5-8]. An association between maternal use of erythromycin in early pregnancy and an increased risk for congenital heart defects has been suggested [9,10] but not verified [8], and a similar effect of nitrofurantoin [9] was also seen. A small study of newer macrolides [11]found no teratogenic effect but had little power to show an effect similar to that postulated for erythromycin. Quinolone derivatives have been implicated in the origin of bone malformations [12]. Two studies, both limited in size, found no teratogenic effect [13,14] Positive effects of antibiotic use have also been described, a reduced rate of preterm births after first trimester use of ampicillin or clotrimazole [15].

Table 36.1. Number of women identified using antibiotics

Total	63 785
Reported use in early pregnancy	33 823
Got prescription later in pregnancy	33 341
Both early and later use	3 379

Type of drug	ATC code	Early use	Later use
Tetracyclines	J01A	1756	223
Doxycycline	J01AA02	1049	140
Chlortetracycline	J01AA03	0	1
Lymecycline	J01AA04	394	49
Metacycline	J01AA05	2	0
Oxytetracycline	J01AA06	23	2
Tetracycline	J01AA07	245	28
Unspecified	J01A	49	3
Amphenicols	J01B	9	2
Chloramphenicol	J01BA01	9	2
Penicillins with extended spectrum	J01CA	4837	5572
Ampicillin	J01CA01	72	30
Amoxicillin	J01CA04	1817	2269
Pivmecillinam	J01CA08	2365	2763
Mecillinam	J01CA11	588	560
Beta-lactamase sensitive penicillin	J01CE	12309	11889
Benzylpenicillin	J01CE01	6	9
Phenoxymethylpenicillin	J01CE02	12297	11864
Unspecified	J01CE	8	22
Beta-lactamase resistant penicillin	J01CF	758	650
Dicloxacillin	J01CF01	29	15
Cloxacillin	J01CF02	4	2
Flucloxacillin	J01CF05	727	634
Penicillin and enzyme inhibitor	J01CR	139	80
Amoxicilllin	J01CR02	138	80
Piperacillin	J01CR05	1	0
Cephalosporins	J01D	2278	3288
Cefalexin	J01DB01	174	302
Cefadroxil	J01DB05	1869	2705
Cefuroxime	J01DC02	123	194
Loracarbef	J01DC08	74	50
Cefotaxime	J01DD01	9	5
Ceftazidime	J01DD02	6	3
Ceftriaxone	J01DD04	2	3
Ceftibuten	J01DD14	54	100
Cefepime	J01DE01	1	0
Monobactams	J01DF	1	3
Aztreonam	J01DF01	1	3
Trimethoprim and sulfonamides	J01E	940	263
Trimethoprim	J01EA01	876	247
Trimethoprim and sulfamethoxasole	J01EE01	53	15
Trimethoprim and sulfadiazeine	J01EE02	3	0
Unspecified	J01E	8	1
Macrolides	J01F	3116	4174
Erythromycin	J01FA01	2504	2751
Spiramycin	J01FA02	6	4

Type of drug	ATC code	Early use	Later use
Roxithromycin	J01FA06	25	20
Clarithromycin	J01FA09	56	4
Azithromycin	J01FA10	54	29
Telitromycin	J01FA15	0	1
Clindamycin	J01FF01	508	1405
Lincomycin	J01FF02	1	1
Unspecified	J01FA	0	1
Aminoglycosides	J01G	6	1
Tobramycin	J01GB01	1	0
Gentamicin	J01GB03	4	1
Netilmicin	J01GB07	1	0
Quinolone derivates	J01M	1002	180
Ofloxacin	J01MA01	7	1
Ciprofloxacin	J01MA02	155	27
Enoxacin	J01MA04	1	0
Norfloxacin	J01MA06	831	135
Levofloxacin	J01MA12	4	12
Moxifloxacin	J01MA14	7	6
Other antibiotics	J01X	5650	10963
Vancomycin	J01XA01	10	4
Fusidic acid	J01XC01	4	0
Metronidazole	J01XD01	507	242
Tinidazole	J01XD02	17	0
Nitrofurantoin	J01XE01	4878	10587
Methenamine	J01XX05	269	202

Use of more than one antibiotic class during early pregnancy occurred in 1819 women and during later part of the pregnancy in 2113 women. Two different antibiotics were used by 1717 women in early pregnancy, three by 96, and four by six. In later pregnancy, the corresponding numbers were 1944, 161, and eight.

Characteristics of Women using Antibiotics

Based on women reporting the drug in early pregnancy (n=33 819, four with unknown maternal age). Each variable is adjusted for all other variables and year of delivery. Comparison with all women who gave birth during the period and with information from the first antenatal care (n=967 742). The odds ratios for maternal age, parity, smoking in early pregnancy, number of previous miscarriages, BMI, subfertility, and country of birth are adjusted for all other variables and are shown in Figure 36.1.

Some further maternal characteristics were analyzed, adjusting for year of delivery, maternal age, parity, smoking, and BMI (Table 36.2).

Maternal characteristics may well vary with the type of disease for which antibiotics were used. One main indication is urinary tract infections, to a large extent treated either with pivmecillinam/mecillinam or with nitrofurantoin. If maternal characteristics were compared between users of these two drugs against all other antibiotics, some differences were seen, reasonably associated with the risk for urinary tract infection (Table 36.3).

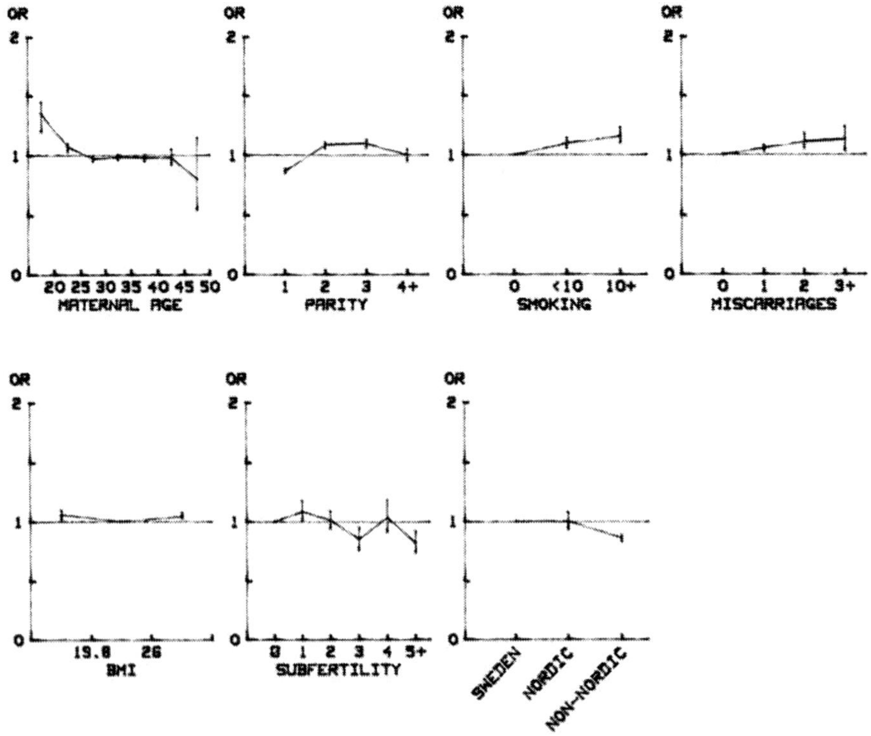

Figure 36.1. Odds ratios for seven maternal characteristics. The odds ratios (OR) for each variable are adjusted for the other variables and year of delivery. Vertical lines mark 95% confidence intervals. For maternal age and parity, each class is compared with all other classes.

Table 36.2. Some further characteristics of women using antibiotics in early pregnancy

Variable studied	Number	OR	95% CI
Education (1996-2001, 18 066 women with drugs, 526 695 in population)			
Unknown	470	-	-
<12 years	2020	0.90	0.85-0.95
12 years	9230	1.00	reference
13-14 years	954	1.00	0.93-1.07
>14 years	5392	1.07	1.03-1.11
Family situation			
Unknown	624	-	-
Co-habiting	31057	1.00	reference
Living alone	1030	1.15	1.08-1.23
Other family situation	1108	1.25	1.16-1.24
Work outside home			
Unknown	4596	-	-
Full time	15360	1.00	reference
Part time	8410	1.01	0.98-1.04
None	5453	0.89	0.86-0.92

Table 36.3. Maternal characteristics for women using antibiotics for urinary tract infections or other antibiotics

Variable studied	Pivmecillinam/nitrofurantoin			Other antibiotics		
	Number	OR	95% CI	Number	OR	95% CI
Maternal age <25 years	1570	1.36	1.28-1.45	4092	1.04	1.01-1.08
Parity 1	3928	1.33	1.27-1.40	9788	0.76	0.74-0.78
Any smoking	828	0.96	0.84-1.11	3430	1.19	1.11-1.27
Any previous miscarriage	1674	1.18	1.11-1.15	5694	1.04	1.01-1.07
Education <12 years	404	1.08	0.96-1.21	1616	0.86	0.81-0.91
Country of birth outside						
Nordic countries	1363	1.14	1.08-1.21	3274	0.78	0.75-0.81
Not working outside home	1466	1.12	1.05-1.20	3987	0.83	0.80-0.86

Note that a proportion of the "other antibiotics" may have been prescribed for urinary tract infections which would reduce the differences between then two groups.

Table 36.4. Concomitant drug use (early pregnancy)

Drug group	Number	OR	95% CI
Drugs for stomach ulcer and reflux	450	1.55	1.41-1.71
Drugs for inflammatory bowel disease	84	0.94	0.75-1.17
Insulin	90	0.74	0.60-0.91
Multivitamins	1755	0.71	0.68-0.75
Folic acid	1349	0.76	0.72-0.81
Antihypertensives	108	0.87	0.71-1.05
Oral contraceptives	142	1.29	1.09-1.52
Progestogens	120	0.85	0.71-1.02
Gonadotropins	65	0.81	0.63-1.04
Systemic corticosteroids	224	1.84	1.62-2.10
Thyroid drugs	365	0.82	0.74-0.91
NSAIDs	838	1.49	1.39-1.60
Opioids	404	2.36	2.13-2.60
Minor analgesics	3291	1.30	1.26-1.35
Drugs for migraine	90	0.96	0.78-1.19
Anticonvulsants	63	0.64	0.50-0.82
Sedatives, hypnotics	195	1.30	1.13-1.50
Antidepressants	378	0.95	0.85-1.05
Drugs for rhinitis	1591	3.77	3.59-3.97
Antiasthmatics	1267	1.20	1.13-1.27
Cough medicine	1031	7.42	6.99-7.89
Antihistamines	2204	1.13	1.08-1.18
For NVP	1568	1.04	0.99-1.09
For allergy	718	1.37	1.27-1.48

As can be expected there is a strong association for drugs given at upper respiratory infections, asthma, and urinary tract infections, including analgesics. Less expected is an association with oral contraceptives and with sedatives and hypnotics.

Table 36.5. Some maternal diagnoses associated with the use of antibiotics

Diagnosis	Drug use in early pregnancy			Drug use later in pregnancy		
	Number	OR	95% CI	Number	OR	95% CI
Pre-existing diabetes	407	0.93	0.85-1.04	479	1.03	0.94-1.13
Chronic hypertension	379	0.99	0.89-1.10	489	1.17	1.07-1.28
Gestational diabetes	327	1.08	0.97-1.21	345	1.08	0.97-1.20
Preeclampsia	1569	1.05	1.00-1.11	1698	1.14	1.08-1.19
Hyperemesis gravidarum	357	1.08	0.97-1.21	486	1.12	1.01-1.24
Placenta previa	387	1.05	0.95-1.16	423	1.04	0.95-1.15
Abruptio placentae	439	1.08	0.98-1.19	467	1.04	0.94-1.14
Antepartum bleeding	497	1.09	1.00-1.20	474	1.02	0.93-1.12
Intrapartum bleeding	718	1.07	0.99-1.15	776	1.05	0.98-1.13
Postpartum bleeding	1914	1.01	0.97-1.06	1904	1.07	1.02-1.13
Delivery induction	3983	1.14	1.10-1.18	4151	1.18	1.14-1.22
Caesarean section	5641	1.10	1.06-1.13	5589	1.08	1.04-1.11

There are thus no strong effects of antibiotic use on any of the pregnancy diagnoses studied but they all have a tendency to have odds ratios slightly above 1. Delivery induction and caesarean section rates are significantly increased both after early and later exposure. These variables were therefore analyzed for pivmecillinam/nitrofurantoin (urinary tract infections) and for other antibiotics (Table 36.6).

Table 36.6. Risk for delivery induction and caesarean section among women who used antibiotics for urinary tract infections or other antibiotics

Drugs used	Delivery induction			Caesarean section		
	Number	OR	95% CI	Number	OR	95% CI
Early exposure						
pivmecillinam/nitrofurantoin	1005	1.26	1.18-1.35	1405	1.20	1.11-1.45
other antibiotics	2978	1.10	1.06-1.15	4236	1.07	1.03-1.10
Later exposure						
pivmecillinam/nitrofurantoin	1730	1.24	1.17-1.30	2421	1.14	1.09-1.19
other antibiotics	2277	1.12	1.07-1.17	3312	1.05	1.01-1.09

The effects are stronger after the antibiotics used for urinary tract infections than after other antibiotics (some of which may have been used for such infections) which suggests that the effects are due to the infections.

Outcome after Maternal use of Antibiotics

Infant Sex

After early exposure to antibiotics, 17 264 male and 16 681 female infants were born (13 with unknown sex), sex ratio 1.06 (95% CI 1.03.1.08). After later exposure, there were 17 387 male and 16 431 female infants (11 with unknown sex), sex ratio 1.06 (95% CI 1.04-1.08). Both sex ratios are thus exactly normal.

Multiple Births

After early exposure to antibiotics, there were 480 twin deliveries, eight triplet deliveries, and one quadruplet delivery. The odds ratio for twinning was 0.95 (95% CI 0.87-1.05). After later exposure, there were 477 twin and three triplet deliveries, OR for twinning = 0.97 (95% CI 0.88-1.06).

Table 36.7. Infant mortality after maternal use of antibiotics

Variable studied	Drug use in early pregnancy			Drug use later in pregnancy		
	Number	OR	95% CI	Number	OR	95% CI
Stillbirth	98	0.86	0.70-1.05	89	0.81	0.65-1.00
Early neonatal death	49	0.97	0.73-1.30	37	0.73	0.53-1.02

Restriction of the analysis to women who had used pivmecillinam/mecillinam or nitrofurantoin resulted in no statistically significant odds ratios.

Table 36.8. Pregnancy duration and infant birth weight at maternal use of antibiotics

Variable studied	Drug use in early pregnancy			Drug use later in pregnancy		
	Number	OR	95% CI	Number	OR	95% CI
<37 weeks	1676	1.04	0.99-1.10	1517	0.96	0.91-1.02
<2500g	1046	1.02	0.96-1.09	941	0.95	0.89-1.01
≥4500g	1416	1.01	0.96-1.07	1454	1.01	0.96-1.07
SGA	716	1.03	0.96-1.11	603	0.91	0.84-0.99
LGA	2111	1.00	0.96-1.05	2313	1.05	1.01-1.10

Table 36.9. Neonatal diagnoses after maternal use of antibiotics

Diagnosis	Drug use in early pregnancy			Drug use later in pregnancy		
	Number	OR	95% CI	Number	OR	95% CI
Hypoglycaemia	1190	0.98	0.92-1.04	1178	1.02	0.96-1.08
pivmecillinam/nitrofurantoin	357	1.27	1.14-1.42	534	1.14	1.05-1.25
other antibiotics	833	0.89	0.83-0.96	644	0.93	0.86-1.01
Respiratory diagnoses	1748	1.04	0.99-1.09	1513	0.97	0.92-1.02
pivmecillinam/nitrofurantoin	425	1.13	1.02-1.24	658	1.04	0.96-1.13
other antibiotics	1323	1.01	0.96-1.07	855	0.93	0.86-0.99
Low Apgar score	687	1.05	0.97-1.13	569	0.99	0.91-1.07
pivmecillinam/nitrofurantoin	172	1.17	1.00-1.36	256	1.07	0.94-1.22
other antibiotics	515	1.01	0.92-1.10	313	0.93	0.83-1.04
CNS diagnoses	209	1.05	0.91-1.20	209	1.05	0.91-1.21
pivmecillinam/nitrofurantoin	57	1.13	0.86-1.49	101	1.22	1.00-1.49
other antibiotics	152	1.02	0.87-1.20	108	0.93	0.77-1.13
Jaundice	1419	1.04	0.99-1.20	1338	1.02	0.96-1.07
pivmecillinam/nitrofurantoin	375	1.16	1.05-1.29	601	1.11	1.02-1.21
other antibiotics	1044	1.00	0.95-1.07	737	0.95	0.88-1.02

The odds ratio for preterm birth after early pregnancy use of pivmecillinam/mecillinam or nitrofurantoin (444 preterm births) was 1.19 (95% CI 1.08-1.31), after early use of other antibiotics (644 preterm births) 1.00 (95% CI 0.94-1.06). In the literature, it has been suggested that use of ampicillin could reduce the risk for preterm birth. Only few such exposures were included but an analysis of all penicillins with extended spectrum when used in early pregnancy (259 preterm births) gave an OR = 1.11 (95% CI =0.98-1.26) and after later use (277 preterm births) an OR = 1.03 (95% CI 0.92-1.17). These data do not favour the mentioned hypothesis.

For the total material of antibiotics, there are no statistically significant effects on the neonatal diagnoses studied, but at least for hypoglycaemia, respiratory diagnoses and low Apgar score (after early exposure), and jaundice, risks after maternal use of drugs for urinary tract infections are increased and higher than those after maternal use of other antibiotics.

Table 36.10. Congenital malformations in infants whose mothers had used antibiotics in early pregnancy

Congenital malformation	Number	OR	95% CI
All malformation	1695	1.05	1.00-1.10
Relatively severe malformation	1178	1.06	1.00-1.12
Chromosome anomalies	64	0.97	0.75-1.24
Without chromosome anomalies			
Any CNS malformation	51	1.20	0.90-1.60
Neural tube defect	16	1.19	0.71-2.01
Eye malformations	43	1.27	0.94-1.72
Ear malformations	70	0.87	0.69-1.11
Orofacial clefts	60	0.95	0.73-1.23
Any cardiovascular defect	396	1.09	0.98-1.21
VSD and/or ASD	202	1.06	0.92-1.22
Pylorostenosis	31	1.20	0.83-1.74
Oesophageal atresia	10	0.97	0.50-1.89
Small bowel atresia	9	1.07	0.49-2.03#
Anal atresia	16	1.24	0.75-2.05
Hypospadias	103	1.06	0.87-1.29
Abdominal wall defect	13	1.45	0.77-2.48#
Diaphragmatic hernia	5	0.69	0.22-1.60#
Kidney agenesis/dysgenesis	10	1.02	0.49-1.88#
Cystic kidney	8	0.61	0.31-1.22
Pes equinovarus	61	1.26	0.97-1.63
Hip (sub)luxation, unstable hip	218	1.03	0.90-1.18
Poly/syndactyly	72	1.04	0.82-1.32
Limb reduction defects	21	1.05	0.68-1.62
Craniostenosis	24	1.21	0.81-1.81

#observed over expected number with exact Poisson 95% confidence interval.

Even though there was a small increase in risk for any malformation and relatively severe malformations, both with marginal statistical significance, no individual malformation type showed a significantly increased odds ratio.

The highest estimate refers to body wall defects. Among these 13 infants, three had an unspecified body wall defect, one had omphalocele, and the remaining nine cases had gastroschisis. The expected number of infants with gastroschisis after maternal exposure to antibiotics in early pregnancy is 2.8, RR = 3.26 (95% CI 1.49-6.19). Among the antibiotics used, three were unspecified (one of them penicillin), one was phenoxymethyl penicillin, one amoxicillin, one pivmecillinam, one cefadroxil, and two nitrofurantoin. This finding can well be random in spite of formal statistical significance or could be due to underlying infection – for it speaks the variation in drugs used.

In order to compare the main group of antibiotics, the odds ratios were calculated for having a relatively severe malformation and for having any cardiovascular defect (Table 37.11).

Table 36.11. Risks of relatively severe malformations or cardiovascular defects after specific antibiotics or groups of antibiotics. The total number of exposed infants is given in parenthesis after the drug name

Antibiotic category	Relatively severe malformation			Any cardiovascular defect		
	Number	OR	95% CI	Number	OR	95% CI
Tetracyclins (1771)	68	1.16	0.91-1.48	27	1.49	0.92-2.40
Penicillins						
- with extended spectrum (4925)	153	0.95	0.81-1.12	47	0.89	0.66-1.19
- β lactamase sensitive (12491)	397	0.99	0.89-1.09	135	1.02	0.86-1.21
- β lactamase resistent (764)	26	1.03	0.69-1.53	9	1.06	0.49-2.02#
- with enzyme inhibitor (139)	3	0.68	0.13-1.83#	1	-	-
Cephalosporins (2317)	90	1.21	0.98-1.50	30	1.21	0.84-1.75
Trimethoprim/sulfa (955)	32	1.02	0.72-1.46	8	0.80	0.35-1.58
Macrolides (3154)	118	1.14	0.95-1.38	51	1.54	1.17-2.04
Quinidine derivates (1014)	36	1.04	0.75-1.46	11	1.00	0.55-1.82
Other:						
Metronidazol (511)	15	0.88	0.53-1.48	4	0.77	0.21-1.57#
Nitrofurantoin (4949)	202	1.29	1.12-1.49	64	1.20	0.93-1.54
Methenamine (276)	11	1.22	0.67-2.24	1	-	-

#observed over expected number with exact Poisson 95% confidence interval

There is only one odds ratio which reaches statistical significance: cardiovascular defects after maternal use of macrolides. This association is mainly based on data for erythromycin: 42 cardiovascular defects, OR = 1.59 (95% CI 1.17-2.17). In a previous publication from the Swedish Medical Birth Register and based on data between July1 1995 and 2001, a still higher OR was found. If the present estimate is made separately for the period 1996-2001 and 2002-2006, the first period gives an OR of 1.80 (95% CI 1.23-2.64) and the second period an OR of 1.31 (95% CI 0.78-2.21). These two odds ratios may, however, both estimate the same 1.59 OR (z=0.96, p=0.25).

There is an increased risk for a relatively severe malformation after maternal use of nitrofurantoin but the effect on cardiovascular defects does not reach statistical significance. It does, however, if the analysis is restricted to ventricular or atrium septum defects: OR = 1.68 (95% CI 1.06-2.69), based on 18 cases.

Trimethoprim

Details will be given of the 32 infants with relatively severe malformations recorded after maternal use of trimethoprim and sulfamethoxasole (30 cases) or trimethoprim (2 cases).

- Corpus callosum agenesi + hydrocephalus
- Corpus callosum agenesis + hypospadias
- Congenital cataract
- Absence of punctum lacrimale
- Cleft lip and palate (2)
- Median cleft palate

- Atrium septum defect
- Ventricular septum defect (2)
- Atrium+ ventricular septum defect
- Endocardial cushion defect + pulmonary valve stenosis
- Laevocardia
- Pylorostenosis (2)
- Oesophageal atresia
- Duodenal atresia
- Anal atresia
- Unspecified body wall defect
- Hypospadias (4)
- Bilateral kidney hypoplasia + tricuspidal valve anomaly
- Cystic kidney+small bowel atresia+pulmonary artery malformation
- Hydronephrosis (2)
- Unilateral absence hand/fingers
- Pes equinovarus
- Poly/syndactyly
- Craniostenosis
- Aplasia cutis congenita

The presence of two infants with agenesis of corpus callosum is suggestive but can obviously be random. No neural tube defects occurred.

Quinolone Derivatives

Among the infants exposed to quinolone derivates in early pregnancy, two had limb reduction defects (expected number 0.6) and two had pes equinovarus (expected number 1.4), none had polydactyly or craniostenosis. An excess of skeletal malformations could thus not be verified. There was one child with a complex malformation: duodenal atresia with a spleen malformation combined with a complex cardiac defect. One infant had a syndrome associated with short statue and with an atrioventricular septal defect with a pulmonary valve stenosis.

SUMMARY

Treatment for urinary tract infections appears associated with a slightly increased risk for pregnancy and neonatal complications including preterm birth. Other antibiotic therapy appears to have little influence on pregnancy or neonatal conditions. The teratogenic risks appear small, also for trimethoprim. Two tentative associations are seen: between treatment with erythromycin and cardiac defects and treatment with nitrofurantoin and ventricular and/or atrium septum defects.

REFERENCES

[1] Li Z, Ren A, Liu J, Pei L, Zhang L, Guo Z, Li Z. Maternal flu or fever, medication use, and neural tube defects: a population-based case-control study in Northern China. *Birth Def Res (Part A)* 2007; 79: 295-300.

[2] Sánchez A, Rogers R, Sheridan PJ. Tetracycline and other tetracycline-derivative staining of the teeth and oral cavity. *Int J Dermatol* 2004; 43: 709-715.

[3] Schardein JL. *Chemially Induced Birth Defects, Revised and Expanded.* Marker Dekker Ltd, 3Rev Ed. 2000.

[4] Czeizel AE, Rockenbauer M, Sørensen HT, Olsen J. The teratogenic risk of trimethoprim-sulfonamides: a population-based case-control study. *Reprod Toxicol* 2001; 15: 637-646.

[5] Czeizel AE, Rockenbauer M, Sørensen HT, Olsen J. A population-based case-control teratologic study of ampicillin treatment during pregnancy. *Am J Obst Gynecol* 2001; 185: 140-147.

[6] Dencker BB, Larsen H, Jensen ES, Schønheyder HC, Nielsen GL, Sørensen HT. Birth outcome of 1886 pregnancies after exposure to phenoxymethylpenicillin in utero. *Clin Microbiol Infect* 2002; 8: 196-201.

[7] Jepsen P, Skriver MV, Floyd A, Lipworth L, Schønheyder HC, Sørensen HT. A population-based study of maternal use of amoxicillin and pregnancy outcome in Denmark. *Br J Pharmacol* 2003; 55:216-221.

[8] Cooper WO, Hernandez-Diaz A, Arbogast PG, Dudley JA, Dyer SM, Gideon PS, Hall KS, Kaltenbach LA, Ray WA. Antibiotics potentially used in response to bioterrorism and the risk of major congenital malformations. *Ped Perinat Epidemiol* 2008; 23: 18-28.

[9] Källén BAJ, Otterblad Olausson P. Maternal drug use in early pregnancy and infant cardiovascular defect. *Reprod Toxicol* 2003; 17: 255-261.

[10] Källén BAJ, Otterblad Olausson P, Danielsson BR. Is erythromycin therapy teratogenic in humans? *Reprod Toxicol* 2005; 20: 209-214.

[11] Bar-Oz B, Diav-Citrin O, Shechtman S, Tellem R, Arnon J, Francetic I, Berkovitch M, Ornoy A. Prgnancy outcome after gestational exposure to the new macrolides: a prospective multi-center observational study. *Europ J Obst Gynecol Reprod Biol* 2008; 141: 31-34.

[12] Wogelius P, Nørgaard M, Gisham M, Pedersen L, Schønheyder HC, Sørensen HT. Further analysis of the risk of adverse birth outcome after maternal use of fluoroquinolones. *Int J Antimicrob Agents* 2005; 26: 323-326.

[13] Schaefer C, Amoura-Elefant E, Vial T, Ornoy A, Garbis H, Robert E, Rodriguez-Pinilla E, Pexieder T, Prapas N, Merlob P. Pregnancy outcome after prenatal quinolone exposure. Evaluation of a case registry of the European Network of Teratology Information Services (ENTIS). *Eur J Obst Gynecaol Reprod Biol* 1996; 69: 83-89.

[14] Loebstein R, Addis A, Ho E, Andreou R, Sage S, Donnenfeld AE, Schick B, Bonati M, Moretti M, Lalkin A, Pastuszak A, Koren G. Pregnancy outcome following gestational exposure to fluoroquinolones: a multicenter prospective controlled study. *Antimicr Agents Chemother* 1998; 1336-1339.

[15] Czeizel A, Puhó EH, Kazy Z. The use of data set of the Hungarian case-control surveillance of congenital abnormalities for evaluation of birth outcomes beyond birth defects. *Cent Eur J Public Health* 2007; 15: 147-153.

Chapter 37

ANTIMYCOTICS USED SYSTEMICALLY

Even though high doses of fluconazole have been reported to cause a typical malformation syndrome, no information exists of the magnitude of risk. For more normal usage, for instance used at vaginal candidiasis, there seems to be no general increase in malformation risk and no association with any specific malformation type. Until more information is availabel, exposure during the first trimester should be avoided but if exposure has occurred there is no reason to discuss a termination of pregnancy. If treatment of more serious infections (e.g., coccidioidal meningitis) has occurred in early pregnancy, a teratogenic risk probably exists which may result in a discussion of a pregnancy termination.

Mainly small studies are available on the use of antimycotics during pregnancy. One such drug, griseofulvin, is a teratogen for cats but only little information is available on its use by pregnant women and it is not, at present, used in Sweden. Much interest has been paid to the possible teratogenic effect of fluconazole and other related antimycotics, based on a number of case histories. The presence of an identifiable dysmorphic phenotype has been suggested associated with high dosage therapy (400-800 mg daily) [1]: cranial synostosis, symphalangism, and long bone anomalies. One TIS study of 226 women exposed to fluconazole found no evidence for teratogenicity [2], a register-based study identified 121 women who had used fluconazole [3] and found no increase in malformation risk. This was verified in a larger similar study [4] based on 1079 exposed women. A study described 156 liveborn infants, five of them malformed, whose mothers had used itraconazole during the first trimester and had been reported to the manufacturer [5].

Table 37.1. Number of women identified using systemic antimycotics

Total	783
Reported use in early pregnancy	641
Got prescription later in pregnancy	149
Both early and later use	7

Type of drug	ATC code	Early use	Later use
Antibiotics	J02AA	12	4
Amphotericin	J02AA01	12	4
Imidazole derivates	J02AB	3	6
Ketoconazole	J02AB02	3	6
Triazole derivates	J02AC	624	138
Fluconazole	J02AC01	562	133
Itraconazole	J02AC02	62	5
Unspecified	J02A	2	2

Characteristics of Women using Systemic Antimycotics

Based on women reporting the drug in early pregnancy (n=641). Each variable is adjusted for all other variables and year of delivery. Comparison with all women who gave birth during the period and with information from the first antenatal care (n=967 742). The odds ratios for maternal age, parity, smoking in early pregnancy, number of previous miscarriages, BMI, subfertility, and country of birth are adjusted for all other variables.

Table 37.2. Maternal characteristics of women who used systemic antimycotics in early pregnancy

Variable studied	Number	OR	95% CI
Maternal age			
<25 years	77	0.69	0.34-0.88
25-34 years	554	1.00	reference
≥35 years	110	1.02	0.81-1.27
Parity			
1	325	1.35	1.14-1.60
≥2	316	1.00	reference
Smoking			
Unknown	13	-	-
No	514	1.00	reference
Yes	54	0.69	0.58-1.22
Previous miscarriage			
No	526	1.00	reference
Yes	115	0.88	0.71-1.09
BMI			
Unknown	46	-	-
<19.8	55	1.00	0.76-1.73
19.8-25.9	411	1.00	reference
≥26	129	0.77	0.63-0.93
Subfertility			
No	599	1.00	reference
Yes	42	0.84	0.61-1.15
Country of birth			
Unknown	4	-	-
Sweden	551	1.00	reference
Other Nordic country	11	0.74	0.41-1.33
Non-Nordic country	75	0.75	0.59-0.96

Some further maternal characteristics were analyzed, adjusting for year of delivery, maternal age, parity, smoking, and BMI (Table 37.3).

Table 37.3. Some further characteristics of women who used systemic antimycotics in early pregnancy

Variable studied	Number	OR	95% CI
Education (1996-2001, 316 women with drugs, 526 695 in population)			
Unknown	5		
<12 years	24	0.78	0.50-1.20
12 years	160	1.00	reference
≥13 years	127	1.12	0.88-1.42
Family situation			
Unknown	6	-	
Co-habiting	585	1.00	reference
Living alone	17	1.17	0.70-1.93
Other family situation	14	0.98	0.55-1.72
Work outside home			
Unknown	69	-	
Full time	232	1.00	reference
Part time	131	0.86	0.68-1.08
None	90	0.94	0.73-1.23

There were thus rather small deviations from expected values: an increased risk of using systemic antimycotics at first parity and a reduced risk at high BMI and among women born outside the Nordic countries.

Table 37.4. Concomitant drug use (early pregnancy)

Drug group	Number	OR/RR	95% CI
Drugs for stomach ulcer and reflux	14	2.24	1.22-3.76#
Insulin	5	2.65	0.81-6.17#
Multivitamins	26	0.83	0.57-1.21
Folic acid	20	0.69	0.44-1.08
Thyroid drugs	7	0.83	0.33-1.70#
Antibiotics	97	5.44	4.49-6.60
NSAIDs	25	1.94	1.31-2.87
Opioids	10	3.33	1.60-6.13#
Minor analgesics	40	0.72	0.69-4.82
Sedatives, hypnotics	7	2.33	0.94-4.81#
Antidepressants	8	1.03	0.44-2.02#
Drugs for rhinitis	17	1.78	1.03-2.84#
Antiasthmatics	25	1.21	0.81-1.81
Cough medicines	7	2.06	0.83-4.24#
Antihistamines	52	1.33	1.00-1.76

#observed over expected number with exact Poisson 95% confidence interval.

The association with drugs for stomach ulcer is reasonably explained by the common gastric side effects of the antimycotics, the high use of antibiotics by mixed infections. It is more difficult to understand the association with drugs used for rhinitis.

Table 37.5. Some maternal diagnoses associated with the use of systemic antimycotics

Diagnosis	Drug use in early pregnancy			Drug use later in pregnancy		
	Number	OR/RR	95% CI	Number	OR/RR	95% CI
Pre-existing diabetes	8	1.02	0.44-2.00#	3	1.47	0.30-4.30#
Chronic hypertension	6	0.87	0.32-1.90#	4	2.18	0.60-5.60#
Gestational diabetes	4	0.78	0.21-1.99#	3	2.17	0.45-6.35#
Preeclampsia	27	0.90	0.61-1.34	9	1.37	0.63-2.30#
Hyperemesis gravidarum	6	5.71	2.10-12.4#	6	3.85	1.41-8.37#
Placenta previa	5	0.73	0.24-1.70#	3	1.72	0.36-5.04#
Abruptio placentae	4	0.52	0.14-1.32#	3	1.60	0.33-4.69#
Antepartum bleeding	5	0.60	0.20-1.41#	4	2.01	0.55-5.15#
Intrapartum bleeding	14	1.05	0.61-1.81	3	0.87	0.18-2.56#
Postpartum bleeding	38	1.06	0.76-1.48	10	1.18	0.56-2.16#
Delivery induction	72	1.09	0.85-1.39	18	1.12	0.68-1.84
Caesarean section	112	1.12	0.91-1.37	28	1.15	0.76-1.74

#observed over expected number with exact Poisson 95% confidence interval.

The only marked anomaly is the association with hyperemesis. Nausea is a relatively common side effect of systemic antimycotics and may contribute to this association.

Outcome after Maternal use of Systemic Antimycotics

Infant Sex

After use of antimycotics in early pregnancy, 334 of the infants born were male and 311 female, sex ratio 1.07 (95% CI 0.92-1.25). After later use, there were 83 male and 66 female infants, sex ratio 1.26 (95% CI 0.91-1.75). The normal sex ratio (1.06) is thus contained in both confidence intervals.

Multiple Births

There were four twin deliveries after early use of systemic antimycotics. OR for twinning was 0.41 (95% CI 0.11-1.06). There were no twin deliveries after later use.

Infant Mortality

After early use of systemic antimycotics there was one stillbirth, after later use two. No early neonatal deaths occurred.

No certain deviations from expected values were thus seen.

Table 37.6. Pregnancy duration and infant birth weight at maternal use of antimycotics

Variable studied	Drug use in early pregnancy			Drug use later in pregnancy		
	Number	OR/RR	95% CI	Number	OR/RR	95% CI
<37 weeks	28	0.90	0.62-1.31	9	1.31	0.60-2.49#
<2500g	14	0.69	0.41-1.18	5	1.14	0.37-2.65#
≥4500g	24	0.94	0.62-1.43	4	0.63	0.17-1.62#
SGA	11	0.80	0.43-1.46	3	0.98	0.20-2.87#
LGA	38	1.09	0.77-1.53	6	0.62	0.23-1.35#

#observed over expected number with exact Poisson 95% confidence interval.

Table 37.7. Neonatal diagnoses after maternal use of antimycotics

Diagnosis	Drug use in early pregnancy			Drug use later in pregnancy		
	Number	OR/RR	95% CI	Number	OR/RR	95% CI
Hypoglycaemia	22	0.97	0.63-1.50	3	0.57	0.12-1.61#
Respiratory diagnoses	28	0.88	0.60-1.28	4	0.57	0.16-1.47#
Low Apgar score	9	0.77	0.40-1.48	2	0.73	0.09-2.65#
CNS diagnoses	5	1.33	0.43-3.11#	0	-	-
Jaundice	19	0.68	0.43-1.09	8	1.36	0.59-2.67#

#observed over expected number with exact Poisson 95% confidence interval.

No significant deviations in neonatal outcome were thus found.

Table 37.8. Congenital malformations in infants whose mothers had used systemic antimycotics in early pregnancy

Congenital malformation	Number	OR	95% CI
All malformation	38	1.28	0.92-1.78
Relatively severe malformation	24	1.19	0.79-1.19
Chromosome anomalies	0	-	-
Without chromosome anomalies			
Any cardiovascular defect	6	0.90	0.33-1.95#
VSD and/or ASD	5	1.40	0.45-3.27#

Among the 24 infants with relatively severe malformations, 20 were exposed to fluconazole and four to itraconazole. The OR for flucanazole was 1.13 (95% CI 0.72-1.76).

In this rather limited material, no certain teratogenic effect can be seen.

SUMMARY

The systemic use of antimycotics at the doses relevant in Sweden seems not to be associated with any major ill effects on pregnancy, delivery, or neonatal conditions, including congenital malformations. The number of exposed cases is, however, limited and associations with specific malformations cannot be excluded. The presence of five infants with ventricular septal defects may be a chance finding.

Table 37.9. Specification of relatively severe malformations and drugs use

Malformation diagnosis	Antimycotic	Other drugs
Cleft lip/palate	fluconazole	norfloxacin
Transposition of great arteries	fluconazole	
Ventricular septum defect	fluconazole	phenoxymethylpenicillin (2 cases)
Ventricular septum defect	fluconazole	
Ventricular septum defect	fluconazole	promethazine, paracetamol
Ventricular septum defect	itraconazole	valaciclovir
Ventricular septum defect	fluconazole	multivitamin, promethazine
Cong. tracheomalacia	fluconazole	
Duodenal atresia	fluconazole	unspecified penicillin
Meckel diverticle	fluconazole	terbutaline, folic acid
Megacolon	fluconazole	
Gastroschisis	fluconazole	
Testis aplasia	fluconazole	ranitidine
Intersex	fluconazole	
Polycystic kidneys	fluconazole	
Polycystic kidneys	fluconazole	paracetamol
Hydronephrosis	itraconazole	phenoxymethylpenicillin, citalopram, naproxen
Hydronephrosis	fluconazole	cough medicine
Hydronephrosis + vesicoureteral reflux	itraconazole	flupentixol
Hypospadias	itraconazole	oxymethazoline (nasal)
Hypospadias	fluconazole	multiviamin
Upper limb anomaly	fluconazole	
Pes calcaneovalgus	fluconazole	folic acid, ciprofloxacin (eye drop)

REFERENCES

[1] Lopez-Rangel E, van Allen MI: Prenatal exposure to fluconazole: an identifiable dysmorphic phenotype. *Birth Def Res (Part A)* 2005; 73: 919-923.

[2] Mastroiacovo P, Mazzone T, Botto LD, Serafini MA, Finardi A, Caramelli L, Fusco D. Prospective assessment of pregnancy outcomes after first-trimester exposure to fluconazole. *Am J Obst Gynecol* 1996; 175: 1645-1650.

[3] Sørensen HT, Nielsen GL, Olesen C, Larsen H, Steffensen FH, Schønheyder HC, Olse J, Czeizel AE. Risk of malformations and other outcomes in children exposed to fluconazole *in utero*. *Br J Clin Pharmacol* 1999; 48: 234-238.

[4] Nørgaard M, Pedersen L, Gislum M, Erichsen R, Søgaard KK, Schønheyder HC, Sørensen HT. Maternal use of fluconazole and risk of congenital malformations: a Danish population-based cohort study. *J Antimicr Chemother* 2008; 62: 172-176.

[5] Bar-Oz B, Moretti ME, Bishai R, Mareels G, van Tittelboom T, Verspeelt J, Koren G. Pregnancy outcome after in utero exposure to itraconazole: a prospective study. *Am J Obst Gynecol* 2000; 183: 617-620.

Chapter 38

TUBERCULOSTATIC DRUGS

Only limited information exists on risks with treatments for tuberculosis in early pregnancy but no clear-cut teratogenicity has been demonstrated for any of the most common drugs used with the exception of an ototoxic effect of streptomycin and related drugs. The present material adds little new information but shows no signs of any marked risk.

Table 38.1. Number of women identified using tuberculostatic drugs

Total	67
Reported use in early pregnancy	40
Got prescription later in pregnancy	36
Both early and later use	9

Type of drug	ATC code	Early use	Later use
Antibiotics	J04AB	29	17
Rifampicin	J04AB02	26	16
Rifabutin	J04AB04	3	1
Hydrazides	J04AC	33	29
Isoniazid	J04AC01	33	29
Other drugs	J04AK	19	15
Pyrazinamide	J04AK01	10	3
Ethambutol	J04AK02	14	14
Combinations	J04AM	1	0
Rifampin + isoniazid	J04AM01	1	0

Drugs from different groups were often combined:		
Antibiotic + hydrazide	12	8
Antibiotics + other	3	2
Hydrazides + other	2	4
Antibiotic + hydrazide + other	12	6

Streptomycin and kanamycin can have ototoxic effects (se Chapter 36). A summary of early studies on tuberculostatics [1] concluded that treatment with isoniazid and ethambutol seemed to carry little risk of a congenital malformation in the infant. Early studies of rifampicin showed a possible association with teratogenesis and notably with limb reduction defects [2]. The general opinion in the literature is that isoniazid, ethambutol, and rifampicin do not have a substantial teratogenic effect and can be used in early pregnancy [3].

Characteristics of Women using Tuberculostatic Drugs

As only 40 women had used such drugs in early pregnancy, a detailed analysis of characteristics could not be made. The only clear-cut deviation referred to country of origin: 30 of the 40 women with known country of birth were born outside the Nordic countries (75%, 95% CI 59-87%) in contrast to 15% among all women who gave birth.

Some of the 40 women using tuberculostatic drugs in early pregnancy also reported other drugs, most commonly pyridoxine (23 women). Two women reported use of thyroid hormones, one use of two antivirus drugs.

Most maternal diagnoses occurred in less than three cases. After early use, there were three instances of preeclampsia (RR=1.89, 95% CI 0.39-5.51). There were three inductions of delivery after later exposure (RR=0.85, 95% CI 0.18-2.4) and six caesarean sections after early exposure (RR = 1.14, 95% CI 0.42-2.48) and four after later exposure (RR = 0.84, 95% CI 0.23-2.15).

Outcome after Maternal use of Tuberculostatic Drugs

Infant Sex

After early exposure to tuberculostatic drugs, 20 male and 20 female infants were born, sex ratio 1.00 (95% CI 0.53-1.90), after later exposure there were 17 males and 18 females, sex ratio 0.94 (95% CI 0.47-1.07). Both confidence intervals thus contain the normal sex ratio of 1.06.

Multiple Births

There were no multiple births.

Infant Mortality

No infant was stillborn or died during the first week of life.

Pregnancy Duration and Infant Birth Weight at Maternal use of Tuberculostatic Drugs

After early exposure to tuberculostatic drugs, there were four preterm births (10%), RR = 2.06 (95% CI 0.57-5.33). There were two infants with low birth weight, RR = 2.50

(95% CI 0.52-7.31). There were no SGA infants. After later exposure, there were two preterm infants, RR =1.20 (95% CI 0.15-4.33) and one low birth weight infant.

Most studied neonatal diagnoses were present in only one infant. Three infants had a low Apgar score after early exposure to tuberculostatic drugs and two had jaundice. The RRs were 3.45 (95% CI 0.71-10.1) and 1.25 (95% CI 0.15-4.52), respectively.

Only one infant had a malformation diagnosis, pes equinovarus. The mother had used a combination of rifampicin, isoniazid, and ethambutol.

SUMMARY

The study material is small due to the rarity of tuberculosis in Sweden – the majority of the cases identified occurred in women born outside the Nordic countries. The small size of the material makes it impossible to exclude even drastic effects, including teratogenesis, but there were no indications of such an effect.

REFERENCES

[1] Schardein JL. *Chemically induced birth defects.* Marcel Dekker, Inc. New York and Basel. 1985, p. 375.

[2] Steen JS, Stainton.Ellis DM. Rifampicin in pregnancy. *Lancet* 1977; ii:604-605 (Letter).

[3] Brost BC, Newman RB. The maternal and foetal effects of tuberculosis therapy. *Obst Gynecol Clin North Am* 1997; 24: 659-673.

Chapter 39

ANTI-VIRUS DRUGS

Nucleosides or nucleotides mainly used for herpes infections seem to carry no risk for foetal damage. An interesting observation is a low frequence of twin deliveries. The present material contributes little to the question of a possibly teratogenic effect of antiretroviral drugs but data in the literature suggest only a low risk. Exposure in early pregnancy is therefore no reason to discuss a termination of pregnancy. Use of antiretroviral drugs in later pregnancy is important in HIV positive women in order to reduce the risk for virus transmission to the child.

Outcome of pregnancies after first trimester exposure for acyclovir has been extensively studied in a pregnancy register kept by the manufacturer [1]. There were 756 such pregnancies in the final report and among 596 liveborn infants, 19 had a congenital defect (3.2%), a rate which was regarded as normal. The types of anomalies showed no specific patterning. A small study did not observe any teratogenic effects of acyclovir [2].

The possible teratogenic risks with antiretroviral drugs used for HIV has been much discussed. Analysis of an Antiretroviral Pregnancy Registry gave 73 women exposed during the first trimester with one infant with a birth defect [3] but an analysis of Medicaid data indicated an increased risk of infant anomalies but this was not associated with first trimester exposure [4]. Case reports of malformed infants born after maternal use of antiretroviral drugs exist [5]. A larger multicentre study in US identified 880 first trimester exposures, the majority treated with zidovudine, lamivudine, or nelfonavir. No increased rate of birth defects was noticed but there were seven cases of hypospadias [6].

Combinations of drugs from different groups were common.

One woman had a combination of nucleoside/nucleotide, protease inhibitor, and nucleoside/nucleotide analogue in early and late pregnancy. A combination of protease inhibitor, nucleoside/nucleotide analogue and a combination drug was used by three women in early and two in later pregnancy. One woman used in late pregnancy a combination of nucleoside/nucleotide analogue, a non-nucleoside analogue, and a combination drug.

Table 39.1. Number of women identified using anti-virus drugs

Total	1427
Reported use in early pregnancy	955
Got prescription later in pregnancy	569
Both early and later use	97

Type of drug	ATC code	Early use	Later use
Nucleosides and nucleotides	J05AB	863	466
Aciclovir	J05AB01	524	345
Idoxuridin	J05AB02	4	0
Ribavirin	J05AB04	0	3
Famciclovir	J05AB09	4	0
Valaciclovir	J05AB11	335	124
HIV-protease inhibitors	J05AE	45	48
Saquinavir	J05AE01	2	0
Indinavir	J05AE02	4	2
Ritonavir	J05AE03	2	2
Nelfinavir	J05AE04	32	27
Lopinavir	J05AE06	7	18
Atazanavir	J05AE08	0	2
Nucleoside or nucleotide analogues	J05AF	51	64
Zidovudine	J05AF01	14	32
Didanosine	J05AF02	14	12
Zalcitabin	J05AF03	5	4
Stavudine	J05AF04	19	14
Abakavir	J05AF06	4	7
Tenofovir+disoproxil	J05AF07	2	2
Non-nucleoside analogues	J05AG	10	6
Nevirapine	J05AG01	6	5
Efavirenz	J05AG03	4	1
Neuraminidase inhibitors	J05AH	1	0
Zanamir	J05AH01	1	0
Combinations	J05AR	34	40
Unspecified	J05A	6	1

Table 39.2. Combinations of anti-virus drugs

	Nucleoside or nucleotide analogue	Non-nucleoside analogue	Combination drugs
Early pregnancy			
Protease inhibitors	16		21
Nucleoside/nucleotide analogue		6	1
Non nucleoside analogue			1
Later pregnancy			
Protease inhibitors	13		30
Nucleoside/nucleotide analogue		2	1
Non nucleoside analogue			1

CHARACTERISTICS OF WOMEN USING ANTIVIRUS DRUGS

This analysis was made on women using nucleosides or nucleotides, mainly for herpes infections. The low number of women using antiretroviral drugs made it only possible to note some characteristics.

Based on women reporting nucleosides or nucleotides in early pregnancy (n=887). Each variable is adjusted for all other variables and year of delivery. Comparison with all women who gave birth during the period and with information from the first antenatal care (n=967 742). The odds ratios for maternal age, parity, smoking early pregnancy, number of previous miscarriages, BMI, subfertility, and country of birth are adjusted for all other variables and are shown in Figure 39.1.

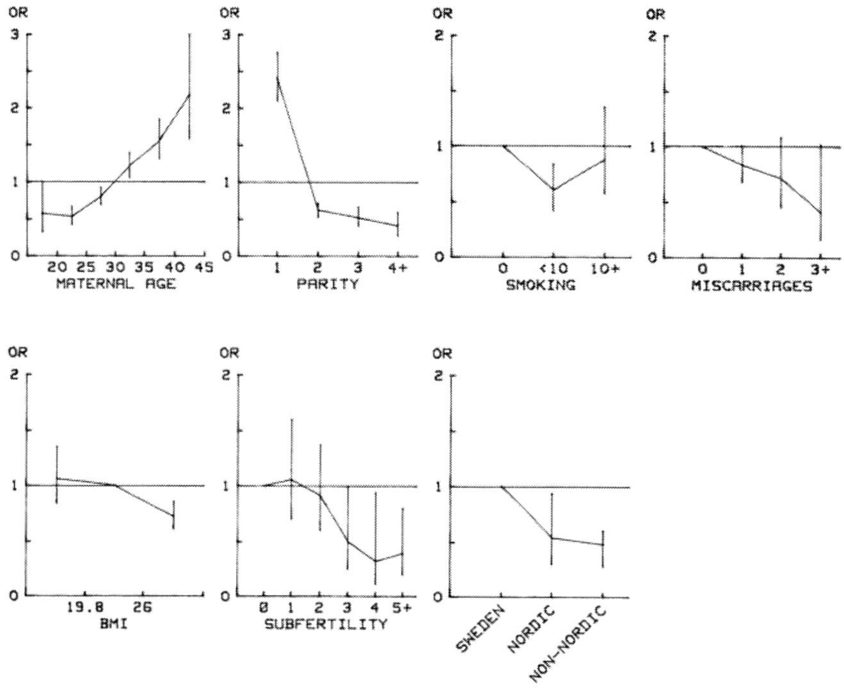

Figure 39.1. Odds ratios for seven maternal characteristics. The odds ratios (OR) for each variable are adjusted for the other variables and year of delivery. Vertical lines mark 95% confidence intervals. For maternal age and parity, each class is compared with all other classes.

Some further maternal characteristics were analyzed, adjusting for year of delivery, maternal age, parity, smoking, and BMI (Table 39.2).

Women who had used antiretroviral drugs in early pregnancy (n=68) were older than expected (OR for 35 years or more = 1.98, 85% CI 3.25). There was a strong excess of women born outside the Nordic countries: n=57 (84%) and five women lived alone and five under other conditions than co-habitation. There was an excess of women who did not work outside home (OR = 2.87, 95% CI 1.52-5.42).

Table 39.3. Some further maternal characteristics of women using nucleosides or nucleotides in early pregnancy

Variable studied	Number	OR	95% CI
Education (1996-2001, 417 women with drugs, 526 695 in population)			
Unknown	10	-	-
<12 years	26	0.84	0.55-13.7
12 years	171	1.00	reference
13-14 years	44	2.00	1.45-2.76
>14 years	166	1.35	1.08-1.69
Family situation			
Unknown	14	-	
Co-habiting	819	1.00	reference
Living alone	26	1.39	0.93-2.09
Other family situation	29	1.14	0.73-1.77
Work outside home			
Unknown	103	-	
Full time	534	1.00	reference
Part time	148	0.76	0.62-0.93
None	102	0.70	0.55-0.90

Table 39.4. Concomitant drug use (early pregnancy), women using nucleosides or nucleotides

Drug group	Number	OR/RR	95% CI
Drugs for stomach ulcer and reflux	7	0.89	0.36-1.83#
Drugs for inflammatory bowel disease	4	1.40	0.38-3.51#
Multivitamins	58	0.95	0.73-1.23
Folic acid	37	0.74	0.53-1.01
Oral contraceptives	4	1.61	0.44-4.11#
Systemic corticosteroids	6	1.02	0.37-2.22
Thyroid drugs	10	0.81	0.44-1.52
Antibiotics	50	1.88	1.42-2.49
NSAIDs	27	1.63	1.11-2.39
Opioids	11	2.63	1.32-4.72
Minor analgesics	59	0.86	0.66-1.12
Neuroleptics	4	1.37	0.37-3.50
Sedatives, hypnotics	11	2.48	1.24-4.43
Antidepressants	15	1.31	0.79-2.70
Drugs for rhinitis	24	1.81	1.21-2.70
Antiasthmatics	53	2.01	1.53-2.66
Cough medicine	8	1.69	0.73-3.33#
Antihistamines	59	1.14	0.88-1.49
For NVP	35	0.89	0.60-1.25
For allergy	24	1.67	1.12-2.50

#observed over expected number with exact Poisson 95% confidence interval.

There is thus an association between nucleosides or nucleotides and antibiotics and also drugs for allergies, including asthma.

Women who used antiretroviral drugs used less than expected multivitamins and folic acid and more than expected antibiotics but numbers were low and statistical significance not reached.

Table 39.5. Some maternal diagnoses associated with the use of nucleosides and nucleotides

Diagnosis	Drug use in early pregnancy			Drug use later in pregnancy		
	Number	OR/RR	95% CI	Number	OR/RR	95% CI
Pre-existing diabetes	8	0.75	0.37-1.50	9	1.33	0.61-2.52#
Chronic hypertension	7	0.69	0.33-1.45	7	1.10	0.44-2.27#
Gestational diabetes	5	0.68	0.22-1.58#	7	1.52	0.61-3.13#
Preeclampsia	46	1.02	0.76-1.37	18	0.72	0.45-1.15
Hyperemesis gravidarum	8	1.01	0.44-1.19#	7	1.35	0.54-2.77#
Placenta previa	6	0.63	0.23-1.36#	8	1.31	0.57-2.59#
Abruptio placentae	7	0.68	0.32-1.43	10	1.52	0.73-2.39#
Antepartum bleeding	9	0.77	0.40-1.49	8	1.15	0.49-2.26#
Intrapartum bleeding	26	1.33	0.89-1.99	14	1.15	0.67-1.98
Postpartum bleeding	54	1.02	0.77-1.34	36	1.23	0.88-1.73
Delivery induction	97	1.03	0.83-1.28	60	1.07	0.82-1.41
Caesarean section	190	1.26	1.07-1.49	106	1.20	0.96-1.49

#observed over expected number with exact Poisson 95% confidence interval.

The only statistically significant excess is in caesarean sections.

Women who were treated with antiretrovirus drugs had an excess of intrapartum bleedings; RR = 3.26 (95% CI 1.20-7.10) after early exposure and 3.05 (95% CI 1.12-1.63) after later exposure. The vast majority (31 of 68 after early and 61 of 65 after later exposure) had a caesarean section.

OUTCOME AFTER MATERNAL USE OF ANTIVIRUS DRUGS

Infant Sex

Among infants born after maternal use of anti-virus drugs, sex ratio is normal. After use of nucleosides/nucleotides in early pregnancy, there were 467 male and 425 female infants born, sex ratio 1.10 (95% CI 0.96-1.25) and after later use 269 male and 243 female infants (in both groups one with unknown sex), sex ratio 1.11 (95% CI 0.93-1.36). The normal sex ratio of 1.06 is thus contained within both confidence intervals. – After antiretroviral drugs there were 37 male and 31 female infants after early exposure and 33 male and 32 female infants after later exposure. The sex ratios were 2.29 (95% CI 0.74-1.96) and 1.03 (95% CI 0.63-1.70), respectively.

Multiple Births

After early exposure for nucleosides or nucleotides there were six twin deliveries (OR 0.41, 95% CI =0.19-0.88), after later exposure also 8 twin deliveries (RR = 1.01, 95% CI 0.44-1.99). The twinning rate is thus significantly low after early exposure. No higher order births were born.

Table 39.6. Pregnancy duration and infant birth weight at maternal use of antivirus drugs

Variable studied	Drug use in early pregnancy			Drug use later in pregnancy		
	Number	OR/RR	95% CI	Number	OR/RR	95% CI
Nucleosides and nucleotides						
<37 weeks	49	1.09	0.81-1.45	13	0.52	0.30-0.89
<2500g	33	1.11	0.79-1.58	11	0.69	0.38-1.25
≥4500g	31	0.99	0.68-1.42	25	1.33	0.89-1.99
SGA	19	0.84	0.53-1.32	12	1.09	0.61-1.93
LGA	47	1.18	0.87-1.60	31	1.19	0.82-1.74
Antiretroviral drugs						
<37 weeks	6	1.84	0.68-4.01#	5	1.52	0.49-3.56#
<2500g	5	2.36	0.77-5.50#	7	3.43	1.38-7.07#
SGA	3	2.05	0.42-6.01#	5	3.85	1.25-8.98#

#observed over expected number with exact Poisson 95% confidence interval.

After nucleoside or nucleotide exposure, the only deviation is thus a reduced risk for preterm birth after later exposure. After exposure to antiretroviral drugs, the risk ratios for preterm birth, low birth weight and SGA are all high even though statistical significance is only reached for low birth weight and SGA after later exposure.

The only infant mortality is seen after early exposure to nucleosides or nucleotides. Three infants were stillborn (RR 0.91, 95% CI 0.19-2.67) and one died before the age of 7 days.

Table 39.7. Neonatal diagnoses after maternal use of anti-virus drugs

Diagnosis	Drug use in early pregnancy			Drug use later in pregnancy		
	Number	OR/RR	95% CI	Number	OR/RR	95% CI
Nucleosides and nucleotides						
Hypoglycaemia	33	0.95	0.67-1.35	14	0.73	0.43-1.23
Respiratory diagnoses	51	1.04	0.78-1.39	21	0.82	0.53-1.26
Low Apgar score	14	0.71	0.42-1.21	12	1.30	0.73-2.31
CNS diagnoses	1	-	-	6	1.34	0.64-3.80#
Jaundice	37	0.95	0.68-1.32	22	1.00	0.65-1.54
Antiretroviral drugs						
Respiratory diagnoses	3	0.91	(0.19-2.67)#	5	1.66	0.54-3.86#

#observed over expected number with exact Poisson 95% confidence interval.

No clear-cut effects were thus seen even.

Table 39.8. Congenital malformations in infants whose mothers had used nucleosides and nucleotides

Congenital malformation	Number	OR	95% CI
All malformation	39	0.87	0.63-1.20
Relatively severe malformation	24	0.79	0.53-1.18
Chromosome anomalies	0	-	-
Without chromosome anomalies			
Any cardiovascular defect	12	1.21	0.63-2.12#
VSD and/or ASD	7	1.28	0.51-2.64#
Unspecified cardiac defect	3	3.45	0.71-10.1#

The "relatively severe" malformations observed are specified in Tables 39.9-10.

Table 39.9. Relatively severe malformations occurred after three different nucleoside/nucleotide drugs

Drug	Number of infants		OR/RR	95% CI
	Malformed	Total		
Aciclovir	12	527	0.64	0.36-1.13
Famciclovir	1	4	-	-
Valaciclovir	11	337	1.02	0.56-1.86

Table 39.10. Specification of malformed infants after maternal use of nucleosides or nucleotides

Malformation	Number	Antivirus drug
Spina bifida	2	aciclovir (2)
Pulmonary valve stenosis	1	aciclovir
Ventricular septum defect	6	aciclovir (2), famciclovir (1), valaciclovir (3)
Ventricular septum defect+ polydactyly	1	valaciclovir
Patent ductus arteriosus	1	valaciclovir
Unspecified cardiac defect	3	aciclovir (1), valaciclovir (2)
Pylorostenosis	1	valaciclovir
Meckel's diverticle	1	aciclovir
Diaphragmatic hernia	1	valaciclovir
Unilateral renal agenesis	1	aciclovir
Testis aplasia	1	valaciclovir
Chondrodystrophy	1	aciclovir (also phenytoin, carbamazepine)
Pes equnovarus	1	aciclovir
Unspecified skin malformation	1	valaciclovir
Syndrome with cleft palate	1	aciclovir

The only remarkable association is between valaciclovir and cardiac defects, notably ventricular septum defects. This may well be random: RR = 2.00, 95% CI 0.80-4.12.

Only one infant had a malformation after maternal early use of anti-virus drugs against HIV: an infant with megacolon, exposed for nelfinavir.

SUMMARY

The group of nucleoside and nucleotide anti-virus drugs is mainly represented by drugs used for herpes infections. There are no signs of ill effects, neither in early, nor in later use. There are only few exposures of such drugs used for other purposes. – The number of pregnancies with use of anti-virus drugs for HIV is small but no major effects are seen. There is an indicated increase in preterm birth, low birth weight and SGA but these effects may well be due to underlying pathology.

REFERENCES

[1] Stone KM, Reiff-Eldridge R, White AD, Cordero JF, Bown Z, Alexander ER, Andrews EB. Pregnancy outcomes following systemic prenatal acyclovir exposure: conclusions from the International Acyclovir Pregnancy Registry, 1984-1999. *Birth Defects Res (Part A)* 2004; 201-207.

[2] Ratanajamit C, Vinther Skriver M, Jepsen P, Chongsuvivatwong V, Olsen J, Sørensen HT. Adverse pregnancy outcome in women exposed to acyclovir during pregnancy: a population-based observational study. *Scand J Infect Dis* 2003; 35: 244-259.

[3] White A, Eldridge R, Andrews E. Birth outcomes following zidovudine exposur in pregnant women: the Antiretroviral Pregnancy Registry. *Acta Paediatr Scand* 1997; 421: 86-88.

[4] Newschaffer CJ, Cocroft J, Anderson CE, Hauck WW, Turner BJ. Prenatal zidovudine use and congenital anomalies in a Medicaid population. *J Acquir Immune Defic Syndr* 2000; 24: 249-256.

[5] Murdaca G, Constantini S, Villa R, Setti M, Puppo F, Indiveri F. A case of transposition of the great arteries in a female infant of a HIV-1-infected woman. Potential teratogenic effects of antiretroviral drugs. *Intern Emerg Med* 2006; 1: 86-88

[6] Watts DH, Li D, Handelsman E, Tilson H, Paul M, Foca M, Vajaranant M, Diaz C, Tuomala R, Thompson B. Assessment of birth defects according to maternal therapy among infants in the women and infants transmission study. *J Acquir Immune Defic Syndr* 2007; 44: 299-305.

Chapter 40

IMMUNOGLOBULINS

Use of immunoglobulins during pregnancy appears to have no ill effects on pregnancy or neonatal diagnoses, including congenital malformations. Use of anti-Rh immunoglobulin during early pregnancy should be avoided but if exposure has occurred this does not motivate a discussion of pregnancy termination.

The main use of gammaglobulin is for hepatitis prophylaxis during travel. Only scattered observations on effects of pregnancy are available. It seems unlikely that a harmful effect could exist. The use of immunoglobulins against Rh antigen (notably before pregnancy) is an adequate way to prevent immunization in pregnancies where that risk exists.

Table 40.1. Number of women identified, treated with immunoglobulins

Total	879
Reported use in early pregnancy	774
Got prescription later in pregnancy	123
Both early and later use	18

Type of drug	ATC code	Early use	Later use
Normal gammaglobulin	J06BA	765	80
Specific immunoglobulins	J06BB	9	43
Against Rh antigen	J06BB01	5	42
Against RSV virus	J06BB02	3	0
Against hepatitis B	J06BB04	1	1

The vast majority of women had thus got normal gammaglobulin in early pregnancy or Rh-prophylaxis before delivery.

CHARACTERISTICS OF WOMEN TREATED WITH IMMUNOGLOBULINS

Based on women reporting the drug in early pregnancy (n=774). Each variable is adjusted for all other variables and year of delivery. Comparison with all women who gave birth during the period and with information from the first antenatal care (n=967

742). The odds ratios for maternal age, parity, smoking in early pregnancy, number of previous miscarriages, BMI, subfertility, and country of birth are adjusted for all other variables and are shown in Figure 40.1.

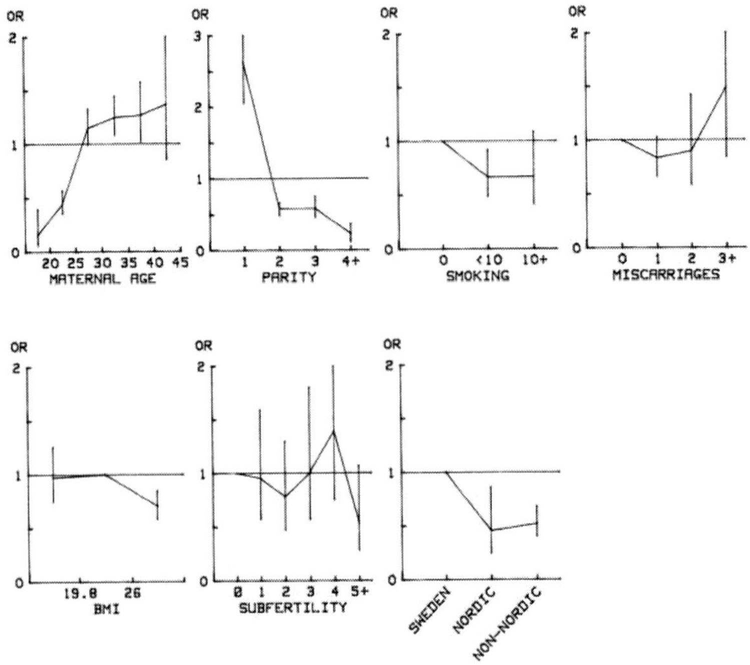

Figure 40.1. Odds ratios for seven maternal characteristics. The odds ratios (OR) for each variable are adjusted for the other variables and year of delivery. Vertical lines mark 95% confidence intervals. For maternal age and parity, each class is compared with all other classes.

Some further maternal characteristics were analyzed, adjusting for year of delivery, maternal age, parity, smoking, and BMI (Table 40.2).

Table 40.2. Some further characteristics of women treated with immunoglobulins in early pregnancy

Variable studied	Number	OR	95% CI
Education (1996-2001, 607 women with drugs, 526 695 in population)			
Unknown	9	-	-
<12 years	37	0.82	0.59-1.18
12 years	273	1.00	reference
13-14 years	40	1.32	1.11-1.59
>14 years	248	1.30	1.10-1.55
Family situation			
Unknown	12	-	
Co-habiting	739	1.00	reference
Living alone	17	0.80	0.49-1.32
Other family situation	3	0.34	0.11-1.00
Work outside home			
Unknown	80		-
Full time	483	1.00	reference
Part time	148	0.84	0.69-1.03
None	60	0.53	0.40-0.70

Women wo got immunoglubilns were thus characterized by low age and first parity. They were less often than expected smokers, of high BMI, and born outside Sweden. They more often than expected worked outside home.

Table 40.3. Concomitant drug use (early pregnancy)

Drug group	Number	OR/RR	95% CI
Drugs for stomach ulcer and reflux	5	0.81	0.26-1.89#
Multivitamins	12	0.61	0.34-1.12
Folic acid	10	0.53	0.29-0.99
Oral contraceptives	4	1.92	0.52-4.92#
Progestogens	7	1.44	0.58-2.97#
Thyroid drugs	5	0.65	0.21-1.52#
Antibiotics	33	1.32	0.94-1.52
NSAIDs	10	0.82	0.44-1.52
Minor analgesics	53	0.89	0.68-1.18
Sedatives, hypnotics	6	2.01	0.76-4.49#
Antidepressants	7	1.04	0.42-2.15#
Drugs for rhinitis	14	1.19	0.70-2.02
Antiasthmatics	29	1.23	0.85-1.78
Cough medicines	6	1.44	0.53-3.14#
Antihistamines	38	0.87	0.63-1.20

#observed over expected number with exact Poisson 95% confidence interval.

No specific associations with concomitant drugs were thus seen.

Table 40.4. Some maternal diagnoses associated with the treatment with immunoglobulins

Diagnosis	Drug use in early pregnancy		
	Number	OR/RR	95% CI
Pre-existing diabetes	6	0.72	0.26-1.57#
Chronic hypertension	6	0.83	0.30-1.83#
Gestational diabetes	6	1.02	0.38-2.22#
Preeclampsia	35	0.90	0.64-1.27
Hyperemesis gravidarum	6	0.95	0.35-2.08#
Placenta previa	6	0.84	0.31-1.82#
Abruptio placentae	8	0.98	0.42-1.93#
Antepartum bleeding	14	1.49	0.88-2.53
Intrapartum bleeding	12	0.90	0.51-1.60
Postpartum bleeding	46	1.02	0.75-1.38
Delivery induction	85	1.09	0.87-1.37
Caesarean section	116	0.94	0.77-1.15

#observed over expected number with exact Poisson 95% confidence interval.

No statistically significant associations thus appeared.

For drug use later in pregnancy, the number of diagnoses is low but no significant deviations from expected values are seen. Delivery induction occurred in 16 cases (OR =1.14, 95% CI 0.66-1.97) and caesarean section in 28 (OR =1.26, 95% CI 0.81-1.94).

Outcome after Maternal Treatment with Immunoglobulins

Infant Sex

After early use there were 389 male and 400 female infants, sex ratio = 0.97 (95% CI 0.85-1.12) and after later use 67 males and 60 female infants, sex ratio 1.12 (95% CI 0.79-1.59). The normal sex ratio (1.06) is thus included in both confidence intervals.

Multiple Births

After early use 15 twin deliveries occurred (OR = 1.36, 95% CI 0.82-2.28) and after later use four (RR = 2.02, 95% CI 0.55-5.17).

Table 40.5. Pregnancy duration and infant birth weight at maternal treatment with immunoglobulins

Variable studied	Drug use in early pregnancy			Drug use later in pregnancy		
	Number	OR/RR	95% CI	Number	OR/RR	95% CI
<37 weeks	30	0.75	0.52-1.08	7	1.17	0.47-2.40#
<2500g	19	0.73	0.47-1.16	6	1.48	0.54-3.22#
≥4500g	16	0.60	0.36-0.98	4	0.80	0.21-2.06#
SGA	17	0.87	0.54-1.41	2	0.80	0.10-2.90#
LGA	29	0.85	0.58-1.25	7	0.87	0.35-1.79#

#observed over expected number with exact Poisson 95% confidence interval.

No significant deviations were seen.

Table 40.6. Infant mortality after maternal treatment with immunoglobulins

Variable studied	Drug use in early pregnancy			Drug use later in pregnancy		
	Number	OR/RR	95% CI	Number	OR/RR	95% CI
Stillbirth	3	0.94	0.19-2.76#	1	-	-
Early neonatal death	3	2.15	0.44-6.28#	0	-	-

#observed over expected number with exact Poisson 95% confidence interval.

The high odds ratio for early neonatal death is thus based on only three cases and may well be random.

After later use of immunoglobulin, an increased risk for low Apgar score and for jaundice is seen. None of the infants with jaundice had a diagnosis indicating blood group incompatibility.

Table 40.7. Neonatal diagnoses after maternal treatment with immunoglobulins

Diagnosis	Drug use in early pregnancy			Drug use later in pregnancy		
	Number	OR/RR	95% CI	Number	OR/RR	95% CI
Hypoglycaemia	26	0.91	0.61-1.36	6	1.26	0.46-2.73#
Respiratory diagnoses	49	1.07	0.80-1.43	5	0.82	0.27-1.91#
Low Apgar score	19	1.07	0.61-1.71	7	2.93	1.18-6.02#
CNS diagnoses	3	0.82	0.22-2.10#	1	-	-
Jaundice	28	0.81	0.55-1.18	11	2.07	1.03-3.70#

#observed over expected number with exact Poisson 95% confidence interval.

Table 40.8. Congenital malformations in infants whose mothers had been treated with immunoglobulins in early pregnancy

Congenital malformation	Number	OR	95% CI
All malformation	34	0.84	0.59-1.18
Relatively severe malformation	19	0.69	0.44-1.09
Chromosome anomalies	0	-	-
Without chromosome anomalies			
Any cardiovascular defect	8	0.97	0.42-1.90#

#observed over expected number with exact Poisson 95% confidence interval.

The following relatively severe malformations were observed (table 40.9):

Table 40.9. Specification of relatively severe malformations in infants whose mothers had been treated with immunoglobulins in early pregnancy

Malformation diagnosis	Number
Encephalocele	1
Septo-optic dysplasia	1
Vitruous opacity	1
Microtia	1
TGV with atrium septum defect	1
Ventricular septum defect	1
Atrium septum defect	1
VSD, ASD, PDA, gallbladder agenesis, ectopic kidney	1
Pulmonal valve stenosis with atrium septum defect	1
Unspecified cardiovascular defect	2
Duodenal atresia	1
Diaphragmatic hernia	1
Hypospadias	1
Hydronephrosis	1
Unilateral renal hypoplasi with ureter stenosis	1
Syndactyly	1
Pes equinovarus	1
Unspecified musculoskeletal malformation	1

SUMMARY

Except for some variations which may be random, pregnancy and delivery outcome appear normal after treatment with immunoglobulins.

References

[1] Ross L. Congenital anomalies in two infants born after gestational gamma-globulin prophylaxis. *Acta Paediatr* 1995;84:1436-7.

Chapter 41

VACCINES

> Vaccines based on attenuated living viruses and used during pregnancy carry a theoretical risk for foetal damage but not even for rubella vaccines there is firm evidence that this occurs. Such vaccinations should be avoided but if they have already been given there is no reason to bring up the question of pregnancy termination. Other vaccines are unlikely to cause foetal damage. On the other hand, vaccine reactions, for instance with high fever, could be a hazard and it is therefore sensible to avoid also such vaccinations when they are not absolutely necessary. The beneficial effect of vaccinations if performed before pregnancy is obvious, notably against some viral infections which may represent pregnancy hazards, well illustrated with rubella.

Vaccines are usually given prophylactically and may prevent an infection which in itself can damage a developing embryo. Lack of adequate vaccinations can therefore represent a hazard [1]. Theoretically, the most likely risk would be with vaccines based on attenuated living viruses. The classical example is rubella which has a strong teratogenic effect in early pregnancy with a typical rubella embryopathy syndrome. Vaccination against rubella which is using living but attenuated virus will prevent rubella during pregnancy but should not be given during pregnancy because of the possibility that the attenuated virus could cause damage to the embryo. Such vaccinations will accidentally occur, however, and published studies show that the risk for the child is then small [2,3] but the number of studied women who had been vaccinated in early pregnancy is limited. Other specific vaccinations have been studied: yellow fever [4,5], smallpox [6,7], oral polio vaccine [8], anthrax [9], or tetanus toxoid [10], none was associated with a significantly increased risk for foetal damage with the possible exception of anthrax vaccine. One study followed children whose mothers had been vaccinated in connexion with travels, including vaccines for hepatitis, polio, yellow fever, meningitis, typhoid [11]. The number of studied women was limited, a total of 131, but no adverse effects were seen.

Table 41.1. Number of women identified who had been vaccinated

Total	1041
Reported use in early pregnancy	849
Got prescription later in pregnancy	195
Both early and later use	3

Type of vaccine	ATC code	Early use	Later use
Vaccines against bacterial infections	J07A	294	42
Vaccine againt cholera	J07AE	162	33
Vaccine against diphteria	J07AF	36	2
Vaccine against haemophilus	J07AG	2	2
Vaccine against pertussis	J07AJ	1	1
Vaccine against pneumococcs	J07AL	2	0
Vaccine against tetanus	J07AM	84	3
Vaccine against meningitis	J07AN	7	0
Vaccine against typhoid	J07AP	8	2
Vaccines against viral infections	J07B	590	158
Vaccine against encephalitis	J07BA	54	2
Vaccine against influenza	J07BB	122	8
Vaccine against hepatitis	J07BC	332	37
Vaccine against measles etc.	J07BD	1	0
Vaccine against parotitis	J07BE	1	0
Vaccine against polio	J07BF	68	4
Vaccine against rabies	J07BG	8	57
Vaccine against rubella	J07BJ	17	52
Vaccine against yellow fever	J07BL	7	0
Combined vaccines against bacterial and viral infections	J07CA	0	1
Vaccine against haemophilus and polio	J07CA01	0	1
Unspecified vaccines	J07	13	0

Forty-eight women had, in early pregnancy, got both a vaccine for bacterial infections and a vaccine for a viral infection. In later pregnancy five women got such a combination.

Characteristics of Women who were Vaccinated in Early Pregnancy

Based on women reporting vaccination in early pregnancy (n=849). Each variable is adjusted for all other variables and year of delivery. Comparison with all women who gave birth during the period and with information from the first antenatal care (n=967 742). The odds ratios for maternal age, parity, smoking in early pregnancy, number of previous miscarriages, BMI, subfertility, and country of birth are adjusted for all other variables and are shown in Figure 41.1.

Some further maternal characteristics were analyzed, adjusting for year of delivery, maternal age, parity, smoking, and BMI (Table 41.2).

These women thus deviate in many aspects from the general population of pregnant women: higher age, first parity, non-smoking, low proportion of women with a high BMI and of women born outside Sweden. They also have a higher education than expected and more often than expected had full-time work outside home. Many of these characteristics are reasonably associated with travel vaccinations and resemble those of women who got immunoglobulins (Chapter 40).

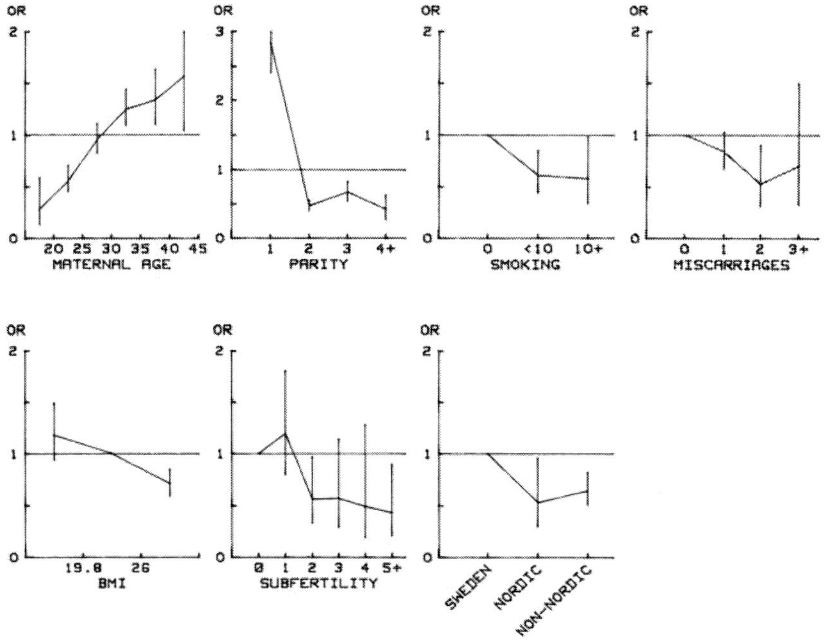

Figure 41.1. Odds ratios for seven maternal characteristics. The odds ratios (OR) for each variable are adjusted for the other variables and year of delivery. Vertical lines mark 95% confidence intervals. For maternal age and parity, each class is compared with all other classes.

Table 41.2. Further maternal characteristics of women who were vaccinated in early pregnancy

Variable studied	Number	OR	95% CI
Education (1996-2001, 518 women with vaccines, 526 695 in population)			
Unknown	13	-	-
<12 years	32	0.92	0.62-1.35
12 years	212	1.00	reference
13-14 years	40	1.52	1.08-2.14
>14 years	221	1.53	1.26-1.86
Family situation			
Unknown	8	-	
Co-habiting	805	1.00	reference
Living alone	16	0.86	0.51-1.45
Other family situation	12	0.66	0.34-1.21
Work outside home			
Unknown	88	-	
Full time	517	1.00	reference
Part time	154	0.88	0.72-1.09
None	82	0.71	0.35-0.92

Table 41.3. Concomitant drug use (early pregnancy)

Drug group	Number	OR/RR	95% CI
Drugs for stomach ulcer and reflux	4	0.54	0.15-1.38#
Insulin	4	1.35	0.37-3.44#
Multivitamins	28	0.85	0.58-1.25
Folic acid	20	0.63	0.40-0.98
Progestogens	5	0.94	0.31-2.20#
Systemic corticosteroids	5	1.37	0.44-3.19#
Thyroid drugs	14	1.34	0.79-2.26
Antibiotics	35	1.32	0.95-1.85
NSAIDs	26	1.58	1.07-2.32
Opioids	4	1.03	0.28-3.63#
Minor analgesics	65	0.94	0.73-1.21
Antidepressants	8	0.81	0.35-1.60#
Drugs for rhinitis	15	1.10	0.66-1.83
Antiasthmatics	22	0.80	0.52-1.22
Antihistamines	55	1.07	0.82-1.41

#observed over expected number with exact Poisson 95% confidence interval.

The only significant increase thus refers to NSAID – probably taken because of side effects of the vaccinations. The women used folic acid (and perhaps also multivitamins) less often than expected.

Table 41.4. Some maternal diagnoses associated with the use of vaccines

Diagnosis	Drug use in early pregnancy			Drug use later in pregnancy		
	Number	OR/RR	95% CI	Number	OR/RR	95% CI
Pre-existing diabetes	11	1.11	0.55-1.99#	3	0.90	0.19-2.64#
Chronic hypertension	7	0.76	0.30-1.56#	4	2.11	0.57-5.39#
Gestational diabetes	6	0.90	0.33-1.95	3	2.10	0.43-1.13#
Preeclampsia	45	1.04	0.77-1.41	7	0.82	0.33-1.69#
Hyperemesis gravidarum	7	0.94	0.38-1.93#	3	1.75	0.31-5.13#
Placenta previa	10	1.17	0.56-2.15	3	1.58	0.33-4.61#
Abruptio placentae	7	0.74	0.30-1.52#	3	1.36	0.28-3.99#
Antepartum bleeding	9	0.85	0.44-1.64	4	1.75	0.48-4.49#
Intrapartum bleeding	14	0.82	0.49-1.40	4	1.06	0.29-2.72#
Postpartum bleeding	47	0.96	0.71-1.29	13	1.26	0.72-2.24
Delivery induction	82	0.89	0.71-1.12	16	0.71	0.42-1.19
Caesarean section	140	0.98	0.82-1.19	25	0.88	0.52-1.23

#observed over expected number with exact Poisson 95% confidence interval.

No statistically significant deviations from expected values are seen.

Outcome after Maternal Vaccination During Pregnancy

Infant Sex

After vaccination in early pregnancy, there were 424 male and 433 female infants born, sex ratio 0.98 (95% CI 0.86-1.12). After vaccination later in pregnancy there were

97 male and 101 female infants, sex ratio 0.96 (95% CI 0.72-1.27). Both sex ratios are thus low but the normal one (1.06) is contained within both confidence intervals.

Multiple Births

After vaccination in early pregnancy, there were eight twin deliveries, OR = 0.58 (95% CI 0.29-1.15). After vaccination in later pregnancy, there were three twin deliveries, RR = 0.97 (95% CI 0.20-2.84). No higher order multiple births occurred.

Table 41.5. Pregnancy duration and infant birth weight at maternal use of

Variable studied	Vaccination in early pregnancy			Vaccination later in pregnancy		
	Number	OR/RR	95% CI	Number	OR/RR	95% CI
<37 weeks	45	1.03	0.76-1.39	9	0.93	0.42-1.76#
<2500g	35	1.21	0.86-1.70	7	1.13	0.45-2.33#
≥4500g	26	0.88	0.60-1.32	2	0.29	0.04-1.05#
SGA	23	1.05	0.69-1.60	1	0.23	0.01-1.29#
LGA	37	1.03	0.93-1.45	5	0.51	0.16-1.18#

#observed over expected number with exact Poisson 95% confidence interval.

These oucomes were thus normal.

Infant Mortality

After vaccination in early pregnancy, four stillbirths and three early neonatal deaths occurred. The RR for stillbirth was 1.25 (95% CI 0.24-3.20) and for early neonatal death 2.47 (95% CI 0.51-7.21), both elevated but none statistically significant.

Table 41.6. Neonatal diagnoses after maternal vaccination

Diagnosis	Drug use in early pregnancy			Drug use later in pregnancy		
	Number	OR/RR	95% CI	Number	OR/RR	95% CI
Hypoglycaemia	26	0.82	0.55-1.21	8	1.13	0.49-2.24#
Respiratory diagnoses	41	0.87	0.63-1.20	8	0.87	0.38-1.71#
Low Apgar score	17	0.94	0.58-1.52	3	1.25	0.26-3.65#
CNS diagnoses	3	0.50	0.10-1.47	0	-	-
Jaundice	33	0.87	0.62-1.24	11	1.34	0.67-2.39#

#observed over expected number with exact Poisson 95% confidence interval.

There were thus no statistically significant deviations in neonatal outcome after vaccinations during pregnancy.

The distribution of "relatively severe" malformations according to vaccine is shown in Table 41.8 and the malformations are further specified in Table 41.9.

Table 41.7. Congenital malformations in infants whose mothers had been vaccinated in early pregnancy

Congenital malformation	Number	OR/RR	95% CI
All malformation	34	0.78	0.55-1.10
Relatively severe malformation	18	0.62	0.39-0.99
Chromosome anomalies	2	1.11	0.13-4.01#
Without chromosome anomalies			
Any cardiovascular defect	4	0.44	0.12-1.12#

#observed over expected number with exact Poisson 95% confidence interval.

Table 41.8. Relatively severe malformations and specific vaccine types

Vaccine against	Number malformed	Number total	OR/RR	95% CI
Cholera	3	164	0.58	0.12-1.69#
Diphteria	1	36	0.83	0.02-4.60#
Tetanus	2	84	0.66	0.08-2.40#
Encephalitis	0	54	0.00	0.00-1.95#
Influenza	2	123	0.47	0.06-1.70#
Hepatitis	10	335	0.92	0.47-1.70
Polio	1	69	2.44	0.06-13.6#

Table 41.9. Specification of relatively severe malformations after maternal vaccination in early pregnancy with vaccine and other drugs given

Malformation diagnosis	Vaccine	Other drugs
Spina bifida, arrhinencephaly, persistent cloaca, abdominal wall defect	hepatitis	
Eyelid and lacrimal duct anomaly	hepatitis	
Branchial cyst or fistula	hepatitis	citalopram
Branchial cyst or fistula	hepatitis	
Cleft lip/palate, VSD, ASD, pulmonary artery malformation., aortic stenosis	cholera	folic acid
Cleft palate with unstable hip	hepatitis	
Ventricukar septum defect	diphteria+polio	chloroquine, proguanil, insulin
Ventricular seprtum defect	tetanus	ceterizine
Ventricular septum defect	cholera	
Pulmonary hypoplasia	hepatitis	
Megacolon	hepatitis	cetirizine, oral contraceptive
Hypospadias	tetanus	unspec. malaria drug
Double ureters	hepatitis	
Polydactyly	influenza	
Syndactyly	influenza	
Ulnar defect with hand reduction	cholera	penicillin, pivmecillinam, codein, paracetamol, gabapentin
Down syndrome	hepatitis	mefloquine, medoxyprogesterone
Down syndrome	hepatitis	terbutaline

There are thus two complex malformations, one after vaccination for hepatitis, the other after vaccination for cholera.

There were seven infants exposed in early pregnancy to vaccine against meningococcs, eight to vaccine against rabies, and 17 to vaccine against rubella. None of the infants had a malformation diagnosis. Exposures to other vaccines occurred in only one or two cases; no infant had a malformation.

SUMMARY

In this rather limited material there are no signs of any foetal harm after maternal vaccination. The material does not exclude teratogenic effects because the number of exposures to each specific vaccine is small.

REFERENCES

[1] Brent RL. Risks and benefits of immunizing pregnant women: The risk of doing nothing. *Reprod Toxicol* 2006; 21: 383-389.

[2] Namael MH, Zlaee M, Naseh N. Congenital rubella syndrome in infants of women vaccinated during or just before pregnancy with measles-rubella vaccine. *Indian J Med* 2008; 127: 551-554.

[3] Minussi L, Mohrdieck R, Bercini M, Ranleri T, Sanseverino MT, Momino W, Callegari-Jacques SM, Schuler-Faccini I. Prospective evaluation of pregnant women vaccinated against rubella in soutehrn Brazil. *Reprod Toxicol* 2008; 25: 120-123.

[4] Robert E, Vial T, Schaefer C, Arnon J, Reuvers M. Exposure to yellow fever vaccine in early pregnancy. *Vaccine 17*: 283-285, 1999.

[5] Suzano CES, Amaral E, Sato HK, Papaiordanou PM. The effects of yellow fever immunization (17DD) inadvertently used in early pregnancy during a mass campaign in Brazil. *Vaccine* 2006; 24: 1421-1426.

[6] Ryan MA, Seward JF; Smallpox Vaccine in Pregnancy Registry Team. Pregnancy, birth, and infant health oucomes from the National Smallpox Vaccine in Pregnancy Registry, 2003-2006. *Clin Infect Dis* 2008; 46 (Suppl. 3): 5221-5226.

[7] Ryan MA, Gumbs GR, Conlin AM, Sevick CJ, Jacobson IG, Snell KJ, Spooner CN, Smith TC; Department of Defense Birth and Infant Health Registry. Evaluation of preterm births and birth defects in liveborn infants of US military women who received smallpos vaccine. *Birth Defect Res (Part A)* 2008; 82: 533-539.

[8] Harjulehto-Mervaala T, Aro T, Hillesmaa VK, Hovi T, Saxén H, Saxén L. Oral polio vaccination during pregnancy: lack of impact on foetal development and perinatal outcome. *Clin Infect Dis* 1994; 18: 414-420.

[9] Ryan M, Smith TC, Sevick CJ, Honner WK, Loach RA, Moore CA, Erickson JD. Birth defects among infants born to women who received anthrax vaccine in pregnancy. *Am J Epidemiol* 2008; 168: 434-442.

[10] Czeizel AE, Rockenbauer M. Tetanus toxoid and congenital abnormalities. *Int J Gynecol Obst* 1999; 64: 253-258.

[11] D'Acremont V, Tremblay S, Genton B. Impact of vaccines given during pregnancy on the offspring of women consulting a travel clinic: A longitudinal study. *J Travel Med* 2008; 15: 77-81.

Chapter 42

Antineoplastic, Immunomodulating and Immunosuppressive Drugs

Oncologic use of antineoplatic drugs, notably folic acid antagonists, carry a high risk for teratogenesis while use as immunosuppressants is less likely to cause damage. Such exposure should be avoided in early pregnancy but if it has occurred it is hardly a reason for discussing a pregnancy termination. Use of interferons and most immunosuppressants are not associated with any marked risk for the embryo with the exception of mycophenolate mofetil which should be avoided. If exposure to mycophenolate mofetil has occurred, a termination of the pregnancy may be considered but there is not enough data to state the magnitude of risk. A weak association between early use of azathioprine and mild cardiac defects may exit but the risk is small and may be due to underlying disease.

These drugs are used at many different pathologies. Among pregnant women, the use of antineoplastic drugs because of malignancy is probably low; most of the use of these drugs is associated with immunological diseases. Oncologic therapy with high doses of antineoplastic drugs and notably aminopterine and methotrexate [1] is associated with a marked teratogenic risk, but a harmful effect of methotrexate when used in lower doses at immunological diseases (e.g., immunological bowel disease or rheumatoid arthritis) is not clearly demonstrated but has been suggested [2].

Immunomodulating drugs have not been shown to carry a teratogenic risk but the number of studied exposed pregnancies is small [3-5].

Table 42.1. Number of women identified using antineoplastic or immunomodulating or -suppressive drugs

Total	821
Reported use in early pregnancy	632
Got prescription later in pregnancy	451
Both early and later use	262

Type of drug	ATC code	Early use	Later use
Antineoplatic agents	L01	90	88
Cyclophosphamide	L01AA01	32	20
Chlorambucil	L01AA02	0	1
Busulfan	L01AB01	1	0
Carmustine	L01AD01	2	0
Lomustine	L01AD02	8	31
Streptozocin	L01AD04	1	0
Methotrexate	L01BA01	19	2
Mercaptopurine	L01BB02	13	8
Tioguanine	L01BB03	1	0
Fludarabine	L01BB05	0	1
Cytarabine	L01BC01	1	0
Fluorouracil	L01BC02	1	3
Vinblastine	L01CA01	1	1
Doxorubicin	L01DB01	3	0
Daumorubicin	L01DB02	3	0
Mitomycin	L01DC03	1	0
Carboplatin	L01XA02	3	0
Unspecified	L01	4	2
Endocrine therapy	L02	14	13
Tamoxifen	L02BA01	3	1
Flutamide	L02BB01	11	12
Immunomodulating agents	L03	54	31
Filgrastin	L03AA02	4	1
Interferon alpha	L03AA04/AB01/AB05	12	10
Lemogastrim	L03AA10	0	9
Thymopentin	L03AB07	17	8
Interferon beta	L03AB08	10	3
Peginterferon alfa-2b	L03AB10	1	0
Glatirameracetate	L03AX13	6	0
Unspecified	L03	4	0
Immunosuppressive agents	L04	477	321
Ciclosporin	L04AA01	95	66
Tacrolimus	L04AA05	12	8
Mycophenolate mofetil	L04AA06	1	1
Etanercept	L04AA11	2	1
Infliximab	L04AA12	1	2
Adalimumab	L04AA17	5	1
Azathioprine	L04AX01	391	267

A combination of an antineoplastic agent and an immunosuppressive agent was used by four women in early pregnancy and by two later in pregnancy.

Most interest has been paid to immunosuppressive drugs, used for instance at immunological bowel disease or rheumatoid arthritis but also after organ transplantation. Tacrolimus has not been associated with a teratogenic risk [6] and this seems to be the case for ciclosporine as well [7]. Mycophenolate mofetil seems to be associated with a considerable teratogenic risk [8-10] while azathioprine is generally regarded as a low-risk drug [11-12] even though an association with mild cardiac defects may exist [13].

Characteristics of Women using Antineoplastic, Immunomodulating or Immunosuppressive Drugs

Based on women reporting the drug in early pregnancy (n=104 for antineoplastic drugs, 531 for immunomodulating or immunosuppressive drugs). Each variable is adjusted for all other variables and year of delivery. Comparison with all women who gave birth during the period and with information from the first antenatal care (n=967 742). The odds ratios for maternal age, parity, smoking in early pregnancy, number of previous miscarriages, BMI, subfertility, and country of birth are adjusted for all other variables (Table 42.2).

Table 42.2. Characteristics of women using antineoplastic, immunomodulating, or immunosuppressive drugs in early pregnancy

Variable studied	Antineoplastic drugs			Immunomodulating/ suppressive drugs		
	Number	OR	95% CI	Number	OR	95% CI
Maternal age						
<25 years	16	0.92	0.51-1.67	66	0.66	0.50-0.86
25-34 years	64	1.00	reference	376	1.00	reference
≥35 years	24	1.59	1.01-2.51	89	1.01	0.80-1.29
Parity						
1	55	1.88	1.25-2.84	295	1.65	1.37-1.97
≥2	49	1.00	reference	236	1.00	reference
Smoking						
Unknown	4	-	-	12	-	-
No	78	1.00	reference	457	1.00	reference
Yes	22	1.81	0.74-4.42	62	1.21	0.69-2.11
Previous miscarriages						
No	73	1.00	reference	426	1.00	reference
Yes	31	1.66	1.08-2.63	105	1.02	0.82-1.28
BMI						
Unknown	10	-	-	37	-	-
<19.8	14	1.91	1.06-3.42	53	1.19	0-89-1.59
19.8-25.9	51	1.00	reference	332	1.00	reference
≥26	29	1.35	0.85-2.53	109	0.80	0.64-0.99
Unwanted childlessness						
No	89	1.00	reference	464	1.00	reference
Yes	15	1.70	0.96-2.99	67	1.52	1.17-1.98
Country of birth						
Unknown	0	-	-			
Sweden	90	1.00	reference	485	1.00	reference
Other Nordic country	5	1.80	0.74-4.37	18	1.29	1.00-1.67
Non-Nordic country	9	0.54	0.28-1.07	17	0.80	0.41-1.58

Some further maternal characteristics were analyzed, adjusting for year of delivery, maternal age, parity, smoking, and BMI (Table 42.3).

Table 42.3. Some further characteristics of women using antineoplastic, immunomodulating, or immunosuppressive drugs

Variable studied	Antineoplastic drugs			Immunomodulating/ immunosuppressive drugs		
	Number	OR	95% CI	Number	OR	95% CI
Education (1996-2001, 46 women with antineoplastic drugs, 162 with immunomodulating or immunosuppressive drugs, 526 695 in population)						
Unknown	1	-	-	2	-	-
<12 years	5	0.62	0.22-1.77	14	0.77	0.43-1.37
12 years	26	1.00	reference	99	1.00	reference
≥13 years	14	0.95	0.45-1.99	38	0.69	0.47-0.96
Family situation						
Unknown	2	-	-	7	-	-
Co-habiting	92	1.00	reference	489	1.00	reference
Living alone	4	0.85	0.27-2.67	18	1.51	0.88-2.59
Other family situation	6	1.56	0.61-4.02	17	0.80	0.41-1.58
Work outside home						
Unknown	17	-	-	57	1.54	0.88-2.59
Full time	41	1.00	reference	240	1.00	reference
Part time	24	1.29	0.70-2.38	134	1.29	1.00-1.67
None	22	1.64	0.89-3.02	100	1.43	1.08-1.90

The number of exposed women is low (notably for antineoplastic drugs) and therefore many estimates uncertain. It can be noted that both groups show less use than expected among young women but only antineoplastic drugs show an excess use in women aged 35 or more. Both types of drugs are used more often in parity 1 than in higher parity. Previous miscarriages are associated with antineoplastic drugs but not with immunomodulating or immunosuppressive drugs, while both groups of women show an excess of a period of unwanted childlessness. Both are associated with not working full time even though this is statistically significant only for immunomodulating or immunosuppressive drugs.

The nine women who had used both drugs for immunological bowel diseases and antineoplastic drugs had used methotrexate (four women) or mercaptopurine (five women). There is an association between allergy, rhinitis and asthma with antineoplastic drugs but not with immunomodulating or immunosuppressive drugs. Both groups have an association with opioids.

Due to the low number of women exposed to antineoplastic drugs, only the risk for delivery induction and for caesarean section is given. The risk for delivery induction is only slightly increased: 11 cases after early exposure and 12 cases after later exposures, RR = 1.12, 95% CI 0.56-2.01 and RR = 1.20, 95% CI 0.62-2.10, respectively. The risk for caesarean section is non-significantly increased both after early and later exposure, for both based on 22 cases and with an OR of 1.53 (95% CI 0.93-2.53) and 1.55 (95% CI 0.95-2.94), respectively.

The following Table gives data on pregnancy diagnoses in women using immunosuppressive drugs (mainly azathioprine) (Table 42.5).

There is thus a clear-cut association with chronic hypertension and a weaker one with preeclampsia. There also seems to be an association with placental abruption. Both delivery inductions and caesarean sections occur in clear excess.

Table 42.4. Concomitant drug use (early pregnancy)

Drug group	Number	OR/RR	95% CI
Antineoplastic drugs			
Drugs for inflammatory bowel disease	9	25.7	11.8-48.8#
Multivitamins	6	0.66	0.24-1.44#
Folic acid	16	2.68	1.53-4-35#
Systemic corticosteroids	6	12.2	4.49-26.7#
Antibiotics	5	1.39	0.45-3.24#
NSAIDs	9	4.46	2.04-8.46#
Opioids	7	9.21	3.70-19.0#
Minor analgesics	13	1.57	0.84-2.69
Drugs for rhinitis	4	2.82	0.77-7.21#
Antiasthmatics	16	4.11	2.35-6.68#
Antihistamines	11	1.87	0.94-2.85#
For NVP	5	1.22	0.40-2.85#
For allergy	6	9.21	3.70-19.0#
Immunomodulating or –suppressive drugs			
Drugs for stomach ulcer and reflux	23	4.94	3.13-7.41#
Drugs for inflammatory bowel disease	161	-	-
Insulin	5	2.78	0.90-6.48#
Multivitamins	28	0.54	0.48-0.64
Folic acid	92	3.00	2.47-3.46
Antihypertensive drugs	34	18.8	13.0-26.2
Systemic corticosteroids	172	-	-
Thyroid drugs	14	1.85	2.01-3.11#
Antibiotics	23	1.37	0.94-1.99
Opioids	11	3.86	1.93-6-91#
NSAIDs	9	0.85	0.44-1.66
Minor analgesics	39	0.94	0.68-1.30
Drugs for migraine	5	3.11	1.01-7.25#
Anticonvulsants	9	5.84	2.67-11.1#
Sedatives, hypnotics	5	2.11	0.69-4.92#
Antidepressants	15	1.87	1.05-3.08#
Drugs for rhinitis	7	0.89	0.36-1.84#
Antiasthmatics	18	1.05	0.66-1.67
Antihistamines	14	0.42	0.25-0.69

#observed over expected number with exact Poisson 95% confidence interval.

Outcome after Maternal use of Antineoplastic Drugs, Immunomodulating or Immunosuppressive Drugs

Infant Sex

After exposure to antineoplastic drugs in early pregnancy, there were 47 male and 60 female infants born, sex ratio 0.78 (95% CI 0.53-1.14) and after later such exposure there were 56 male and 49 female infants, sex ratio 1.14 (95% CI 0.78-1.69). After early exposure to immunomodulating or immunosuppressive drugs, there were 281 male and 257 female infants, sex ratio 1.09 /95% CI 0.92-1.30) and after later exposure 194 male and 162 female infants, sex ratio 1.20 (95% CI 0.97-1.48). The normal sex ratio of 1.06 is thus contained in all confidence intervals.

Table 42.5. Pregnancy diagnoses among women who used immunosuppressive drugs (mainly azathioprine)

Diagnosis	Drug use in early pregnancy			Drug use later in pregnancy		
	Number	OR/RR	95% CI	Number	OR/RR	95% CI
Pre-existing diabetes	10	1.68	0.81-3.10#	9	2.12	0.97-4.02
Chronic hypertension	22	4.18	2.63-6.33#	16	4.16	2.38-6.75#
Gestational diabetes	5	1.28	0.41-2.98#	2	0.72	0.09-2.60#
Preeclampsia	41	1.94	1.41-2.67	26	1.72	1.15-2.57
Hyperemesis gravidarum	6	1.33	0.49-2.90#	2	0.61	0.07-2.20#
Placenta previa	7	1.38	0.55-2.84	3	0.79	0.11-2.32#
Abruptio placentae	13	2.26	1.21-3.87#	5	1.26	0.41-2.93#
Antepartum bleeding	7	1.14	0.46-2.35#	4	0.94	0.26-2.41#
Intrapartum bleeding	13	1.25	0.72-2.18	8	1.05	0.45-2.06#
Postpartum bleeding	30	1.10	0.76-1.60	16	0.85	0.51-1.41
Delivery induction	104	2.77	2.23-3.45	71	2.69	2.06-3.50
Caesarean section	159	2.51	2.08-3.03	109	2.40	1.91-3.01

#observed over expected number with exact Poisson 95% confidence interval.

Multiple Births

After early exposure to antineoplastic drugs there were three twin deliveries and after later exposure four. After early exposure for immunomodulating or immunosuppressive drugs, there were seven twin deliveries (RR = 0.89, 95% CI 0.42-1.88) and after later exposure four twin deliveries (RR = 0.73, 95% CI 0.27-1.94).

After exposure to antineoplastic drugs, there was only one perinatal death: a stillbirth after early exposure. After early exposure to immunomodulating or immunosuppressive drugs, there were three stillbirths (RR = 1.50, 95% CI 0.31-4.38) and one early neonatal death.

Table 42.6. Pregnancy duration and infant birth weight at maternal use of antineoplastic or immunomodulating or immunosuppressive drugs

Variable studied	Drug use in early pregnancy			Drug use later in pregnancy		
	Number	OR/RR	95% CI	Number	OR/RR	95% CI
Antineoplastic drugs						
<37 weeks	14	2.55	1.40-4.29	8	1.71	0.74-3.38
<2500g	11	2.62	1.31-4.69	7	3.41	1.37-7.04#
≥4500g	4	1.05	0.29-2.70#	2	0.46	0.06-1.65#
SGA	5	1.63	0.53-3.81#	3	1.43	0.29-4.17#
LGA	5	0.95	0.31-2.21#	4	0.63	0.17-1.60#
Immunomodulating or -suppressive drugs						
<37 weeks	87	3.72	2.99-4.62	64	4.18	3.25-5.38
<2500g	62	3.98	3.10-5.10	34	3.22	2.30-4.51
≥4500g	14	0.74	0.44-1.26	7	0.52	0.25-1.09
SGA	32	2.64	1.85-3.76	15	1.85	1.10-3.11
LGA	19	0.73	0.46-1.15	13	0.71	0.41-1.24

By and large the patterns for the two groups of drugs are very similar even though precision in the estimates is larger for the immunomodulating or immunosuppressive drugs than for antineoplastic drugs, especially after later exposure.

Table 42.7. Neonatal diagnoses among infants whose mothers had used antineoplastic, immunomodulating, or immunosuppressive drugs

Diagnosis	Drug use in early pregnancy			Drug use later in pregnancy		
	Number	OR/RR	95% CI	Number	OR/RR	95% CI
Antineoplastic drugs						
Hypoglycaemia	10	2.58	1.24-4.75#	10	2.70	1.29-4.96#
Respiratory diagnoses	10	1.82	0.87-2.43#	6	1.15	0.42-2.50#
Low Apgar score	7	3.27	1.32-6.74#	1	-	-
CNS diagnoses	4	6.90	1.88-17.7#	1	-	-
Jaundice	9	2.33	1.07-4.43#	8	1.98	0.85-3.89#
Immunomodulating or –suppressive drugs						
Hypoglycaemia	38	2.05	1.48-2.85	20	2.50	0.95-2.35
Respiratory diagnoses	39	1.55	1.12-2.16	24	1.39	0.91-2.11
Low Apgar score	16	1.57	0.95-2.61	8	1.17	0.50-2.30#
CNS diagnoses	2	0.56	0.07-2.05	2	0.72	0.09-2.60#
Jaundice	44	1.98	1.46-2.69	36	2.41	1.72-3.38

#observed over expected number with exact Poisson 95% confidence interval.

For both groups of drugs, clear-cut effects on neonatal conditions can be seen notably after early exposure.

Congenital Malformations in Infants whose Mothers had used Antineoplastic, immunomodulating, or Immunosuppressive Drugs in Early Pregnancy

A total of 35 infants with congenital malformations were identified. Among them only one had been exposed to an antineoplastic drug: the infant had ventricular and atrium septum defects and the mother had used cyclophosphamide in early pregnancy. One infant had been exposed to an immunomodulating drug. It had a minor anomaly, undescended testis, and the mother had got thymopentin. The remaining 33 malformed infants had been exposed to immunosuppressive drugs and are summarized below (Table 42.8).

Table 42.8. Congenital malformations in infants whose mothers used immunosuppressive drugs in early pregnancy

Congenital malformation	Number	OR	95% CI
All malformation	33	1.53	1.07-2.17
Relatively severe malformation	22	1.53	1.00-2.34
Chromosome anomalies	1	0.88	-
Without chromosome anomalies			
Any cardiovascular defect	10	1.96	0.94-3.61#
VSD and/or ASD	8	2.69	1.16-3.51#

Four specific drugs were associated with congenital malformations

Table 42.9. Number of malformations in infants whose mothers used specific drugs

Drug	Number exposed	Number malformed
Cyclosporine	96	6
Tacrolimus	12	2
Mycophenolate mofetil	1	1
Azathioprine	396	26

Table 42.10. Specific malformations and immunosuppressive drug used

Malformation diagnosis	Immunosuppressive drug	Prednisolone	Note
Branchial cyst/fistula	ciclosporine	yes	
Branchial cyst/fistula	azathioprine	no	
Cleft palate, unstable hip	azathioprine	no	
Ventricular septum defect	azathioprine	yes	2 cases
Ventricular septum defect	azathioprine	no	
Ventricular septum defect	ciclosporine	no	
Atrium septum defect	azathioprine	yes	2 cases
Atrium septum defect	tacrolimus,azathioprine	no	
Ventricular and atrium septum defect	azathioprine	no	
Unspecified cardiac defect	azathioprine,ciclosporine	yes	
Pylorostenosis	azathioprine	yes	
Oesophageal atresia, eye mal-formation, cardiac defect	tacrolimus, mycophenolate mofetil	yes	
Megacolon	azathioprine	no	
Hydronephrosis	azathioprine	yes	
Hypospadias	azathioprine	no	
Ovarian cyst	azathioprine	no	
Pes equinovarus	azathioprine	yes	
Polydactyly	azathioprine	no	
Craniostenosis	ciclosporine	no	
Down syndrome	azathioprine	no	

Among the eight infants with atrium or ventricular septum defect, thus four had ventricular defects, three atrium defects, and one both conditions.

Summary

Women who use these drugs have an increased risk of pregnancy complications and their infants of neonatal complications. Much of the drug use occurred at immunological bowel disease and a direct effect of the diseases may explain the associations. There is also a slight increase in the risk of a congenital malformation which is mainly associated with the use of azathioprine and which seems to be due to ventricular and/or atrium septum defects. The possibility cannot be excluded that the underlying disease causes also this effect.

REFERENCES

[1] Schardein J. *Chemically Induced Birth Defects*. Marcel Dekker, Inc. New York and Basel, 1985.

[2] Østensen M. Antirheumatische Therapie und Reproduktion. *Z Rheumatol* 2006; 65: 217-224.

[3] Sandberg-Wohlheim M, Frank D, Goodwin TM, Giesser B, Lopez-Bresnahan M, Stam-Moraga M, Chang P, Francis GS. Pregnancy outcome during treatment with interferon beta-1a in patients with multiple sclerosis. *Neurology* 2005; 65: 802-806.

[4] Boskovic R, Wide R, Wolpin J, Bauer DJ, Koren G. The reproductive effects of beta interferon therapy in pregnancy: a longitudinal cohort. *Neurology* 2005; 65: 807-811.

[5] Exposure to interferon during pregnancy. *Prescrire Int* 2007; 16: 22.

[6] Jain AB, Reyes J, Marcos A, Mazariegos G, Eghtesad B, Fontes PA, Cacciarelli TV, Marsh JW, de Vera ME, Rafail A, Fung JJ. Pregnancy after liver transplantation with tacrolimus immunosuppression: a single center's experience update at 13 years. *Transplantation* 2003; 76: 827-832.

[7] Bar-Oz B, Hackman R, Einarson T, Koren G. Pregnancy outcome afer cyclosporine therapy during pregnancy: a meta-analysis. *Transplantation* 2001; 71: 1051-1055.

[8] Källén B, Westgren M, Åberg A, Otterblad Olausson P. Pregnancy outcome after maternal organ transplantation in Sweden. *BJOG* 2005; 112: 904-909.

[9] Pisoni CN, D'Cruz DP. The safety of mycophenolate mofetil in pregnancy. *Expert Opin Drug Saf* 2008; 7: 219-222.

[10] Carey JC, Martinez L, Balken E, Leen-Mitchell M, Robertson J. Determination of human teratogenicity by the astute clinician method: Review of illustrative agents and a proposal of guidelines. *Birth Defects Res (Part A)* 2009; 85: 63-68.

[11] Goldstein LH, Dolinsky G, Greenberg R, Schaefer C, Cohen-Kerem R, Diav-Citrin O, Malm H, Reuvers-Lodewijks ME, Rost can Tonningen-van Driel MM, Arnon J, Ornoy A, Clementi M, di Gianantonio E, Koren G, Braunstein R, Berkovitch M. Pregnancy outcome of women exposed to azathioprine during pregnancy. *Birth Defects Res (Part A)* 2007; 79: 696-701.

[12] Langagergaard V, Pedersen L, Gislum M, Nørgard B, Sørensen HT. Birth outcome in women treated with azathioprine or mercaptopurine during pregnancy: A Danish nationwide cohort study. *Aliment Pharmacol Ther* 2007; 25: 73-81.

[13] Cleary BJ, Källén B. Early pregnancy azathioprine use and pregnancy outcomes. *Birth Def Res (Part A)* 2009; 85: 647-654.

Chapter 43

NON-STEROID ANTIINFLAMMATORY DRUGS

Use of non-steroid antiinflammatory drugs in late pregnancy carries a risk for pregnancy and foetal complications and should be avoided. When used in early pregnancy, a moderately increased risk for certain malformations and notably cardiovascular defects may occur and this effect seems to be strongest for propionic acid derivates, notably naproxen, but there may also be a difference between long-term and temporary use of the drugs. Notably long-term use should be avoided but if exposure has occurred this does not motivate a discussion on termination of pregnancy.

Non-steroid antiinflammatory drugs (NSAID) have a multitude of different uses. Originally much used at rheumatic diseases, their use has spread and they have become general analgesics and antipyretics leading to a more temporary usage. They affect prostaglandin synthesis which could influence pregnancy and foetal development. An increased risk of miscarriage has been described [1], even though evidence for this is imperfect. NSAID drugs have been associated with the origin of malformations [1], notably cardiovascular defects [2,3]. An association between ibuprofen and gastroschisis [4,5], and between naproxen and orofacial clefts [6] has been suggested. The support for the latter two associations is still weak.

When used in late pregnancy, NSAID has been associated with an increased risk for various complications: premature closure of ductus arteriosus [7], foetal kidney toxicity leading to kidney failure and oligohydramnios [8], increased risk for bleeding at delivery, and weakening of contractions. Topical use of NSAID is expected to have fewer effects than systemic use but ductus arteriosus constriction after such treatment has been described [9].

Table 43.1. Number of women identified using

Total	18683
Reported use in early pregnancy	16223
Got prescription later in pregnancy	2757
Both early and later use	297

Type of drug	ATC code	Early use	Later use
For systemic use			
Acetic acid derivates	M01AB	2664	609
Indometacin	M01AB01	71	22
Sulindac	M01AB02	4	0
Tolmetin	M01AB03	4	0
Diclofenac	M01AB05	2516	584
Ketorolac	M01AB15	0	1
Aceclofenac	M01AB16	7	1
Diclofenac with misoprostol	M01AB55	69	1
Oxicams	M01AC	136	16
Piroxicam	M01AC01	37	6
Tenoxicam	M01AC02	77	4
Lornoxicam	M01AC05	4	0
Meloxicam	M01AC06	19	5
Propionic acid derivates	M01AE	13261	2072
Ibuprofen	M01AE01	10397	1718
Naproxen	M01AE02	2420	311
Ketoprofen	M01AE03	456	46
Fenbufen	M01AE05	1	0
Dexibuprofen	M01AE14	9	1
Unspecified	M01AE	75	10
Coxibs	M01AH	174	25
Celecoxib	M01AH01	76	10
Rofeocoxib	M01AH02	93	15
Etoricoxih	M01AH05	7	0
Other non-steroid ant-inflammatory drugs			
Nabumetone	M01AX01	50	7
Ketorolac	M01AX03	4	0
Azapropazone	M01AX04	1	2
Glucosamine	M01AX05	6	2
For local use			
Ketoprofen	M02AA10	86	41
Salicylic acid	M02AC	4	5

Characteristics of Women using NSAID Drugs Systemically in Early Pregnancy

Based on women reporting the drug in early pregnancy (n=1622, one missing maternal age). Each variable is adjusted for all other variables and year of delivery. Comparison with all women who gave birth during the period and with information from the first antenatal care (n=967 742). The odds ratios for maternal age, parity, smoking in early pregnancy, number of previous miscarriages, BMI, subfertility, and country of birth are adjusted for all other variables and are shown in Figure 43.1.

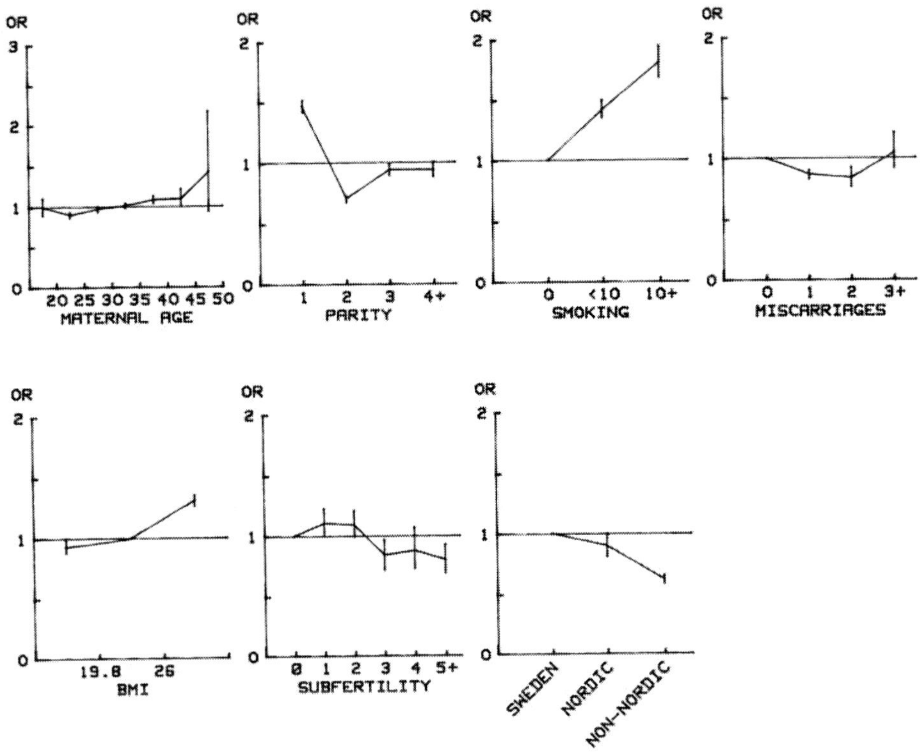

Figure 43.1. Odds ratios for seven maternal characteristics. The odds ratios (OR) for each variable are adjusted for the other variables and year of delivery. Vertical lines mark 95% confidence intervals. For maternal age and parity, each class is compared with all other classes.

Some further maternal characteristics were analyzed, adjusting for year of delivery, maternal age, parity, smoking, and BMI (Table 43.2).

Table 43.2. Some further characteristics of women using NSAID in early pregnancy

Variable studied	Number	OR	95% CI
Education (1996-2001, 7262 women with drugs, 526 695 in population)			
Unknown			
<12 years	855	0.90	0.83-0.97
12 years	3928	1.00	reference
13-14 years	398	0.95	0.85-1.05
>14 years	1973	0.87	0.82-0.92
Family situation			
Unknown	258	-	
Co-habiting	14814	1.00	reference
Living alone	420	1.00	0.90-1.10
Other family situation	600	1.17	1.06-1.28
Work outside home			
Unknown	1971	-	-
Full time	8164	1.00	reference
Part time	3720	1.02	0.98-1.06
None	2237	0.78	0.74-0.82

Women using NSAID thus have a near-normal age distribution but there is an excess of parity 1 and a low number of parity 2 women. They smoke more than expected and there is an increased usage of NSAID among over-weight women while previous miscarriage or subfertility has no clear-cut association with NSAID use. Women born outside the Nordic countries use less NSAID than women born in Sweden.

Table 43.3. Concomitant drug use (early pregnancy)

Drug group	Number	OR/RR	95% CI
Drugs for stomach ulcer and reflux	317	2.07	1.85-2.32
Drugs for inflammatory bowel disease	101	2.30	1.89-2.79
Insulin	30	0.49	0.34-0.70
Multivitamins	520	0.77	0.71-0.85
Folic acid	475	0.68	0.62-0.75
Oral contraceptives	123	1.97	1.65-2.31
Progestogens	35	0.41	0.30-0.57
Gonadotropins	26	0.59	0.40-0.86
Systemic corticosteroids	140	2.19	1.85-2-58
Thyroid drugs	148	0.65	0.55-0.77
Antibiotics	771	1.55	1.44-1.67
Opioids	25	0.41	0.30-0.60
Minor analgesics	3626	2.98	2.88-3.09
Migraine drugs	207	4.16	3.64-4.75
Anticonvulsants	37	0.73	0.53-1.01
Neuroleptica	25	0.41	0.28-0.60
Sedatives, hypnotics	183	2.02	1.75-2.35
Antidepressants	301	1.21	1.07-1.35
Drugs for rhinitis	406	1.72	1.55-1.90
Antiasthmatics	457	0.78	0.71-0.86
Cough medicines	190	2.23	1.93-2.57
Antihistamines	1087	1.08	1.02-1.15

Table 43.4. Some maternal diagnoses associated with the use of NSAID drugs

Diagnosis	Drug use in early pregnancy			Drug use later in pregnancy		
	Number	OR/RR	95% CI	Number	OR/RR	95% CI
Pre-existing diabetes	200	0.83	0.72-0.96	40	1.03	0.75-1.41
Chronic hypertension	210	0.97	0.85-1.12	41	1.15	0.85-1.57
Gestational diabetes	159	0.95	0.81-1.12	29	1.14	0.79-1.64
Preeclampsia	910	1.11	1.03-1.19	153	1.16	0.98-1.36
Hyperemesis gravidarum	183	1.00	0.86-1.16	36	1.22	0.88-1.70
Placenta previa	203	0.99	0.86-1.14	36	1.08	0.78-1.50
Abruptio placentae	233	1.01	0.89-1.16	34	0.94	0.66-1.32
Antepartum bleeding	229	0.95	0.83-1.09	42	1.11	0.82-1.52
Intrapartum bleeding	389	1.02	0.92-1.04	76	1.07	0.88-1.39
Postpartum bleeding	945	1.02	0.95-1.09	158	1.03	0.87-1.21
Delivery induction	2075	1.13	1.07-1.18	364	1.11	0.99-1.25
Caesarean section	2935	1.08	1.03-1.12	557	1.17	1.06-1.29

Most concomitant drugs are used less often than expected but for some the opposite is seen: drugs for stomach ulcer and reflux, drugs for inflammatory bowel disease, systemic corticoids, antibiotics, and analgesics including drugs for migraine. There is also an excess of sedatives, hypnotics, and antidepressants, drugs for symptoms of common cold, and antihistamines. The associations may partly be due to similar indications for the drugs (e.g., analgesics), to side effects of the drugs (e.g., drugs for stomach ulcer and reflux), or co-morbidity (e.g., psychoactive drugs).

There are thus few significant deviations from expected values: preeclampsia, delivery inductions, and caesarean sections are moderately increased.

Outcome after Maternal use of Non-steroid Antiinflammatory Drugs

Infant Sex

After early exposure to NSAID; there were 8512 male and 7918 female infants born (four with unknown sex), sex ratio 1.07 (95% CI 1.04-1.11), and after later exposure there were 1423 male and 1366 female infants born, sex ratio 1.04 (95% CI 0.97-1.12). Both sex ratios are thus close to the normal one (1.06).

Multiple Births

After early exposure for NSAID there were 213 twin deliveries and 5 triplet deliveries. The OR for twinning was 0.86 (95% CI 0.75-0.99). After later exposure, there were 32 twin deliveries (no triplet delivery). The OR for twinning was 0.83 (95% CI 0.59-1.18). There is thus a moderate reduction in twinning after use of NSAID.

Table 43.5. Pregnancy duration and infant birth weight at maternal use of

Variable studied	Drug use in early pregnancy			Drug use later in pregnancy		
	Number	OR/RR	95% CI	Number	OR/RR	95% CI
<37 weeks	904	1.09	1.02-1.17	161	1.17	1.00-1.38
<2500g	609	1.13	1.04-1.23	103	1.11	0.91-1.36
≥4500g	673	1.03	0.95-1.12	113	1.07	0.88-1.30
SGA	412	1.06	0.96-1.17	60	0.89	0.68-1.15
LGA	981	1.08	1.01-1.16	150	0.96	0.81-1.14

A weak increase of the risk for preterm birth and low birth weight is thus seen.

Table 43.6. Infant mortality after maternal use of NSAID

Variable studied	Drug use in early pregnancy			Drug use later in pregnancy		
	Number	OR/RR	95% CI	Number	OR/RR	95% CI
Stillbirth	45	0.73	0.54-0.98	8	0.85	0.37-1.67#
Early neonatal death	24	1.00	0.70-1.38	8	2.27	0.98-4.48#

#observed over expected number with exact Poisson 95% confidence interval.

If anything, the stillbirth rate is lower than expected, notably after early exposure. The risk for early neonatal death is increased after later exposure but is not quite statistically significant.

Table 43.7. Neonatal diagnoses after maternal use of NSAID

Diagnosis	Drug use in early pregnancy			Drug use later in pregnancy		
	Number	OR/RR	95% CI	Number	OR/RR	95% CI
Hypoglycaemia	630	1.01	0.93-1.10	124	1.05	0.88-1.27
Respiratory diagnoses	847	1.01	0.94-1.08	128	0.94	0.79-1.13
Low Apgar score	317	0.98	0.88-1.10	49	0.92	0.69-1.22
CNS diagnoses	111	1.01	0.84-1.23	21	0.94	0.61-1.45
Jaundice	784	1.12	1.04-1.21	147	1.20	1.01-1.42

The only anomaly in neonatal pathology is a moderate increase in the risk for jaundice.

Table 43.8. Congenital malformations in infants whose mothers had used NSAID drugs in early pregnancy

Congenital malformation	Number	OR/RR	95% CI
All malformation	818	1.04	0.97-1.12
Relatively severe malformation	566	1.06	0.98-1.16
Chromosome anomalies	28	0.88	0.58-1.25
Without chromosome anomalies			
Any CNS malformation	25	1.29	0.86-1.92
Neural tube defects	7	1.14	0.54-2.42#
Eye malformations	16	1.02	0.62-1.69
Ear malformations	32	1.02	0.62-1.69
Orofacial clefts	40	1.34	0.97-1.88
Isolated cleft palate	12	1.03	0.57-1.88
Cleft lip with or without cleft palate	28	1.51	1.03-2.20
Any cardiovascular defect	203	1.15	1.00-1.33
VSD and/or ASD	100	1.16	0.96-1.41
Unspecified cardiac defect	14	0.83	0.47-1.44
Pylorostenosis	14	1.10	0.65-1.87
Oesophageal atresia	4	0.79	0.22-2.03#
Small gut atresia	9	2.10	0.96-3.98#
Anal atresia	10	1.48	0.71-2.72#
Abdominal wall defect	8	1.69	0.73-1.33#
Diaphragmatic hernia	3	0.82	0.17-2.38#
Hypospadias	52	1.20	0.92-1.56
Severe kidney malformation	20	1.89	1.21-2.96
Pes equinovarus	21	0.87	0.56-1.34
(Sub)luxation of hip. unstable hip	99	0.93	0.76-1.14
Poly/syndactyly	24	0.72	0.48-1.07
Limb reduction defects	6	0.60	0.27-1.34#
Craniostenosis	8	0.87	0.38-1.72#

#observed over expected number with exact Poisson 95% confidence interval.

Among infants with abdominal wall defects, there were five with gastroschisis and three with omphalocele. Both malformations occur in a slight but statistically non-significant excess.

Table 43.9. Relatively severe malformations according to group of NSAID

NSAID group	Number of infants		OR/RR	95% CI
	malformed	total		
Acetic acid derivates	78	2701	0.87	0.69-1.10
Oxicams	5	137	1.14	0.37-2.65#
Propionic acid derivates	479	13439	1.11	1.01-1.21
Coxibs	8	176	1.44	0.62-2.84#
Other NSAIDs	1	62	0.49	0.01-2.74#

#observed over expected number with exact Poisson 95% confidence interval.

Table 43.10. Specification of malformations after maternal use of oxicams, coxibs, or other NSAIDs

Oxicams
Spina bifida, branchial cyst/fistula, unspecified multiple malformations
Patent ductus arteriosus
Megacolon
Hypospadias
Craniostenosis, hypospadias, unspecified brain malformation, patent ductus arteriosus
Marfan syndrome
Coxibs
Anencephaly
Ventricular septum defect
Ventricular septum defect and patent ductus arteriosus
Choanal atesia
Duodenal atresia, megacolon
Pylorostenosis
Malformation syndrome involving the limbs
Ivemark syndrome (spleen malformation, cardiac defect)
Other NSAIDs
Craniostenosis

There were thus three infants with cardiac defects after exposure to coxibs and two central nervous system malformations after exposure to oxicams.

Propionic acid derivates appear to carry a higher risk than acetic acid derivates even though the difference between the groups may be random. Within the group of propionic acid derivates, naproxen appears to show an association with cardiovascular defects, hypospadias and orofacial clefts. Among then ten orofacial clefts, seven were cleft lip/palate: RR = 2.56 (95 % 1.03-5.28). The association with severe kidney malformations appears only for ibuprofen. In all three instances, the difference between the two drugs may be random.

SUMMARY

Use of NSAIDs seems to be associated with an increased risk for preeclampsia, induced delivery, caesarean section, and preterm birth. There seems to be an association between early use of NSAIDs and a slightly increased risk for congenital malformations. Two associations with more clear-cut risks can be identified. One is cardiovascular defects, hypospadias, and orofacial clefts (notably cleft lip/palate) linked to the use of propionic acid derivates and especially naproxen. The other is a link with severe kidney defects, also most noticeable for propionic acid derivates but this time with ibuprofen.

Table 43.11. Some specific malformations according to main group of NSAID

NSAID	Number of infants		OR	95%CI
	malformed	total		
Any cardiovascular malformation				
Acetic acid derivates	30	2701	1.02	0.70-1.49
Propionic acid derivates	171	13439	1.19	1.02-1.39
Ibufren	123	10547	1.09	0.91-1.31
Naproxen	44	2440	1.68	1.24-2.46
Ketoprofen	5	464	1.08	0.35-2.513
Orofacial cleft				
Acetic acid derivates	6	2701	1.03	0.38-2.24#
Propionic acid derivates	34	13439	1.43	1.02-2.02
Ibuprofen	24	10547	1.29	0.86-1.93
Naproxen	10	2440	2.28	1.09-4.19#
Hypospadias				
Acetic acid derivates	7	2701	0.87	0.35-1.79#
Propionic acid derivates	50	13439	1.27	0.95-1.68
Ibuprofen	36	10547	1.16	0.83-1.63
Naproxen	14	2440	1.92	1.13-3.26
Severe kidney malformation				
Acetic acid derivates	2	2701	1.10	0.13-3.99#
Propionic acid derivates	18	13439	2.07	1.23-3.27#
Ibuprofen	15	10547	2.20	1.23-3.62#
Naproxen	1	2440	0.61	0.02-3.42#

REFERENCES

[1] Nielsen GL, Sørensen HT, Larsen H, Pedersen L. Risk of adverse birth outcome and miscarriage in pregnant users of non-steroid anti-inflammatory drugs: population based observational study and case-control study, *BMJ* 2001; 322: 266-269.

[2] Ericson A, Källén BAJ. Nonsteoidal anti-inflammatory drugs in early pregnancy. *Reprod Toxicol* 2001; 15: 371-375.

[3] Ofori B, Oracichi D, Blais, Rey E, Bérard A. Risk of congenital anomalies in pregnant users of non-steroidal anti-inflammatory drugs: A nested case-control study. *Birth Defect Res (Part B)* 2006; 77: 268-279.

[4] Werler MM, Mitchell AA, Shapiro S. First trimester medication use in relation to gastroschisis. *Teratology* 1992; 45: 361-367.

[5] Torfs CP, Katz EA, Bateson TF, Lam PK, Curry CJ. Maternal medications and environmental exposures as risk factors for gastroschisis. *Teratology* 1996; 54: 84-92.

[6] Källén B. Maternal drug use and infant cleft lip/palate with special reference to corticoids. *Cleft Palate Craniofac J* 2003; 40: 6224-628.

[7] Koren G, Florescu A, Costei AM, Boskovic R, Moretti ME. Nonsteroidal antiinflammatory drugs during third trimester and the risk of premature closure of the ductus arteriosus: a meta-analysis. *Ann Pharmacother* 2006; 40: 824-829.

[8] Boubred F, Vendemmia M, Garcia-Meric P, Buffat C, Millet V, Simeoni U. Effects of maternally administered drugs on the foetal and neonatal kidney. *Drug Saf* 2006; 29: 397-419.

Chapter 44

MUSCLE RELAXING DRUGS

Use of muscle relaxing agents appears not to be associated with any significant increase in pregnancy or neonatal complications and the weak effects seen (e.g., a moderate increase in preeclampsia risk) can well be due to concomitant drug use or underlying pathology. In general there is no increase in the rate of relatively severe malformations and the finding of two infants with limb reduction defects among 47 exposed to orphenadrine may well be random. Even though use of these drugs if possible should be avoided during early pregnancy, there is no reason to discuss a pregnancy termination if exposure has ocurred.

In the Collaborative Perinatal Project [1] data on some muscle relaxants were given: among 83 exposed infants only two had a congenital malformation, 22 of these exposures referred to methocarbamol. Little further information is found in the literature.

Table 44.1. Number of women identified using muscle relaxing drugs

Total	1039
Reported use in early pregnancy	872
Got prescription later in pregnancy	189
Both early and later use	28

Type of drug	ATC code	Early use	Later use
Centrally acting agents	M03A	8	3
Pancuronium	M03AC01	0	1
Rocuronium	M03AC09	0	1
Botulinum toxin	M03AX01	8	1
Peripherally acting agents	M03B	865	186
Carisoprodol	M03BA02	123	10
Carisoprodol+paracetamol+codeine	M03BA52	0	2
Methocarbamol	M03BA03	4	0
Chlorzoxazone	M03BB02	243	120
Chlorzoxazone+acetyl salicylic acid+ dextropropoxyphene	M03BB53	386	37
Orphenadrine	M03BC01	11	6
Orphenadrine+paracetamol	M03BC51	35	2
Baclofen	M03BX01	10	5

A combination of a centrally and a peripherally acting agent occurred at one early exposure.

Characteristics of Women using Muscle Relaxing Drugs

Based on women reporting the drug in early pregnancy (n=872). Each variable is adjusted for all other variables and year of delivery. Comparison with all women who gave birth during the period and with information from the first antenatal care (n=967 742). The odds ratios for maternal age, parity, smoking in early pregnancy, number of previous miscarriages, BMI, subfertility, and country of birth are adjusted for all other variables.

Table 44.2. Characteristics of women using muscle relaxing drugs in early pregnancy

Variable studied	Number	OR	95% CI
Maternal age			
<25 years	123	0.85	0.69-1.04
25-34 years	546	1.00	reference
≥35 years	196	1.30	1.09-1.54
Parity			
1	361	1.12	0.97-1.30
≥2	511	1.00	reference
Smoking			
Unknown	34	-	-
No	624	1.00	reference
Yes	214	2.59	2.01-3.33
Previous miscarriage			
No	678	1.00	reference
Yes	194	0.97	0.82-1.15
Body Mass Index			
Unknown	97	-	-
<19.8	60	1.08	0.32-1.42
19.8-25.9	405	1.00	reference
≥26	310	1.70	2.46-1.97
Period of unwanted childlessness			
No	806	1.00	reference
Yes	66	1.08	0.84-1.30
Maternal country of birth			
Unknown	7	-	-
Sweden	760	1.00	reference
Other Nordic country	26	1.03	0.69-1.52
Non-Nordic country	79	0.55	0.43-0.69

Some further maternal characteristics were analyzed, adjusting for year of delivery, maternal age, parity, smoking, and BMI (Table 44.3).

Table 44.3. Some further characteristics of women using muscle relaxing drugs in early pregnancy

Variable studied	Number	OR	95% CI
Education (1996-2001, 544 women with drugs, 526 695 in population)			
Unknown	13		
<12 years	92	1.16	0.90-1.48
12 years	313	1.00	reference
≥13 years	130	0.64	0.52-0.80
Family situation			
Unknown	24	-	-
Co-habiting	775	1.00	reference
Living alone	41	1.24	0.89-1.73
Other family situation	29	1.40	0.96-2.04
Work outside home			
Unknown	158	-	-
Full time	321	1.00	reference
Part time	197	1.19	0.99-1.44
None	193	1.51	1.24-1.83

There is thus an increased usage of these drug at high maternal age, first parity, and by smoking women and women with a high BMI. High education appears to reduce the use of these drugs and these women work less often than expected outside home and are less often than expected born outside the Nordic countries.

Table 44.4. Concomitant drug use (early pregnancy)

Drug group	Number	OR/RR	95% CI
Drugs for stomach ulcer and reflux	30	3.09	2.08-4.41#
Multivitamins	23	0.81	0.54-1.23
Folic acid	21	0.68	0.44-1.05
Oral contraceptives	5	1.60	0.52-3.72#
Systemic corticosteroids	8	2.17	0.94-4.28#
Thyroid drugs	9	0.74	0.38-1.42#
Antibiotics	39	1.28	0.93-1.26
NSAIDs	136	8.57	7.31-10.0
Opioids	114	15.4	12.7-18.5
Minor analgesics	253	4.00	3.49-4.57
Anticonvulsants	5	1.67	0.54-5.90#
Neuroleptics	5	1.46	0.47-3.41#
Sedatives, hypnotics	46	7.50	5.48-10.0#
Antidepressants	55	4.28	3.31-5.54
Drugs for rhinitis	13	1.14	0.67-1.94
Antiasthmatics	48	1.56	1.16-2.08
Antihistamines	76	1.57	1.24-1.98
For NVP	46	1.24	0.92-1.67
For allergy	32	2.31	1.64-3.25

#observed over expected number with exact Poisson 95% confidence interval.

The strongest associations refer to analgesics and NSAIDs but also to sedatives, hypnotics and antidepressants. There is also an association with drugs used for stomach ulcer and reflux and also with antihistamines used for allergy.

Table 44.5. Some maternal diagnoses associated with the use of muscle relaxing drugs. Only use in early pregnancy as only few exposures occurred later in pregnancy

Diagnosis	Drug use in early pregnancy		
	Number	OR/RR	95% CI
Pre-existing diabetes	18	1.35	0.89-2.15
Chronic hypertension	17	1.40	0.86-2.27
Gestational diabetes	13	1.31	0.76-2.28
Preeclampsia	57	1.36	1.03-1.78
Hyperemesis gravidarum	16	1.55	0.95-2.55
Placenta previa	15	1.26	0.75-2.12
Abruptio placentae	17	1.31	0.80-2.12
Antepartum bleeding	22	1.59	1.04-2.43
Intrapartum bleeding	28	1.44	0.99-2.10
Postpartum bleeding	52	1.04	0.78-1.39
Delivery induction	125	1.36	1.12-1.66
Caesarean section	219	1.66	1.42-1.95

#observed over expected number with exact Poisson 95% confidence interval.

The number of exposures during later pregnancy was so low that most complications only occurred 1-2 times. Preeclampsia was, however, present in 12 instances (RR = 1.23, 95% CI 0.63-2.14), delivery induction in nine (OR = 0.82, 95% CI 0.42-1.61) and caesarean section in 50 (OR = 1.63, 95% CI 1.17-2.26).

There is thus a tendency for an increased risk of pregnancy complications, only significant for preeclampsia and antepartum bleeding and resulting in an increased rate of delivery inductions and caesarean sections.

Outcome after Maternal use of Muscle Relaxing Drugs

Infant Sex

Among infants whose mothers had used muscle relaxing drugs in early pregnancy there were 464 males and 420 females, a sex ratio of 1.10 (95% CI 0.97-1.26). After later use there were 92 males and 99 females, sex ratio 0.93 (95% CI 0.70-1.23). The normal sex ratio of 1.06 is thus contained in both confidence intervals.

Multiple Births

After early use there were 12 twin deliveries (OR = 0.87, 95% CI 0.49-1.55) and after later use only two (RR = 0.67, 95% CI 0.08-2.42).

Infant Mortality

There were no stillbirths but three early neonatal deaths after early exposure (RR = 1.92, 95% CI 0.40-5.60) and no deaths after later exposure.

Table 44.6. Pregnancy duration and infant birth weight at maternal use of muscle relaxing drugs

Variable studied	Drug use in early pregnancy			Drug use later in pregnancy		
	Number	OR/RR	95% CI	Number	OR/RR	95% CI
<37 weeks	60	1.31	1.00-1.72	9	0.92	0.42-1.75#
<2500g	31	1.00	0.69-1.44	7	1.15	0.45-2.37#
≥4500g	32	0.84	0.59-1.20	6	0.71	0.26-1.55#
SGA	28	1.29	0.88-1.91	4	0.97	0.26-2.47#
LGA	59	1.05	0.80-1.38	11	0.81	0.43-1.52

The only marginally significant deviation is thus in an increased risk of preterm birth after early drug use.

Table 44.7. Neonatal diagnoses after maternal use of muscle relaxing drugs

Diagnosis	Drug use in early pregnancy			Drug use later in pregnancy		
	Number	OR/RR	95% CI	Number	OR/RR	95% CI
Hypoglycaemia	35	0.97	0.69-1.37	5	0.66	0.21-1.54#
Respiratory diagnoses	50	1.03	0.74-1.38	6	0.62	0.23-1.34#
Low Apgar score	19	0.98	0.62-1.56	1	0.27	0.01-1.49#
CNS diagnoses	7	1.25	0.50-2.58#	0	-	-
Jaundice	46	1.26	0.93-1.71	4	0.50	0.14-1.27#

#observed over expected number with exact Poisson 95% confidence interval.

Thus, no neonatal diagnoses occurred in excess.

Table 44.8. Congenital malformations in infants whose mothers had used muscle relaxing drugs in early pregnancy

Congenital malformation	Number	OR	95% CI
All malformation	63	1.48	1.14-1.91
Relatively severe malformation	34	1.14	0.80-1.62
Chromosome anomalies	2	0.96	0.12-3.47#
Without chromosome anomalies			
Orofacial cleft	4	2.33	0.63-5.95#
Any cardiovascular defect	10	1.06	0.51-1.95#
VSD and/or ASD	6	1.32	0.48-2.87#
Poly/syndactyly	3	1.62	0.33-4.74#
Pes equinovarus	3	1.82	0.37-5.31#

#observed over expected number with exact Poisson 95% confidence interval.

There is thus an excess of any malformation but not of relatively severe malformations. Among infants with the minor anomalies which were not included in the latter group, there were nine with undescended testicle, seven with hip (sub)luxation or unstable hip, four with nevus, and four with preauricular tags.

Among the ten cardiac defects, there were five with ventricular septum defect (one with polydactyly and one with pes equinovarus), one with atrium septum defect, one with an unspecified septum defect, one with patent ductus arteriosus, and two with unspecified cardiac defects.

Table 44.9. Other relatively severe malformations in infants whose mothers used muscle relaxing drugs in early pregnancy

Malformation	Number
Hydrocephalus	1
Congenital ptosis and skull/face malformation	1
Lacrimal duct stenosis	1
Prominent ear	1
Cleft lip/palate	3
Median cleft palate	1
Oesophageal atresia	1
Pylorostenosis	1
Renal dysplasia with ectopic ureter	1
Hydronephrosis	3
Hypospadias	1
Testis anomaly	1
Hand/finger reduction and deformity	1
Fibula and foot reduction	1
Polydactyly	2
Pes equinovarus	2
Down syndrome	1
Fragile X syndrome	1

Some of these are thus really minor anomalies.

Table 44.10. Number of infants with any congenital malformation according to drug used

Muscle relaxing drug	Number of infants		OR/RR	95% CI
	malformed	total		
Carisoprodol	4	182	0.64	0.17-1.64#
Methocarbamol	0	4	-	-
Chlormezanone	1	5	-	-
Chlorzoxazone	23	217	1.05	0.69-1.62
Orphenadrine	4	47	2.50	0.68-6.40#
Baclofen	2	10	6.25	0.76-22.6#

#observed over expected number with exact Poisson 95% confidence interval

Among the four infants born after exposure to orphenadrine, two had limb reduction defects, one had oesophageal atresia, and one had a ventricular septum defect. The two infants born after exposure to baclofen had ventricular septum defect and median cleft palate, respectively.

SUMMARY

Use of muscle relaxing agents is strongly associated with use of analgesics or NSAID. Except for a moderate increase in the risk of preeclampsia and possibly of preterm birth, no major ill effects on pregnancy or neonatal period was seen There was a statistically significant increase in malformation risk but this is mainly due to unusually many mild and variable conditions without any specificity to type. No certain risk increase is seen among relatively severe malformations. An interesting observation is the occurrence of two limb reduction defects among 47 infants exposed to orphenadrine but this may well be random.

References

[1] Heinonen OP, Slone D, Shapiro S. *Birth Defects and Drugs in Pregnancy.* Publishing Sciences Group, Inc. Littleton, MA.

Chapter 45

Other Drugs for Musculoskeletal Diseases

If a woman has been treated with colchicine before or in early pregnancy, this seems not to represent any major risk for foetal damage but foetal diagnosis with karyotyping can be suggested. Biphosphonates should be avoided during pregnancy but if exposure has occurred this is hardly a reason for discussing a termination of the pregnancy. More information on these relatively rare expsoures is needed.

Table 45.1. Number of women identified using other drugs for musculoskeletal disease

Total	60
Reported use in early pregnancy	42
Got prescription later in pregnancy	24
Both early and later use	6

Type of drug	ATC code	Early use	Later use
Antigout drugs	M04	20	5
Allopurinol	M04AA01	12	3
Colchicine	M04AC01	8	2
Drugs for treatment of bone diseases (biphosphonates)	M05BA	17	15
Etidronic acid	M05BA01	1	1
Clodronic acid	M05BA02	14	13
Alendronic acid	M05BA04	3	1
Other drugs	M09	5	4
Hyaluronic acid	M09AX01	1	0
Chondroitin sulfate	M09AX03	4	4

A few women had used drugs for musculoskeletal problems which belong to other drug categories than those mentioned in previous chapters. The most debated one among these drugs is colchicine, a substance with an effect on the mitotic spindle. In Sweden it is mainly used for gout but is also used for Mediterranean fever. One study of 225 colchicine-exposed pregnancies found no increase in the rate of foetal abnormalities [1].Another study [2] investigated 901 pregnancies where one of the partners had Mediterranean fever. A slightly increased rate of numerical and structural chromosome anomalies was found but it was not statistically significant. An early paper reported two colchicine-exposed infants among 54 with Down syndrome [3]. Biphosphonates used during pregnancy could affect foetal bone development but limited experience so far does not show any risk [4].

The number of exposures is so low that an analysis is relatively meaningless. None of the 42 infants exposed in early pregnancy had a congenital malformation registered. The expected number is 1.8 but the upper confidence limit of the RR is 2.

Summary

There are no signs of a teratogenic effect of these drugs but the number of exposures is so low that no certain conclusions can be drawn, notably for individual drugs.

References

[1] Rabinovitch O, Zemer D, Kukia E, Sohar E, Mashiach S. Colchicine treatment in conception and pregnancy: two hudred thirty-one pregnancies in patients with familial Mediterranean fever. *Am J Reprod Immunol* 1992; 28: 245-246.

[2] Barkenstadt M, Weisz B, Cuckle H, Di-Castro M, Guetta E, Barkai G. Chromosomal abnormalities and birth defects among couples with colchicine treated familial Mediterranean fever, *Am J Obst Gynecol* 2005; 193: 1513-1516.

[3] Ferreira NR. Frota-Pessoa O. Trisomy after colchicine treatment. *Lancet* 1969;1:1161-2.

[4] Djokanovic N, Klieger-Grossman C, Koren G. Does treatment with biphosphonates endanger the human pregnancy? *J Obstet Gynaecol Can* 2008; 30: 1146-1148.

Chapter 46

ANALGESICS (EXCLUDING DRUGS FOR MIGRAINE)

Opioid analgetics can cause neonatal withdrawal and other symptoms and should be avoided towards the end of the pregnancy. There seems to be no certain teratogenic effect with such drugs. Acetylsalicylic acid can increase maternal and foetal bleeding but can also have some beneficial effects. Use of minor analgesics, mainly acetylsalicylic acid and paracetamol, seems not to be associated with any teratogenic risk and especially the postulated association with gastroschisis cannot be substantiated in prospective studies. Small deviations in pregnancy outcome may be due to co-morbidity and concomitant drug use.

Use of analgesics during late pregnancy can be associated with neonatal symptoms including withdrawal symptoms, notably after the use of opioids. Late use of acetylsalicylic acid has been linked to an increased risk for bleeding at delivery and in the infant but treatment with this drug has also been tried in order to reduce thromboembolic complications [1]. No certain increased risk for congenital malformations has been seen after opioids [2] but the relative risk was higher after codeine than after other such drugs. A few small studies of buphrenophine showed no teratogenic effect but this drug gave neonatal withdrawal symptoms when used in late pregnancy [3]. The teratogenic risk of acetylsalicylic acid in early pregnancy has been much discussed and some authors found associations with some congenital malformations, neural tube defects, gastroschisis, and cleft lip and palate [4]. Most of these studies were retrospective case-control studies. Other studies found no such effects [5]. It has been suggested that maternal use of paracetamol should markedly increase the risk for gastroschisis [6] but a large Danish study could not confirm this and found no other signs of teratogenicity [7]. A small study on metamizole [8] found no teratogenic effect: among 98 infants exposed during the first trimester, three had congenital malformations.

Analgesics are often used for short periods in association with fever or other temporary illness and it may therefore be difficult to demonstrate specific effects on malformations with a short organogenetic period.

Table 46.1. Number of women identified using analgesics

Total	85587
Reported use in early pregnancy	74668
Got prescription later in pregnancy	14324
Both early and later use	3405

Type of drug	ATC code	Early use	Later use
Opioids	N02A	4725	2578
Morphine	N02AA01	121	37
Morphine + spasmolytic	N02AG01	116	78
Hydromorphone + spasmolytic	N02AG04	19	3
Oxycodone	N02AA05	11	0
Codeine + paracetamol/ASA	N02AA59	935	786
Ketobemidone	N02AB01	28	7
Ketobemidone + spasmolytic	N02AG02	138	44
Pethidine	N02AB02	22	1
Fentanyl	N02AB03	2	1
Methadone	N02AC02	38	18
Dextropropoxyphene	N02AC04	1293	928
Dextropropoxyphene + paracetamol/ASA	N02AC54	1399	508
Pentazocine	N02AD01	4	0
Buprenorphine	N02AE01	64	59
Tramadol	N02AX02	772	213
Salicylate acid derivates	N02BA	8246	779
Acetylsalicylic acid (ASA)	N02BA01	2101	235
ASA + caffeine/metoclopramide	N02BA51	6218	546
Diflunisal	N02BA11	3	2
Pyrazolones	N02BB	56	18
Metamizole	N02BB02	6	2
Phenazone + caffeine	N02BB51	49	16
Anilides	N02BE	65285	12110
Paracetamol (acetaminophen)	N02BE01	62564	11031
Paracetamol + codeine	N02BE51	3325	1317
Unspecified analgesics	N02	50	3

Table 46.2. Combinations of different classes of analgesics

	Early use			Later use		
	Salicylates	Pyrazolones	Anilides	Salicylates	Pyrazolones	Anilides
Opioids	83	2	1563	27	1	936
Salicylates		4	1934			160
Pyrazolones			13			3

A combination of opioids, salicylates, and anilides was used by 35 women in early pregnancy and by 17 in later pregnancy. A combination of salicylates, pyrazolones, and anilides was used by two women in early pregnancy.

Characteristics of Women using Analgesics

Based on women reporting the drug in early pregnancy (n=74 661, seven missing maternal age). Each variable is adjusted for all other variables and year of delivery.

Comparison with all women who gave birth during the period and with information from the first antenatal care (n=967 742). The odds ratios for maternal age, parity, smoking in early pregnancy, number of previous miscarriages, BMI, subfertility, and country of birth are adjusted for all other variables and are shown in Figure 46.1.

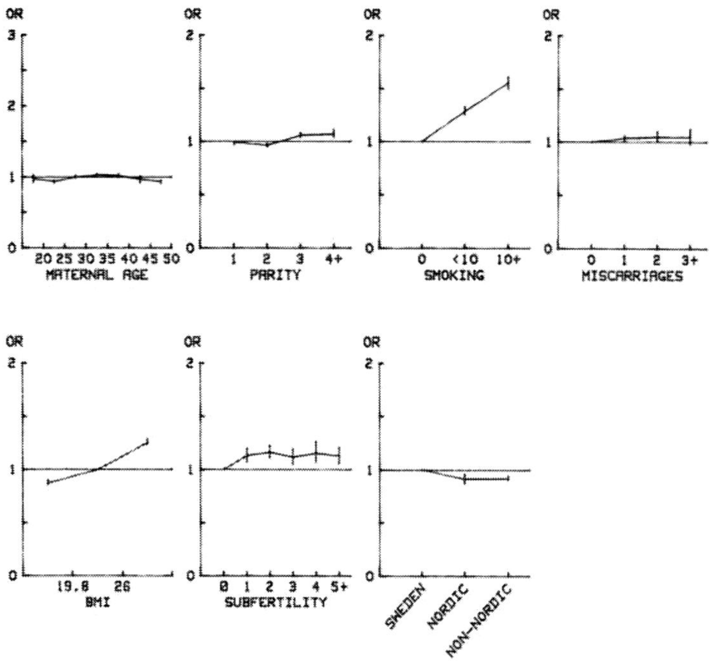

Figure 46.1. Odds ratios for seven maternal characteristics. The odds ratios (OR) for each variable are adjusted for the other variables and year of delivery. Vertical lines mark 95% confidence intervals. For maternal age and parity, each class is compared with all other classes.

Some further maternal characteristics were analyzed, adjusting for year of delivery, maternal age, parity, smoking, and BMI (Table 46.3).

Table 46.3. Some further characteristics of women using analgesics

Variable studied	Number	OR	95% CI
Education (1996-2001, 39158 women with drugs, 526 695 in population)			
Unknown	972	-	-
<12 years	5054	1.04	1.01-1.08
12 years	20406	1.00	reference
13-14 years	2075	0.97	0.92-1.01
>14 years	10651	0.93	0.91-0.96
Family situation			
Unknown	528	-	
Co-habiting	68604	1.00	reference
Living alone	2147	1.06	1.01-1.12
Other family situation	2153	1.10	1.05-1.16
Work outside home			
Unknown	9802	-	
Full time	33172	1.00	reference
Part time	18310	1.10	1.08-1.12
None	12838	1.04	1.01-1.06

The women using analgesics deviate rather little from other women who gave birth. They smoke more and there is an increased usage with increasing BMI. A rather weak association with unwanted childlessness is seen and a slightly lower use among women, not born in Sweden. There is a slight association with low educational level, non-cohabiting, and not working full time outside the home.

Table 46.4. Concomitant drug use (early pregnancy)

Drug group	Number	OR/RR	95% CI
Drugs for stomach ulcer and reflux	1031	1.59	1.49-1.70
Drugs for inflammatory bowel disease	216	1.09	0.94-1.25
Insulin	101	0.35	0.28-0.42
Multivitamins	2913	0.98	0.94-1.02
Folic acid	2486	0.82	0.79-0.86
Oral contraceptives	372	1.44	1.29-1.61
Progestogens	294	0.83	0.74-0.94
Gonadotropins	116	0.58	0.48-0.70
Systemic corticosteroids	335	1.16	1.03-1.29
Thyroid drugs	594	0.56	0.51-0.61
Antibiotics	3266	1.41	1.36-1.46
NSAIDs	3965	3.25	3.14-3.36
Drugs for migraine	664	3.53	3.25-3.84
Anticonvulsants	128	0.54	0.45-0.65
Neuroleptics	206	0.75	0.65-0.86
Sedatives, hypnotics	781	2.24	2.08-2.42
Antidepressants	1007	0.96	0.90-1.03
Drugs for rhinitis	2430	2.58	2.47-2.69
Antiasthmatics	2299	0.90	0.86-0.94
Cough medicines	1359	4.40	4.15-4.67
Antihistamines	6589	1.56	1.52-1.61
For NVP	5448	1.71	1.66-1.76
For allergy	1319	1.69	1.03-1.15

Table 46.5. Some maternal diagnoses associated with the use of analgesics

Diagnosis	Drug use in early pregnancy			Drug use later in pregnancy		
	Number	OR/RR	95% CI	Number	OR/RR	95% CI
Pre-existing diabetes	854	0.81	0.75-0.87	179	0.81	0.70-0.94
Chronic hypertension	930	0.98	0.92-1.05	215	1.06	0.92-1.22
Gestational diabetes	760	1.03	0.95-1.11	142	0.96	0.81-1.13
Preeclampsia	3846	1.10	1.06-1.13	807	1.21	1.12-1.30
Hyperemesis gravidarum	819	1.01	0.94-1.09	173	1.02	0.87-1.19
Placenta previa	923	1.01	0.95-1.09	196	1.04	0.90-1.20
Abruptio placentae	1024	1.02	0.95-1.09	193	0.93	0.80-1.08
Antepartum bleeding	1087	1.01	0.95-1.08	209	1.00	0.87-1.15
Intrapartum bleeding	1739	1.07	1.01-1.12	377	1.03	0.93-1.25
Postpartum bleeding	4251	1.02	0.98-1.05	804	1.01	0.94-1.09
Delivery induction	8744	1.08	1.05-1.11	2069	1.29	1.23-1.36
Caesarean section	13015	1.10	1.08-1.12	3017	1.27	1.22-1.32

The strongest associations are seen with other drugs used for pain, notably NSAIDs, drugs for migraine, and corticosteroids. There are also strong associations with drugs used for infections but not for asthma. Some other drug categories are also associated with analgesic use: drugs for stomach ulcer and reflux, oral contraceptives, sedatives and hypnotics (but not antidepressants), and antihistamines.

There is thus a slightly increased risk for preeclampsia, notably after later exposure. After use of acetylsalicylic acid the OR was slightly higher (1.49, 95% CI 1.13-1.98) than after use of paracetamol (OR = 1.18, 95% CI 1.09-1.28) or dextropropoxyphene (OR = 1.19, 95% CI 0.90-1.58). The explanation may be the use of acetyl salicylic acid at incipient preeclampsia. There was no significantly increased risk of bleeding before, during or after delivery after later use of acetylsalicylic acid but the OR for intraparum bleeding was 1.39 (95% CI 0.95-2.04).

OUTCOME AFTER MATERNAL USE OF ANALGESICS

Infant Sex

After use of analgesics in early pregnancy, there were 38 956 male and 36 900 female infants born (27 with unknown sex). The sex ratio was exactly the normal one, 1.06 (95% CI 1.04-1.07). After later exposure there were 7 499 male and 7 042 female infants born, sex ratio also 1.06 (95% CI 1.03-1.10).

Multiple Births

After early exposure, there were 1 192 twin and 18 triplet deliveries. The OR for a twin delivery was 0.89 (95% CI 0.78-1.02). After later exposure there were 216 twin and two triplet deliveries. OR for a twin delivery was 1.06 (95% CI 0.92-1.22).

Table 46.6. Pregnancy duration and infant birth weight at maternal use of analgesics

Variable studied	Drug use in early pregnancy			Drug use later in pregnancy		
	Number	OR/RR	95% CI	Number	OR/RR	95% CI
<37 weeks	3801	1.05	1.01-1.08	813	1.19	1.11-1.28
<2500g	2430	1.05	1.00-1.09	516	1.17	1.07-1.28
≥4500g	3093	0.97	0.94-1.01	540	0.87	0.80-0.95
SGA	1628	1.02	0.97-1.08	344	1.16	1.03-1.29
LGA	4717	1.00	0.97-1.04	951	1.00	0.93-1.07

There are thus small risk increases for preterm birth and low birth weight and after later exposure also for SGA. These effects are probably due to co-morbidity and concomitant use of other drugs.

Table 46.7. Infant mortality after maternal use of analgesics

Variable studied	Drug use in early pregnancy			Drug use later in pregnancy		
	Number	OR	95% CI	Number	OR/RR	95% CI
Stillbirth	238	0.89	0.78-1.02	42	0.93	0.68-1.26
Early neonatal death	98	0.83	0.68-1.02	17	0.83	0.51-1.35

Thus, if anything, the risk estimates were low even though none reached statistical significance.

Table 46.8. Neonatal diagnoses after maternal use of analgesics

Diagnosis	Drug use in early pregnancy			Drug use later in pregnancy		
	Number	OR/RR	95% CI	Number	OR/RR	95% CI
Hypoglycaemia	2656	0.97	0.93-1.01	593	1.04	0.95-1.13
Respiratory diagnoses	3895	1.04	1.00-1.07	734	1.10	1.02-1.19
Low Apgar score	1490	1.03	0.98-1.09	279	1.08	0.96-1.22
CNS diagnoses	462	0.99	0.90-1.09	134	1.29	1.09-1.54
Jaundice	3231	1.06	1.02-1.10	754	1.25	1.15-1.34

The increased risk for CNS diagnoses after later exposure was analyzed for different drugs or drug groups (Table 46.9).

Table 46.9. The risk for CNS diagnosis according to analgesic used in later pregnancy

Drug or drug group	Number with CNS diagnosis	Total number	OR/RR	95% CI
All opioids	42	2610	2.31	1.70-3.14
Opiates	17	832	2.73	1.59-4.39#
Dextropropoxyphene	17	1443	1.75	1.02-2.79#
Tramadol	2	216	1.20	0.15-4.35#
Methadone	2	18	13.3	1.61-48.2#
Acetylsalicylic acid	4	789	0.63	0.17-1.61#
Paracetamol	105	12294	1.17	0.96-1.42#

None of the minor analgesics thus had an effect on the risk of CNS diagnoses but for all opioids such effects are seen although confidence intervals are large except for dextropropoxyphene.

The high OR for buprenorphine is thus based on only six malformed infants. Among them two had ventricular septum defects (one of them with absence of the proximal part of vena cava inferior), one had atrium septum defect, and one had both ventricular and atrium septum defects. One infant had hypospadias and the sixth had a pes calcaneovalgus.

Among infants exposed to acetylsalicylic acid, there were three with neural tube defects (RR = 0.83, 95% CI 0.17-2.42), 94 with cardiovascular defects (OR = 1.05, 95% CI 0.85-1.29), ten with orofacial clefts (OR = 0.63, 95% CI 0.34-1.17) and five with pylorostenosis (RR = 0.78, 95% CI 0.25-1.81). There were three infants with abdominal wall defects, one with omphalocele and two with gastroschisis (which is one more than expected).

Paracetamol represented the majority of exposures to analgesics and odds ratios specific for paracetamol exposure differ only little from those estimated for all analgesics. For one condition, pylorostenosis, the odds ratios increased from 1.25 to 1.39 and became formally statistically significance: 95% CI = 1.08-1.80. A causal association seems unlikely. As paracetamol has been linked to gastroschisis, the body wall defects were analyzed separately for omphalocele and gastroschisis. Among the 15 infants with body wall defects, seven had omphalocele (RR = 0.98, 95% CI 0.40-2.03) and eight had gastroschisis (RR = 0.95, 95% CI 0.41-1.82).

Table 49.10. Congenital malformations in infants whose mothers had used analgesics in early pregnancy

Congenital malformation	Number	OR	95% CI
All malformation	3676	1.03	0.99-1.06
Relatively severe malformation	2551	1.04	1.00-1.08
Chromosome anomalies	157	1.03	0.88-1.22
Without chromosome anomalies			
Any CNS malformation	98	1.04	0.85-1.28
Neural tube defects	30	1.01	0.70-1.46
Eye malformations	82	1.08	0.86-1.36
Ear malformations	170	0.94	0.81-1.11
Orofacial clefts	137	0.98	0.82-1.17
Any cardiovascular defect	877	1.09	1.02-1.17
Relatively severe cardiac defects[a]	149	0.94	0.80-1.11
VSD and/or ASD	460	1.09	0.99-1.21
Unspecified cardiovascular defects	83	1.04	0.83-1.31
Pylorostenosis	69	1.25	0.98-1.61
Oesophageal atresia	18	0.78	0.48-1.27
Small gut atresia	15	0.78	0.46-1.31
Anal atresia	33	1.05	0.73-1.51
Hypospadias	209	0.96	0.83-1.11
Kidney agenesis/dysgenesis	13	0.61	0.35-1.06
Cystic kidneys	32	1.06	0.73-1.53
Abdominal wall defects	20	1.04	0.65-1.64
Diaphragmatic hernia	20	1.16	0.73-1.83
Pes equinovarus	108	0.98	0.80-1.20
Poly/syndactyly	164	1.08	0.92-1.27
Limb reduction defects	51	1.14	0.85-1.53
(Sub)luxation of hip, unstable hip	464	1.00	0.91-1.10
Craniostenosis	43	0.97	0.71-1.32

[a]Comprises truncus arteriosus, transposition of great vessels, tetralogy of Fallot, hypoplastic left heart syndrome, endocardial cushion defect, Ebstein anomaly, coarctatio of aorta.

Table 46.11. Relatively severe malformations according to drug or drug group used

Drug or drug group	Number with malformation	Total number	OR/RR	95% CI
Opioids	177	4805	1.13	0.97-1.31
Morphine	9	241	1.12	0.51-2.12#
Dextropropoxyphene	94	2700	1.02	0.83-1.26
Codeine combinations	34	950	1.18	0.83-1.66
Ketobemidone	6	174	1.09	0.40-2.38#
Buprenorphine	6	66	2.99	1.10-6.50#
Acetylsalicylic acid	266	8371	0.94	0.83-1.06
Paracetamol	2223	66300	1.04	1.00-1.09

SUMMARY

Analgesics are used at a large number of different conditions and together with other drugs. Many of the weak effects, apparent because of the large number of exposures, may well be secondary to such associations. There is a clear-cut (and expected) effect on CNS disturbances by maternal use of opioids during later pregnancy but this is not seen after minor analgesics. The risk for a congenital malformation after early exposure is low and no support is obtained for a specific association between paracetamol and gastroschisis or between acetylsalicylic acid and any specific malformation. An observed malformation risk after exposure to bruphenorphine needs confirmation.

REFERENCES

[1] James AH, Brancazio LR, Price T. Aspirin and reproductive outcomes. *Obstet Gynecol Surv* 2008; 63: 49-57.

[2] Heinoen, OP, Slone D, Shapiro S. *Birth Defects and Drugs in Pregnancy*. Publishing Sciences Group, Inc. Littleton, MA.

[3] Lacroix I, Berrebi A, Chaumerliac C, Lapeyre-Mestre M, Montastruc JL, Damase-Michel C. Buprenorphine in pregnant opioid-dependent women: first results of a prospective study. *Addiction* 2004; 99: 209-214.

[4] Kozer E, Nikfar S, Costei A, Boskivic R, Nulman I, Koren G. Aspirin consumption during the first trimester of pregnancy and congenital malformations: a meta-analysis. *Am J Obst Gynecol* 2002; 187: 1623-1630.

[5] Nørgård B, Puhó E, Czeizel A, Skriver MV, Sørensen HT. Aspirin use during early pregnancy and the risk of congenital abnormalities: A population-based case-control study. *Amer J Obst Gynecol* 2005; 192: 922-923.

[6] Werler MM, Sheehan JE, Mitchell AA. Maternal medication use and risks of gastroschisis and small intestinal atresia. *Am J Epidemiol* 2002; 155: 26-31.

[7] Rebordosa C, Kogevinas M, Horváth-Puhó A, Nørgård B, Morales M, Czeizel AE, Vilstrup H, Sørensen HT, Olsen J. Acetaminophen use during pregnancy: effects on risk for congenital abnormalities. *Amer J Obst Gynecal* 2008; 198: 178e1-178.e7.

[8] Bar-Oz B, Clementi M, Di Giantonio E, Greenberg R, Beer M, Merlob P, Arnon J, Ornoy A, Zimmerman DM, Berkovitch M. Matamizol (dipyrone, optalgin) in pregnancy, is it safe? A prospective comparative study. *Europ J Obstet Gynecol Reprod Biol* 2005; 119: 176-179.

Chapter 47

DRUGS FOR MIGRAINE

Ergot alkaloids should be avoided during pregnancy but no certain teratogenic effect is seen. The use of triptans during pregnancy appears to be free of teratogenic risks but more information on eletriptan is needed.

Ergotamine and related substances have an old reputation as abortificants due to uterine contraction. Little evidence exists for a teratogenic effect. One study [1] found signs of a teratogenic effect at a dose level of 1.5 mg ergotamine but none at 0.3 mg. This was mainly based on the occurrence of three exposed cases of spina bifida. Other studies found no significant excess risk [2,3]. A number of studies on the use of triptans, notably sumatriptan, during pregnancy [3-5], and reviews [6,7] agree that no teratogenic risk is apparent.

Table 47.1. Number of women identified using drugs for migraine

Total	3051
Reported use in early pregnancy	2624
Got prescription later in pregnancy	607
Both early and later use	180

Type of drug	ATC code	Early use	Later use
Ergot alkaloids	N02CA	439	117
Dihydroergotamine	N02CA01	117	91
Methylsergide	N02CA04	1	0
Ergotamine+coffein	N02CA52	35	4
Ergotamine+chlorcyclizine+coffein	N02CA72	286	17
Selective5HT1-receptor agonists	N02CC	2161	454
Sumatriptan	N02CC01	1850	341
Naratriptan	N02CC02	19	5
Zolmitriptan	N02CC03	204	84
Rizatriptan	N02CC04	106	33
Almotriptan	N02CC05	1	1
Eletriptan	N02CC06	6	1
Other drugs for migraine	N02X	58	43
Pizotifen	N02CX01	58	43
Unspecified	N02C	7	0

In early pregnancy, 32 women used both an ergot alkaloid and a 5HT1-receptor agonist and eight used both a 5HT1-receptor agonist and pizotifen. Corresponding numbers at later use was two and four.

Characteristics of Women using Drugs for Migraine

Based on women reporting the drug in early pregnancy (n=2624). Each variable is adjusted for all other variables and year of delivery. Comparison with all women who gave birth during the period and with information from the first antenatal care (n=967 742). The odds ratios for maternal age, parity, smoking in early pregnancy, number of previous miscarriages, BMI, subfertility, and country of birth are adjusted for all other variables and are shown in Figure 47.1.

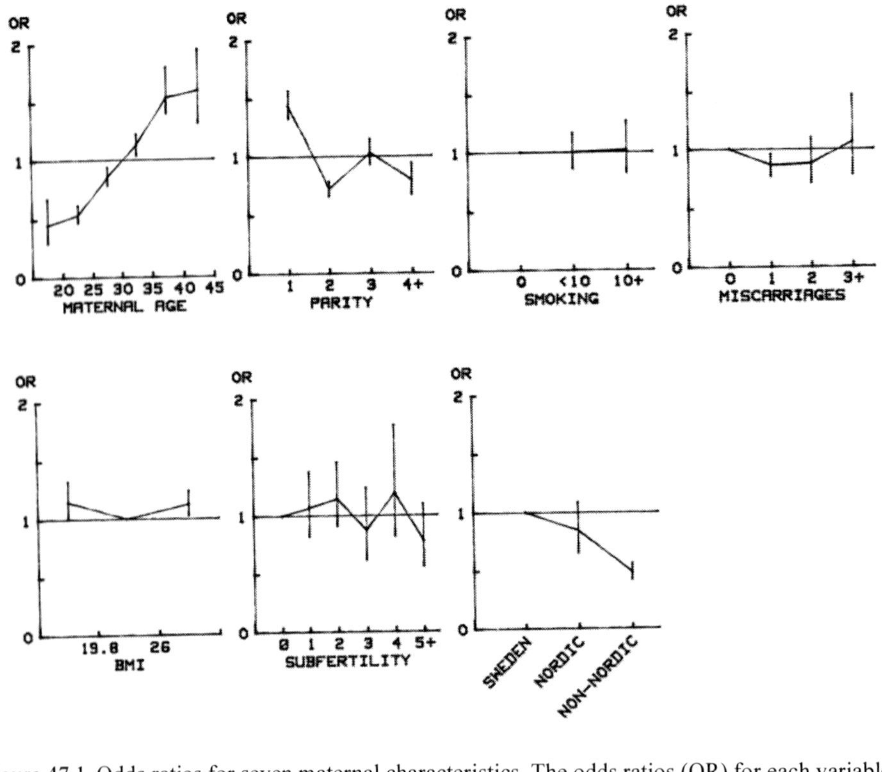

Figure 47.1. Odds ratios for seven maternal characteristics. The odds ratios (OR) for each variable are adjusted for the other variables and year of delivery. Vertical lines mark 95% confidence intervals. For maternal age and parity, each class is compared with all other classes.

Some further maternal characteristics were analyzed, adjusting for year of delivery, maternal age, parity, smoking, and BMI (Table 47.2).

Table 47.2. Some further characteristics of women using drugs for migraine

Variable studied	Number	OR	95% CI
Education (1996-2001, 1410 women with drugs, 526 695 in population)			
Unknown	17	-	-
<12 years	135	0.92	0.76-1.11
12 years	742	1.00	reference
13-14 years	92	1.05	0.84-1.30
≥14 years	516	0.85	0.75-0.97
Family situation			
Unknown	4	-	-
Co-habiting	2423	1.00	reference
Living alone	65	1.05	0.81-1.35
Other family situation	65	1.09	0.83-1.44
Work outside home			
Unknown	297	-	-
Full time	1342	1.00	reference
Part time	619	0.99	0.89-1.10
None	345	0.81	0.71-0.92

The use of drugs for migraine increased with age and was higher at first than at later parities. There was a slightly increased use both at low and high BMI and less use by women born outside the Nordic countries.

Table 47.3. Concomitant drug use (early pregnancy)

Drug group	Number	OR/RR	95% CI
Drugs for stomach ulcer and reflux	78	3.34	2.69-4.15
Drugs for inflammatory bowel disease	11	1.15	0.97-2.01#
Multivitamins	57	0.48	0.37-0.62
Folic acid	79	0.72	0.57-0.90
Antihypertensives	85	9.18	7.64-11.0
Oral contraceptives	13	1.58	0.84-2.70#
Progestogens	8	0.53	0.27-1.04#
Systemic corticosteroids	13	1.24	0.71-2.15#
Thyroid drugs	40	1.07	0.78-1.47
Antibiotics	78	0.95	0.71-1.19
NSAIDs	205	4.14	3.63-4.73
Opioids	108	8.36	7.06-9.90
Minor analgesics	590	3.10	2.90-3.45
Anticonvulsants	9	1.12	0.51-2.13#
Neuroleptics	7	0.76	0.31-1.57#
Sedatives, hypnotics	42	3.25	2.42-4.36
Antidepressants	101	3.00	2.47-3.46
Drugs for rhinitis	65	1.64	1.28-2.09
Antiasthmatics	143	1.69	1.43-2.00
Antihistamines	188	1.21	1.04-1.40
For NVP	127	1.06	0.89-1.27
For allergy	66	1.53	1.20-1.95

#observed over expected number with exact Poisson 95% confidence interval.

As expected there are strong associations with analgesics and NSAIDs. The association with antihypertensives is explained by the use of beta-blocking drugs as migraine prophylaxis. As will be seen further down there is no certain association with pre-existing hypertension. There are also associations with drugs used for allergy: antihistamines, drugs for rhinitis, and antiasthmatics. Sedatives, hypnotics, and antidepressants are also used more than expected.

Table 47.4. Some maternal diagnoses associated with the use of drugs for migraine

Diagnosis	Drug use in early pregnancy			Drug use later in pregnancy		
	Number	OR/RR	95% CI	Number	OR/RR	95% CI
Pre-existing diabetes	25	0.67	0.45-1.00	10	1.03	0.49-1.89#
Chronic hypertension	42	1.25	0.92-1.70	15	1.58	0.89-2.01#
Gestational diabetes	27	1.04	0.70-1.52	9	1.31	0.60-2.48#
Preeclampsia	186	1.47	1.26-1.71	43	1.44	1.05-1.97
Hyperemesis gravidarum	29	1.04	0.72-1.50	10	1.29	0.62-2.37#
Placenta previa	30	0.93	0.64-1.33	10	1.14	0.53-2.69#
Abruptio placentae	37	1.05	0.76-1.46	11	1.16	0.58-2.08#
Antepartum bleeding	36	0.93	0.67-1.30	13	1.34	0.71-2.29#
Intrapartum bleeding	57	0.97	0.74-1.27	24	1.45	0.96-2.19
Postpartum bleeding	160	1.03	0.88-1.21	32	0.92	0.64-1.31
Delivery induction	344	1.21	1.08-1.36	81	1.18	0.93-1.51
Caesarean section	493	1.12	1.01-1.23	135	1.35	1.04-1.53

#observed over expected number with exact Poisson 95% confidence interval.

The only abnormality among the maternal diagnoses listed is an excess of preeclampsia. This may be the explanation to the increased rate of delivery inductions and caesarean sections.

Outcome after Maternal use of Drugs Against Migraine

Infant Sex

After use in early pregnancy there were 1 393 male and 1 262 female infants born (one with unknown sex). The sex ratio was 1.10 (95% CI 1.02-1.19). After later use, there were 314 male and 305 female infants, sex ratio 1.03 (95% CI 0.88-1.20). The normal sex ratio (1.06) is thus contained within both confidence intervals.

Multiple Births

After use in early pregnancy there were 30 twin deliveries and one triplet delivery. The OR for a twin delivery was 0.70 (95% CI 0.49-1.00). After later use, there were 11 twin deliveries, RR = 1.12 (95% CI 0.56-2.01).

Table 47.5. Pregnancy duration and infant birth weight at maternal use of drugs for migraine

Variable studied	Drug use in early pregnancy			Drug use later in pregnancy		
	Number	OR/RR	95% CI	Number	OR/RR	95% CI
<37 weeks	139	1.05	0.89-1.25	38	1.30	0.93-1.81
<2500g	84	1.00	0.80-1.24	19	1.02	0.64-1.61
≥4500g	113	1.05	0.87-1.27	22	0.84	0.55-1.29
SGA	64	1.08	0.84-1.39	9	0.71	0.31-1.38#
LGA	163	1.06	0.90-1.25	38	0.97	0.70-1.36

#observed over expected number with exact Poisson 95% confidence interval.

No certain deviations from expected values are thus seen.

Table 47.6. Infant mortality after maternal use of drugs for migraine

Variable studied	Drug use in early pregnancy			Drug use later in pregnancy		
	Number	OR/RR	95% CI	Number	OR/RR	95% CI
Stillbirth	8	0.80	0.35-1.58#	1	-	-
Early neonatal death	4	0.95	0.21-2.43#	1	-	-

#observed over expected number with exact Poisson 95% confidence interval.

No increase in perinatal mortality was seen.

Table 47.7. Nonatal diagnoses after maternal use of drugs for migraine

Diagnosis	Drug use in early pregnancy			Drug use later in pregnancy		
	Number	OR/RR	95% CI	Number	OR/RR	95% CI
Hypoglycaemia	94	0.94	0.76-1.16	17	0.69	0.43-1.12
Respiratory diagnoses	135	0.97	0.82-1.16	18	0.59	0.37-0.93
Low Agar score	56	1.03	0.79-1.34.	7	0.61	0.29-1.27
CNS diagnoses	17	0.97	0.60-1.56	3	0.64	0.13-1.86#
Jaundice	116	1.04	0.86-1.26	35	1.35	0.96-1.60

#observed over expected number with exact Poisson 95% confidence interval.

No increase in the risk for the tabulated diagnoses is seen. The rate of respiratory diagnoses after later exposure is actually significantly low.

There is only one remarkable figure in the Table and that is three cases of oesophageal atresia. This can obviously be a random phenomenon. All three were exposed to sumatriptan.

The high odds ratio for eletriptan is thus based on two malformed infants among six exposed and may, in spite of formal statistical significance, be random. One of the infants had a ventricular septum defect, the other megacolon.

Table 47.8. Congenital malformations in infants whose mothers had used drugs against migraine in early pregnancy

Congenital malformation	Number	OR	95% CI
All malformation	125	0.97	0.81-1.16
Relatively severe malformation	90	1.02	0.82-1.26
Chromosome anomalies	4	0.67	0.18-1.71#
Without chromosome anomalies			
Any CNS malformation	6	1.78	0.65-3.88#
Eye malformations	4	1.58	0.43-4.05#
Orofacial clefts	2	0.42	0.05-1.50#
Any cardiovascular defect	26	0.92	0.62-1.35
VSD and/or ASD	18	1.20	0.75-1.90
Oesophageal atresia	3	3.80	0.78-11.1#
Pylorostenosis	3	1.53	0.32-4.47#
Hypospadias	5	0.66	0.21-1.53#
Poly/syndactyly	7	1.28	0.51-2.63#
Limb reduction defects	3	1.79	0.37-5.22#
Hip (sub)luxation, unstable hip	14	0.81	0.48-1.37

#observed over expected number with exact Poisson 95% confidence interval.

Table 47.9. Relatively severe malformations divided after type of drugs for migraine

Drug or drug group	Number of infants		OR	95% CI
	malformed	total		
Ergot alkaloids	12	447	0.77	0..43-1.37
5HT1-receptor agonists	77	2187	1.07	0.85-1.35
Sumatriptan	66	1872	1.05	0.82-1.35
Zolmitriptan	6	206	0.97	0.36-2.11#
Rizatriptan	4	107	1.27	0.34-3.24#
Eletriptan	2	6	8.33	1.01-30.1#
Other	2	55	1.14	0.14-4.10#

#observed over expected number with exact Poisson 95% confidence interval.

SUMMARY

The pregnancy and neonatal outcomes after maternal use of drugs for migraine are to a large extent normal. An increased risk for preeclampsia is seen and an increased rate of delivery inductions and caesarean sections. No neonatal ill effects are seen. There are only weak signs of teratogenic effects. One is the occurrence of three cases of oesophageal atresia after exposure to sumatriptan, the other the occurrence of two malformed infants among six exposed to eleptriptan. Both these observations may well be random.

REFERENCES

[1] Ács N, Bánhidy F, Puhó E, Czeizel AE. A possible dose-dependent teratogenic effect of ergotamine. *Reprod Toxicol* 2006; 22: 551-552.

[2] Heinonen OP. Slone D, Shapiro S. *Birth Defects and Drugs in Pregnancy*. Publishing Scoences Group, Inc. Littleton, MA. 1977.

[3] Källén B, Lygner PE. Delivery outcome in women who used drugs for migraine during pregnancy with special reference to sumatriptan. *Headache* 2001; 41. 351-356.

[4] Reiff-Eldridge R, Heffner CR, Aphross SA, Tennis PS, White AD, Andrews EB. Monitoring pregnancy outcomes after prenatal drug exposure through prospective pregnancy registries: a pharmaceutical company commitment. *Amer J Obst Gynecol* 2000; 182: 159-163.

[5] Olesen C, Hald Steffensen F, Sørensen HT, Lauge Nielsen G, Olsen J. Pregnancy outcome following prescription for sumatriptan. *Headache* 2000; 40: 20-24.

[6] Fox AW, Chambers CD, Anderson PO, Diamond ML, Spierings EL. Evidence-based assessment of pregnancy outcome after sumatriptan exposure. *Headache* 2002; 42: 8-15.

[7] Evans EW, Lorber KC. Use of 5-HT1 agonists in pregnancy. *Ann Pharmacother* 2008; 42: 543-549.

Chapter 48

ANTICONVULSANT DRUGS

> The use of anticonvulsants during pregnancy is associated with adverse pregnancy and neonatal outcomes. Most prominent is an increased risk for a congenital malformation but also long term effects on child cognitive development have been demonstrated. These risks are markedly higher after the use of valproic acid than after other anticonvulsants even though only little information is available on the most recently introduced drugs. If possible, valproic acid should be avoided during pregnancy and if exposure has occurred in early pregnancy, intense foetal diagnosis is recommended in order to identify possible spina bifida. Women with epilepsy and treated with anticonvulsants and planning pregnancy should be informed of the relatively moderate risk increase associated with the drug use and if possible monotherapy should be used. – So far little is known whether the use of anticonvulsants as mode stabilizers is associated with similar risks but it seems prudent to avoid them, notably valproic acid.

The association between maternal epilepsy and use of anticonvulsant drugs with an increased risk for congenital malformations in the offspring is well known and documented in many studies. The first study of this problem, based on 262 pregnancies, found no association [1]. An observation of a high rate of epileptic mothers among infants with orofacial cleft [2] suggested an association and further studies verified a number of ill effects of anticonvulsant use on the growth of the foetus [3], an increased risk for major malformations and minor anomalies [4] and an impaired neurological development of the infant [5]. Among major malformations, special importance has been paid to spina bifda since the demonstration that use of valproic acid carries a relatively high risk for this malformation [6] but also carbamazepine appears to have a similar effect [7]. The typical minor anomalies form a syndrome with, for instance, facial anomalies and reductions of the distal finger phalanges. It has been named the phenytoin or valproic acid syndrome but has been observed also after other anticonvulsants. Many review articles have been published. In one of the latest of these [8] it was suggested that teratogenic effects and effects on adverse cognitive outcome were seen after valproic acid but that it was doubtful that it was valid for other anticonvulsants. A similar conclusion was reached in a recent study of cognitive function at three years of age after fetal exposure to anticonvulsants [9].

Table 48.1. Number of women identified using anticonvulsants

Total	2920
Reported use in early pregnancy	2603
Got prescription later in pregnancy	1709
Both early and later use	1392

Type of drug	ATC code	Early use	Later use
Barbiturates	N03AA	30	16
Phenobarbital	N03AA02	20	8
Primidone	N03AA03	10	8
Hydantoin derivates	N03AB	156	92
Phenytoin	N03AB02	156	92
Succinimide derivates	N03AD	23	10
Ethosuximide	N03AD01	23	10
Benzodiazepine derivates	N03AE	112	57
Clonazepam	N03AE01	112	57
Clobazam	N05BA09	4	1*
Carboxamide drivates	N03AF	1290	789
Carbamazepine	N03AF01	1268	773
Oxcarbamazepine	N03AF02	22	16
Fatty acid derivates	N03AG	602	417
Valproc acid	N03AG01	573	390
Vigabatrin	N03AG04	34	30
Other anticonvulsants	N03AX	641	485
Lamotrigine	N03AX09	520	409
Topiramate	N03AX11	34	21
Gabapentin	N03AX12	81	49
Levatiracetam	N03AX14	23	19
Unspecified	N03A	1	0

*In Sweden clobazam is a licenced drug used as anticonvulsant.

Number of anticonvulsants used

Number of anticonvulsants	Early use	Later use
One	2353	1550
Two	231	150
Three	17	9
Four	2	0

Thus, 90-91% of all anticonvulsants were used in monotherapy and only few women used more than two anticonvulsant drugs.

Anticonvulsants have always been used for some other conditions than epilepsy. During recent years, the use as mode stabilizers at antidepressive treatments has become common and a recent review stresses the possibility of teratogenesis [10].

Characteristics of Women Using Anticonvulsants

Based on women reporting the drug in early pregnancy (n=2603). Each variable is adjusted for all other variables and year of delivery. Comparison with all women who gave birth during the period and with information from the first antenatal care (n=967 742). The odds ratios for maternal age, parity, smoking in early pregnancy, number of previous miscarriages, BMI, subfertility, and country of birth are adjusted for all other variables and are shown in Figure 48.1.

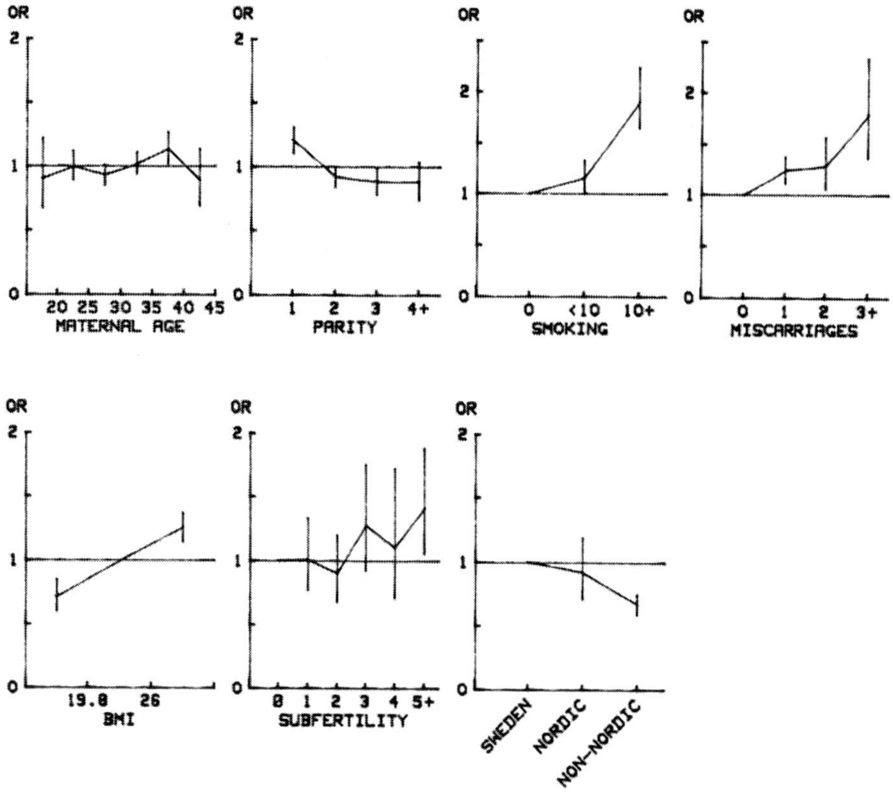

Figure 48.1. Odds ratios for seven maternal characteristics. The odds ratios (OR) for each variable are adjusted for the other variables and year of delivery. Vertical lines mark 95% confidence intervals. For maternal age and parity, each class is compared with all other classes.

Some further maternal characteristics were analyzed, adjusting for year of delivery, maternal age, parity, smoking, and BMI (Table 48.2).

Women using anticonvulsants thus smoke more than expected, have an increased BMI, have had more previous miscarriages and slightly more often subfertility problems. They are under-represented among women born outside the Nordic countries. Their educational level is lower than expected and they have more often than expected other family situations than co-habitation and an increased rate of working only half-time or not at all outside home.

There is a very strong association with the use of folic acid. Other associations of some interest are with oral contraceptives, opioids and various psychoactive drugs including antidepressants. Only 4% of the women reported the use of antidepressants and may have used the anticonvulsants as mode stabilizers. Many drugs are reported significantly less often than expected, e.g., antibiotics, minor analgesics and antihistamines.

Table 48.2. Some further characteristics of women using anticonvulsants

Variable studied	Number	OR	95% CI
Education (1996-2001, 1214 women with drugs, 526 695 in population)			
Unknown	35	-	-
<12 years	202	1.49	1.26-1.76
12 years	648	1.00	reference
13-14 years	54	0.74	0.56-0.98
≥14 years	284	0.71	0.61-0.82
Family situation			
Unknown	47	-	
Co-habiting	2320	1.00	reference
Living alone	108	1.65	1.35-2.02
Other family situation	106	1.46	1.17-1.83
Work outside home			
Unknown	383	-	-
Full time	978	1.00	reference
Part time	622	1.32	1.18-1.48
None	598	1.72	1.53-1.93

Table 48.3. Concomitant drug use (early pregnancy)

Drug group	Number	OR/RR	95% CI
Drugs for stomach ulcer and reflux	36	1.53	1.10-2.13
Drugs for inflammatory bowel disease	4	0.53	0.15-1.37
Insulin	16	1.59	0.97-2.61
Multivitamins	124	0.72	0.62-0.83
Folic acid	1185	20.8	19.6-22.1
Antihypetensives	16	1.65	0.94-2.67#
Oral contraceptives	22	2.59	1.62-3.91#
Progestogens	9	0.74	0.39-1.43
Gonadotropins	5	0.67	0.22-1.56#
Systemic corticosteroids	13	1.32	0.70-2.25#
Thyroid drugs	46	1.26	0.94-1.69
Antibiotics	47	0.55	0.41-0.73
NSAIDs	36	0.72	0.51-1.00
Opioids	42	2.75	2.04-3.70
Minor analgesics	104	0.46	0.38-0.56
Neuroleptics	35	3.53	2.56-4.85
Sedatives, hypnotics	76	5.82	4.09-7.21
Antidepressants	110	3.12	2.63-3.82
Drugs for rhinitis	23	0.60	0.40-0.89
Antiasthmatics	93	1.06	0.86-1.31
Cough medicines	14	0.97	0.57-1.84
Antihistamines	99	0.62	0.51-0.76

#observed over expected number with exact Poisson 95% confidence interval.

There is an association with pre-existing diabetes, most apparent after later use. For many pregnancy complications an increased risk is seen, notably preeclampsia, placental abruption and bleeding associated with delivery. Both delivery induction and caesarean section occurs at an increased frequency.

Table 48.4. Some maternal diagnoses associated with the use of anticonvulsants

Diagnosis	Drug use in early pregnancy			Drug use later in pregnancy		
	Number	OR/RR	95% CI	Number	OR/RR	95% CI
Pre-existing diabetes	45	1.19	0.88-1.61	37	1.41	1.01-1.97
Chronic hypertension	36	1.09	0.78-1.52	30	1.30	0.90-1.87
Gestational diabetes	28	1.07	0.74-1.56	21	1.22	0.74-1.88
Preeclampsia	158	1.27	1.08-1.49	102	1.21	0.99-1.48
Hyperemesis gravidarum	28	1.00	0.69-1.45	22	1.13	0.74-1.72
Placenta previa	52	1.00	0.71-1.43	23	1.03	0.68-1.56
Abruptio placentae	50	1.43	1.07-1.90	37	1.52	1.09-2.11
Antepartum bleeding	44	1.16	0.86-1.58	33	1.32	0.93-1.87
Intrapartum bleeding	73	1.28	1.02-1.62	56	1.36	1.04-1.77
Postpartum bleeding	171	1.16	0.99-1.35	108	1.39	0.94-1.39
Delivery induction	399	1.55	1.39-1.93	267	1.55	1.35-1.77
Caesarean section	599	1.51	1.37-1.66	415	1.55	1.38-1.74

OUTCOME AFTER MATERNAL USE OF ANTICONVULSANTS

Infant Sex

After early use of anticonvulsants there were 1359 male and 1277 female infants, sex ratio 1.06 (95% CI 0.99-1.15). After later use there were 886 male and 843 female infants, sex ratio 1.05 (95% CI 0.96-1.16). Both sex ratios were thus close to the normal sex ratio (1.06).

Multiple Births

After early use of anticonvulsants there were 32 twin deliveries and one triplet delivery. The OR for a twin delivery was 0.82 (95% CI 0.58-1.17). After later use there were 20 twin deliveries, OR = 0.79 (95% CI 0.51-1.24). Thus twinning rate was low but this could be random.

Table 48.5. Pregnancy duration and infant birth weight at maternal use of anticonvulsants

Variable studied	Drug use in early pregnancy			Drug use later in pregnancy		
	Number	OR/RR	95% CI	Number	OR/RR	95% CI
<37 weeks	194	1.53	1.32-1.78	116	1.39	1.15-1.68
<2500g	136	1.68	1.41-2.01	72	1.32	1.04-1.68
≥4500g	113	1.05	0.87-1.27	70	0.98	0.77-1.25
SGA	95	1.63	1.33-2.01	59	1.53	1.18-2.00
LGA	149	0.94	0.79-1.11	96	0.90	0.73-1.12

There is thus an increased risk for preterm birth, low birth weight, and SGA.

Table 48.6. Infant mortality after maternal use of anticonvulsants

Variable studied	Drug use in early pregnancy			Drug use later in pregnancy		
	Number	RR	95% CI	Number	RR	95% CI
Stillbirth	16	1.74	0.93-2.83	14	2.22	1.21-3.72
Early neonatal death	8	1.91	0.83-3.77	3	1.14	0.23-3.32

There is thus an increased risk for intrauterine death while an increased risk for early neonatal death is uncertain.

Table 48.7. Neonatal diagnoses after maternal use of anticonvulsants

Diagnosis	Drug use in early pregnancy			Drug use later in pregnancy		
	Number	OR/RR	95% CI	Number	OR/RR	95% CI
Hypoglycaemia	159	1.66	1.42-1.96	103	1.61	1.32-1.97
Respiratory diagnoses	238	1.82	1.59-2.08	141	1.76	1.48-2.09
Low Apgar score	100	1.91	1.57-2.33	75	2.40	1.91-3.01
CNS diagnoses	43	2.51	1.87-3.37	34	2.87	2.05-4.01
Jaundice	88	0.79	0.64-0.98	59	0.79	0.61-1.02

A markedly increased risk for all neonatal diagnoses studied except for jaundice was thus seen.

Table 48.8. Congenital malformations in infants whose mothers had used anticonvulsants in early pregnancy

Congenital malformation	Number	OR	95% CI
All malformation	221	1.86	1.62-2.13
Relatively severe malformation	164	2.01	1.72-2.35
Chromosome anomalies	3	0.61	0.13-1.78#
Without chromosome anomalies			
Any CNS malformation	10	3.13	1.50-5.71#
Neural tube defects	4	3.57	0.97-9.14#
Orofacial clefts	14	3.07	1.68-5.15
Any cardiovascular defect	53	1.91	1.46-2.51
VSD and/or ASD	31	1.07	1.45-2.96
Small bowel atresia	3	4.55	0.94-13.3#
Anal atresia	4	3.92	1.07-10.0#
Pylorostenosis	5	2.16	0.70-5.05#
Diaphragmatic hernia	5	8.06	2.62-18.8#
Hypospadias	28	3.52	2.34-5.08#
Severe kidney malformations	4	1.00	0.27-2.55#
Pes equinovarus	11	2.74	1.37-4.90#
Poly/syndactyly	12	2.26	1.17-3.95#
Limb reduction defects	3	1.88	0.39-5.48#
Hip (sub)luxation, unstable hip	22	1.33	0.87-2.02
Craniostenosis	6	4.20	1.84-9.13

#observed over expected number with exact Poisson 95% confidence interval.

Most congenital malformations occur more often than expected even though only few are numerous enough to show statistically significant risks: CNS malformations, orofacial clefts, cardiac defects, anal atresia, hypospadias, pes equinovarus, poly/syndactyly, and craniostenosis. Two of the infants with anal atresia also had oesophageal atresia. Most of these malformations have previously been described in association with maternal use of anticonvulsants.

If all infants exposed to valproic acid (in mono- or polytherapy) are studied, 67 among 580 infants had a relatively severe malformation: OR = 4.13 (95% CI 3.24-5.26). Among the 2056 infants that were not exposed to valproic acid, 97 had a relatively severe malformation: OR =1.48 (95% CI 1.21-1.82). There is thus a drastic difference between the two groups, but also in the absence of valproic acid, an increased risk of a malformation is seen. If this study is restricted to monotherapies, both odds ratios go down: for valproic acid (n=49) to 3.56 (95% CI 2.68-4.73) and for other anticonvulsants than valproic acid (n=81) to 1.36 (95% CI 1.08-1.70).

There is a clear-cut difference between the effects of anticonvulsants in monotherapy and in polytherapy. Among 2 363 infants whose mothers had used anticonvulsant monotherapy, 130 had a relatively severe malformation, 5.5% with an odds ratio of 1.77 (95% CI 1.48-3.11). There were 34 infants with such malformations among 273 exposed to anticonvulsants in polytherapy, 12.5%, and with a risk ratio of 3.75 (95% CI 2.60-5.24).

Table 48.9 specifies the number of "relatively severe" malformations after specific anticonvulsants when used in monotherapy.

Table 48.9. Relatively severe malformations after specific anticonvulsants in monotherapy

Anticonvulsant drug	Number of infants		OR/RR	95%CI
	malformed	total		
Phenobarbital or primidone	3	31	2.97	0.61-8.08#
Phenytoin	8	127	1.82	0.79-3.59#
Ethosuximide	2	23	2.47	0.30-8.92#
Clonazepam	3	66	1.24	0.26-3.62#
Carbamazepine	50	1138	1.37	1.03-1.82
Oxcarbamazepine	2	24	3.18	0.38-11.5#
Valproic acid	49	484	3.56	2.68-4.73
Vigabatrin	1	15	2.04	0.05-11.4#
Lamotrigine	12	394	1.01	0.57-1.81
Topiramate	7	35	5.74	2.31-11.8#
Gabapentin	1	66	0.51	0.01-2.84#
Levatiracetam	1	24	1.45	0.04-8.07#

#observed over expected number with exact Poisson 95% confidence interval.

The only three drugs which show statistically significant overrisks are thus carbamazepine, valproic acid, and topiramate. For other drugs, risk estimates are usually increased but confidence intervals are wide and include 1.0.

Topiramate

Among the seven malformed infants, one had ventricular septum defect, one atrium septum defect, polydactyly and syndactyly, one had ventricular and atrium septum defects and split hand and foot, one had coarctation of aorta, one pylorostenosis, one had a hand deformity and polydactyly, and one diaphragmatic hernia.

Carbamazepine and valproic acid

Table 48.10 compares congenital malformations after maternal use of carbamazepine or valproic acid in monotherapy (1 278 and 580 infants, respectively).

Table 48.10. Congenital malformations after maternal use of carbamazepine or valproic acid in monotherapy

Malformation	Carbamazepine			Valproic acid		
	Number malformed	OR/RR	95% CI	Number malformed	OR/RR	95% CI
Any CNS malfornation	4	3.13	0.75-8.00#	5	7.46	2.42-17.4#
Neural tube defects	0	-	-	3	12.0	2.47-35.1#
Any cardiac defect	11	0.92	0.51-1.67	16	3.27	1.87-5.30#
Orofacial clefts	4	2.01	0.55-5.15#	5	5.88	1.91-13.7#
Hypospadias	5	1.35	0.44-3.15#	16	10.5	6.02-17.1#
Pes equiinovarus	4	2.61	0.71-6.69#	4	6.35	1.73-16.3#
Poly/syndactyly	5	2.08	0.68-4.86#	1	1.15	0.03-6.40#

#observed over expected number with exact Poisson 95% confidence interval.

For specific malformations, statistically significant effects are thus only seen with valproic acid in monotherapy.

Among the four CNS malformations after carbamazepine, two had agenesis of corpus callosum, one in association with septo-optic dysplasia. One had hydrocephaly and the fourth had a reduction malformation of the brain. Among the four orofacial clefts after carbamazepine, three were median cleft palate and one cleft lip/palate. Among the two infants exposed to valproic acid and with CNS malformations but not spina bifida, one had agenesis of corpus callosum and one had holoprosencephaly.

Lamotrigine

The total malformation risk was not increased after lamotrigine in monotherapy but among the 12 infants with relatively severe malformations, three had orofacial clefts, one cleft palate and two cleft lip/palate, the RR = 5.00, 95% CI 1.03-1.46.

Gabapentin

The only malformed infant exposed to gabapentin in monotherapy had a reduction of ulna and the hand.

Summary

Women using anticonvulsants, the majority of whom have epilepsy, show a number of pregnancy complications, an increased risk for preterm birth and small-for-gestational age, intrauterine deaths and neonatal symptoms except for jaundice. There is an increased risk for congenital malformations, stronger after anticonvulsants in polytherapy than in monotherapy and stronger with valproic acid than with other anticonvulsants. After valproic acid, there is an increased risk of any CNS malformation and notably of spina bifida, for orofacial clefts, cardiovascular defects, hypospadias, and pes equinovarus. Some other tentative associations are seen: between lamotrigine use and orofacial clefts and between use of topiramate and various relatively severe malformations. Data for most recent anticonvulsants are few, notably when used in monotherapy.

REFERENCES

[1] Janz D, Fuchs U. Sind antiepileptische Medikamente während der Schwangerschaft schädlich? *Deutch Med Wschr* 1964; 89: 241-243.

[2] Meadow SR. Congenital abnormalities and anticonvulsant drugs. *Proc Roy Soc Med* 1970; 63: 48-49.

[3] Wide K, Winbladh B, Tomson T, Källén B. Body dimensions of infants exposed to antiepileptic drugs in utero: observations spanning 25 years. *Epilepsia* 2000; 41: 854-861.

[4] Hanson JW, Myrianthopoulos NC, Sedgwick Harvey MA, Smith DW. Risks to the offspring of women treated with hydantoid anticonvulsants, with emphasis on the foetal hydantoin syndrome. *J Pediatr* 1976; 89: 662-668.

[5] Adab N, Tudor Smith C, Vinten J, Williamson PR. Winterbottom JB. Common antiepileptic drugs in pregnancy in women with epilepsy (Review). Cochrane Library number CD004848. *The Cochrane Library* 2008; issue 1: 1-38.

[6] Robert E, Guibaud P. Maternal valproic acid and congenital neural tube defect. *Lancet* 1982; ii: 937.

[7] Källén AJB. Maternal carbamazepine and infant spina bifida. *Reprod Toxicol* 1994; 8: 203-205.

[8] Harden CL. Antiepileptic drug teratogenesis: what are the risks for congenital malformations and adverse cognitive outcomes? *Int Review Neurobiol* 2008; 83: 205-213.

[9] Meador KJ, Bakeer GA, Browning N, Clayton-Smith J, Combs-Cantrell D, Cohen M, Kalayjian LA, Kanner A, Liporace JD, Pennell PB, Privitera M, Loring DW for the NEAD Study Group. Cognitive function at 3 years of age after fetal exposure to antiepileptic drugs. *New Engl J Med* 2009; 360: 1597-1605.

[10] Nguyen HT, Sharna V, McIntyre RS. Teratogenesis associated with antibipolar agents. Adv Ther 2009. *E-pub ahead of print.*

Chapter 49

ANTI-PARKINSON DRUGS

Very little information exists on pregnancy outcome after maternal use of anti-parkinson drugs in early pregnancy but the available data indicate no increased risk for a congenital malformation or other adverse outcome. If exposure has occurred, there is so far no reason to discuss a termination of pregnancy. Further data are badly needed.

Very little is known about the use of anti-parkinson drugs during pregnancy. In one recent article [1] it is mentioned that 35 pregnancies exposed to such drugs have been recorded in the literature without any malformations being observed.

Table 49.1. Number of women identified using anti-parkinson drugs

Tota	177
Reported use in early pregnancy	61
Got prescription later in pregnancy	29
Both early and later use	13

Type of drug	ATC code	Early use	Later use
Trihexyphenidyl	N04AA01	3	0
Biperiden	N04AA02	10	9
Metixene	N04AA03	7	1
Orphenadrine	N04AB02	24	9
Levodopa+decarboxylase inhibitor	N04BA02	12	8
Amantadine	N04BB01	2	0
Selegiline	N04BD01	4	3

One woman used two drugs, biperiden and levodopa with decarboxylase inhibitor, both in early and later pregnancy.

CHARACTERISTICS OF WOMEN USING ANTI-PARKINSON DRUGS

Based on women reporting the drug in early pregnancy (n=61). Each variable is adjusted for all other variables and year of delivery. Comparison with all women who gave birth during the period and with information from the first antenatal care (n=967

742). The odds ratios for maternal age, parity, smoking in early pregnancy, number of previous miscarriages, BMI, subfertility, and country of birth are adjusted for all other variables (Table 49.2).

Table 49.2. Characteristics of women using anti-parkinson drugs in early pregnancy

Variable studied	Number	OR	95% CI
Maternal age			
<25 years	19	0.37	0.15-0.90
25-34 years	39	1.00	reference
≥35 years	23	3.07	1.78-5.29
Parity			
1	36	0.37	0.15-0.90
≥2	25	1.00	reference
Smoking			
Unknown	1	-	-
No	37	1.00	reference
Yes	23	6.47	2.79-15.0
Previous miscarriage			
No	51	1.00	reference
Yes	10	0.62	0.30-1.26
BMI			
Unknown	8	-	-
<19.8	5	1.58	0.60-4.17
19.8-25.9	28	1.00	reference
≥26	20	1.37	0.76-2.48
Country of birth			
Sweden	54	1.00	reference
Other Nordic country	2	0.85	0.21-3.35
Non-Nordic country	5	0.59	0.24-1.47

Only one woman reported unwanted childlessness (2 years).

Table 49.3. Some further characteristics of women using anti-parkinson drugs in early pregnancy

Variable studied	Number	OR	95% CI
Education (1996-2001, 38 women with drugs, 526 695 in population)			
Unknown	1	-	-
<12 years	8	2.20	0.93-5.18
12 years	17	1.00	reference
≥13 years	12	1.08	0.50-2.36
Family situation			
Unknown	1	-	
Co-habiting	49	1.00	reference
Living alone	4	1.27	0.35-3.26#
Other family situation	7	4.55	2.11-9.78#
Work outside home			
Unknown	9	-	
Full time	23	1.00	reference
Part time	12	1.43	0.69-2.99
None	17	2.31	1.10-4.85

#observed over expected number with exact Poisson 95% confidence interval.

Some further maternal characteristics were analyzed, adjusting for year of delivery, maternal age, parity, smoking, and BMI (Table 49.3).

The women who had anti-parkinson drugs were thus older than expected, less often of first parity, and smokers. These women were more often than expected living in atypical family situations and were more often than expected not working outside home.

Table 49.4. Concomitant drug use (early pregnancy)

Drug group	Number	OR/RR	95% CI
Multivitamins	3	1.21	0.25-3.54#
Folic acid	4	1.99	0.54-5.10#
Minor analgesics	4	0.76	0.21-1.95#
Anticonvulsants	3	15.0	3.09-43.8#
Sedatives, hypnotics	8	6.67	2.88-13.1#
Antidepressants	9	5.49	2.51-10.4#
Antihistamines	5	1.12	0.36-2.62#

#observed over expected number with exact Poisson 95% confidence interval.

There is thus a strong excess use of psychoactive drugs. The three exposures for anticonvulsants were: phenytoin, clonazepam, and valproic acid, respectively. The exposures for neuroleptics were represented by many different drugs: zuclopenthixol (n=9), haloperidol (n=7), flupentixol (n=4), and perphenazine (n=4) were the most common ones.

One woman had also used a dopamine agonist, pramipexole.

Table 49.5. Maternal diagnoses associated with the use of anti-parkinson drugs

Diagnosis	Drug use in early pregnancy			Drug use later in pregnancy		
	Number	OR/RR	95% CI	Number	OR/RR	95% CI
Preeclampsia	4	1.14	0.31-2.91#	3	1.74	0.36-5.10
Delivery induction	10	1.31	0.63-2.41#	7	1.75	0.70-3.60
Caesarean section	15	1.40	0.74-2.65	11	1.71	0.86-3.07

#observed over expected number with exact Poisson 95% confidence interval.

The specific maternal pregnancy diagnoses were few due to the limited number of exposed women. No statistically significant deviations from expected numbers are seen.

Outcome after Maternal use of Anti-parkinson Drugs

Infant Sex

After early exposure, there were 29 male and 32 female infants born, sex ratio 0.91 (95% CI 0.54-1.50) and after later exposure 14 male and 15 female infants, sex ratio 0.93 (95% CI 0.43-1.98). Both ratios are thus low but the normal sex ratio (1.06) lies within the confidence intervals.

Multiple Births

There were no twin deliveries.

Pregnancy Duration and Infant Birth Weight at Maternal use of Anti-parkinson Drugs

None of the observed numbers of the studied variables deviated significantly from expected values but numbers were low. There were five preterm infants (RR = 1.11, 95% CI 0.36-2.59) after early exposure and four infants with a birth weight <2500g (RR = 0.74, 95% CI 0.15-2.15) and only two SGA infants.

None of the infants died perinatally.

Table 49.6. Neonatal diagnoses after maternal use of anti-parkinson drugs

Diagnosis	Drug use in early pregnancy			Drug use later in pregnancy		
	Number	RR	95% CI	Number	RR	95% CI
Hypoglycaemia	5	1.56	0.51-3.65	2	1.09	0.13-3.93
Respiratory diagnoses	5	1.28	0.42-2.98	3	1.68	0.35-4.90

Only three infants with congenital malformations were identified (RR = 1.05, 95% CI 0.22-3.08) (Table 49.7).

Table 49.7. Specification of the malformations present after maternal use of anti-parkinson drugs

Congenital malformation	Anti- parkinson drug	Other drugs
Ventricular septum defect	metixene	-
Ventricular septum defect	orphenadrine	haloperidol, alprazolam
Hypospadias	orphenadrine	haloperidol, phenytoin

Two cases of ventricular septum defect among 61 infants may well be random and this is also true for two relatively major malformations among 24 infants also exposed to orphenadrine. Both were also exposed to haloperidol and there were only a total of six infants exposed to this combination. Also this may be random, however.

Summary

The low number of exposed women makes all results uncertain but there seems to be no major deviation in pregnancy or neonatal outcome or an increase in congenital malformation risk. Further data are needed.

References

[1] Hagell P, Odin P, Vinge E. Pregnancy in Parkinson´s disease: a review of the literature and a case report. *Mov Disord* 1999; 13: 34-38.

Chapter 50

ANTIPSYCHOTIC DRUGS

Some antipsychotic drugs, notably dixyrazine and prochlorperazine, have been used as antiemetics and the pregnancy outcome is then basically normal. When antipsychotic drugs are used for a psychiatric indication, pregnancy and neonatal deviations are seen. It is difficult to say how much of this is due to drug effects and how much is due to underlying psychiatric conditions. A weak teratogenic effect is seen, notably from thioxanthene derivates, but numbers are low and it is not certain that the effect of the different drugs actually differ. There is still uncertainty whether lithium use is associated with an increased risk for cardiac defects but if so the risk is relatively low. If possible, use of antipsychotic drugs during pregnancy should be avoided but if early exposure has occurred there is no reason to discuss a pregnancy termination.

Antipsychotic drugs have different uses. Even though most of them are used at various psychiatric conditions, in Sweden at least two of them have as major indication as antiemetics: dixyrazine and prochlorperazine. Lithium is mainly used as mode stabilizer at mano-depressive disease.

Early discussions were carried out on the possible teratogenic effect of phenothiazine drugs [1,2]. In a TIS study of 179 infants exposed to haloperidol or penfluridol, there were six with a congenital malformation, two of them with limb reduction defects [3]. Another small study on 75 infants exposed to olanzapine found only one with a malformation [4] and in another with 60 exposures for olanzapine, 36 for quetiapine, six for clozapine, and 49 for risperidone no increased risk for a congenital malformation was seen [5]. A case report exists of an infant with an atrioventricular canal defect and a unilateral clubfoot born after maternal use of olanzapine [6]. A review of experiences with risperidone during pregnancy [7] identified 68 prospectively ascertained exposures with a known outcome which included induced and spontaneous abortion. A recent review [8] concluded that there was not enough data available to draw conclusions on the possible teratogenicity of antipsychotic drugs but that an association with neonatal complications exists.

One study, based on 45 exposures to typical and 25 to atypical antipsychotics claimed a difference with regard to birth weight: an increased risk for low birth weight after typical and an increased risk for heavier infants after atypical antipsychotics [9].

Table 50.1. Number of women identified using antipsychotic drugs

Total	4153
Reported use in early pregnancy	3145
Got prescription later in pregnancy	1987
Both early and later use	979

Type of drug	ATC code	Early use	Later use
Drugs mainly used for NVP			
Phenothiazines with piperazine structure	N05AB01/02	2473	1643
Dixyrazine	N05AB01	2254	1555
Prochlorperazine	N05AB04	248	98
Anti-psychotic drugs mainly used for psychiatric indications			
Phenothiazines with aliphatic side chains	N05AA	56	24
Chlorpromazine	N05AA01	6	4
Levomepromazine	N05AA02	50	20
Phenothiazines with piperazine structure	N05AB	105	46
Fluphenazine	N05AB02	15	5
Perphenazine	N05AB03	90	41
Phenothiazines with piperidine structure	N05AC	32	16
Thioridazine	N05AC02	32	16
Butyrophenone derivates	N05AD	77	32
Haloperidol	N05AD01	75	32
Trifluperidol	N05AD02	1	1
Melperone	N05AD03	1	0
Thioxanthene derivates	N05AF	187	103
Flupentixol	N05AF01	111	65
Chlorprothixene	N05AF03	6	2
Zuclopenthixol	N05AF05	70	36
Diazepines and oxazepines	N05AH	117	71
Clozapine	N05AH02	24	13
Olanzapine	N05AH03	91	57
Quetiapine	N05AH04	2	1
Other antipsychotic drugs	N05AX	60	36
Risperidone	N05AX08	58	35
Lithium	N05AN01	81	30

A previous survey of pregnancy outcome after maternal use of antipsychotics based on the Swedish Medical Birth Register has been published [10]. That study covered the period July 1, 1995 to the end of 2005 and is thus to a large extent based on the same material as that presented here. A statistically significant increased risk for a congenital malformation was found with an OR of 1.52 (95% CI 1.05-2.19) for relatively severe malformations.

Lithium has been regarded as a putative teratogen [11], notably due to an association with cardiovascular defects [12,13]. This association is, however, only tentative [14].

There were 606 women who had, in early pregnancy, used antipsychotic drugs excluding those drugs which were primarily used at NVP and lithium. The corresponding number for later use was 323.

Six women used a combination of lithium and another antipsychotic drug both during early pregnancy and later, and nine women used a combination of dixyrazine or prochlorperazine and an antipsychotic drug in early and three in later pregnancy.

Characteristics of Women using Drugs for Antipsychotic Drugs

Based on women reporting the drug in early pregnancy (n=2473 using dixyraxine or prochlorperazine and 671 using other antipsychotics, one of the latter missing maternal age). Each variable is adjusted for all other variables and year of delivery. Comparison with all women who gave birth during the period and with information from the first antenatal care (n=967 742). The odds ratios for maternal age, parity, smoking in early pregnancy, number of previous miscarriages, BMI, subfertility, and country of birth are adjusted for all other variables and are shown in Figure 50.1.

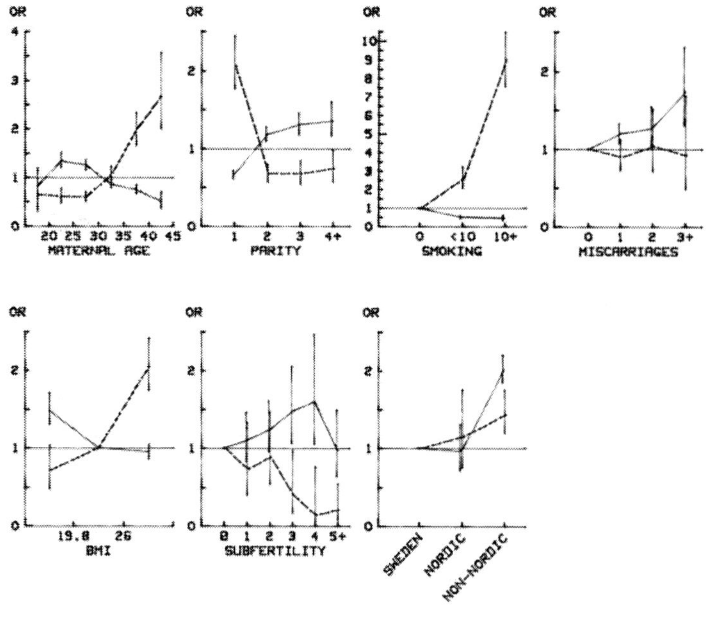

Figure 50.1. Odds ratios for seven maternal characteristics. The odds ratios (OR) for each variable are adjusted for the other variables and year of delivery. Vertical lines mark 95% confidence intervals. For maternal age and parity, each class is compared with all other classes. Unbroken graphs refer to women who used dixyrazine or prochlorperazine, dashed graphs to women using other antipsychotics.

Some further maternal characteristics were analyzed, adjusting for year of delivery, maternal age, parity, smoking, and BMI (Table 50.2).

The maternal characteristics of the two groups of drugs thus differ markedly for nearly all characteristics shown. The only exception is that for both there is an increased use among women born outside the Nordic countries. Interestingly, both previous miscarriages and a period of subfertility are associated with the use of dixyrazine or prochlorperazine. The typical characteristics of women using other antipsychotics are high maternal age, first parity, heavy smoking, and high BMI. Educational level did not differ much but family situation and work situation did, most pronounced for women using other drugs than dixyrazine or prochlorperazine.

Table 50.2. Some further characteristics of women using antipsychotic drugs

Variable studied	Number	OR	95% CI
Women using dixyrazine or prochlorperazine			
Education (1996-2001, 981 women with drugs, 526 695 in population)			
Unknown	34	-	-
<12 years	147	1.44	1.19-1.76
12 years	496	1.00	Reference
13-14 years	40	0.75	0.54-1.03
≥14 years	264	0.91	0.78-1.07
Family situation			
Unknown	41	-	
Co-habiting	2264	1.00	Reference
Living alone	81	1.68	1.33-2.11
Other family situation	87	1.44	1.14-1.82
Work outside home			
Unknown	305	-	
Full time	918	1.00	Reference
Part time	589	1.12	1.00-1.25
None	665	1.76	1.58-1.96
Women using other antipsychotics			
Education (1996-2001, 345 women with drugs, 526 695 in population)			
Unknown	16	-	-
<12 years	72	1.52	1.15-1.99
12 years	165	1.00	Reference
13-14 years	18	0.94	0.70-1.27
≥14 years	74	0.97	0.93-1.28
Family situation			
Unknown	18	-	-
Co-habiting	127	1.00	Reference
Living alone	76	3.08	2.39-3.96
Other family situation	50	2.34	1.67-3.29
Work outside home			
Unknown	153	-	-
Full time	129	1.00	Reference
Part time	103	2.24	1.71-2.94
None	286	6.54	5.25-8.15

Women using dixyrazine or prochlorperazine use drugs for stomach ulcer and reflux and also antihistamines for NVP more than expected which is natural when the main indication is NVP. There is an increased use of folic acid, psychoactive drugs including opioids, and antihistamines for allergy. Women using other antipsychotic drugs use thyroid drugs more than expected and show a very marked excess of the use of other psychoactive drugs, anticonvulsants, and antihistamines.

An association between hyperemesis gravidarum and use of dixyrazine or prochlorperazine is evident. Other pregnancy complications are not increased in frequency after these drugs with the possible exception of gestational diabetes but the use of delivery inductions is increased.

Table 50.3. Concomitant drug use (early pregnancy)

Drug group	Dixyrazine or prochlorperazine			other antipsychotics		
	Number	OR/RR	95% CI	Number	OR/RR	95% CI
Drugs for stomach ulcer and reflux	146	7.02	6.06-8.12	7	0.91	0.37-1.87#
Drugs for inflammatory bowel disease	7	0.94	0.38-1.94#	1	-	-
Insulin	5	0.57	0.19-1.34#	3	0.73	0.17-2.42#
Multivitamins	156	0.77	0.66-0.89	30	0.83	0.17-2.42
Folic acid	193	1.34	1.16-1.56	24	0.79	0.53-1.19
Antihypertensives	8	0.92	0.40-1.82#	8	1.71	0.74-3.36#
Oral contraceptives	6	0.72	0.26-1.57#	3	1.33	0.27-3.88#
Progestogens	6	0.68	0.25-1.49#	1	-	-
Gonadotropins	3	0.60	0.12-1.76#	0	-	-
Systemic corticosteroids	16	1.74	0.99-2.82#	1	-	-
Thyroid drugs	35	1.02	0.73-1.42	33	3.66	2.61-5.13
Antibiotics	86	1.03	0.80-1.27	13	0.55	0.33-0.93
NSAIDs	20	0.45	0.29-0.69	5	0.31	0.13-0.70
Opioids	32	2.41	1.72-3.39	7	1.39	0.56-2.87#
Minor analgesics	150	0.76	0.64-0.89	32	0.48	0.34-0.68
Drugs for migraine	7	1.04	0.42-2.14#	0	-	-
Anticonvulsants	9	1.18	0.54-2.24#	26	9.52	6.22-14.0#
Sedatives, hypnotics	43	4.39	3.30-5.86	149	16.8	14.2-19.7
Antidepressants	87	2.87	2.33-3.53	196	19.9	17.6-22.6
Drugs for rhinitis	35	1.00	0.71-1.39	4	0.38	0.15-0.98#
Antiasthmatics	78	1.02	0.81-1.27	30	1.24	0.86-1.29
Antihistamines	902	8.60	8.03-9.21	70	2.07	1.62-2.64
For NVP	835	9.93	9.27-10.6	57	2.31	1.77-3.03
For allergy	147	3.91	3.35-4.57	18	1.70	1.07-2.70

#observed over expected number with exact Poisson 95% confidence interval.

Also after the use of other antipsychotics, an association with hyperemesis gravidarum and with many other pregnancy complications is seen. A significantly increased frequency of delivery induction and caesarean sections occurs.

Outcome after Maternal use of Antipsychotic Drugs

Infant Sex

The sex ratio was significantly low after early use of dixyraxine of prochlorperazine: 1201 male and 1335 female infants, sex ratio 0.90 (95%CI 0.83-0.97). Also after later use, the sex ratio was low but this could be random: 833 male and 848 female infant (one infant with unknown sex), sex ratio 0.98 (95% CI 0.89-1.08). The latter confidence interval thus includes the normal sex ratio (1.06). The low sex ratio agrees with what is seen with NVP.

Table 50.4. Some maternal diagnoses associated with the use of antipsychotic drugs

Diagnosis	Drug use in early pregnancy			Drug use later in pregnancy		
	Number	OR/RR	95% CI	Number	OR/RR	95% CI
Dixyrazine or prochlorperazine						
Pre-existing diabetes	34	1.09	0.77-1.53	14	0.62	0.36-1.05
Chronic hypertension	33	1.19	0.84-1.69	13	0.64	0.37-1.11
Gestational diabetes	32	1.50	1.06-2.14	12	0.81	0.45-1.43
Preeclampsia	110	1.06	0.88-1.29	16	0.85	0.51-1.40
Hyperemesis gravidarum	83	3.46	2.81-4.28	39	2.27	1.66-3.11
Placenta previa	34	1.27	0.90-1.79	16	0.85	0.51-1.40
Abruptio placentae	35	1.17	0.83-1.64	17	0.81	0.50-1.31
Antepartum bleeding	43	1.35	1.00-1.84	18	0.83	0.52-1.33
Intrapartum bleeding	51	1.01	0.76-1.34	31	0.86	0.60-1.23
Postpartum bleeding	145	1.10	0.93-1.30	88	1.01	0.82-1.26
Delivery induction	319	1.29	1.14-1.45	204	1.18	1.02-1.37
Caesarean section	399	1.09	0.98-1.22	265	1.06	0.93-1.21
Other antipsychotic drugs						
Pre-existing diabetes	22	1.69	1.09-2.61	11	1.42	0.71-2.54#
Chronic hypertension	20	1.64	1.04-2.10	10	1.48	0.71-2.72#
Gestational diabetes	10	1.02	0.49-1.88#	9	1.74	0.80-3.31#
Preeclampsia	47	1.23	0.96-1.66	24	1.17	0.71-1.78
Hyperemesis gravidarum	22	2.34	1.33-3.58	12	2.14	1.10-3.73#
Placenta previa	20	1.82	1.16-2.87	9	1.47	0.67-2.79#
Abruptio placentae	23	1.85	1.21-2.84	11	1.52	0.76-2.72#
Antepartum bleeding	22	1.71	1.11-2.63	11	1.56	0.78-2.79#
Intrapartum bleeding	27	1.45	0.97-2.15	17	1.58	0.96-2.60
Postpartum bleeding	51	1.25	0.93-1.68	22	1.08	0.69-1.67
Delivery induction	107	1.31	1.05-1.63	51	1.11	0.82-1.52
Caesarean section	164	1.28	1.07-1.54	92	1.37	1.07-1.34

#observed over expected number with exact Poisson 95% confidence interval.

After early use of other antipsychotic drugs, the sex ratio was if anything high. After early use there were 375 male and 300 female infants (one with unknown sex), sex ratio 1.25 (95% CI 1.07-1.46) and after later use 188 male and 156 female infants (one with unknown sex), sex ratio 1.21 (95% CI 0.98-1.49).

Multiple Births

After early use of dixyrazine or prochlorperazine, there were 62 twin and one triplet delivery. The odds ratio for twinning was 1.81 (95% CI 1.41-2.33). After later use, there were 38 twins, odds ratio 1.74 (95% CI 1.25-2.40).The high twinning rate is also typical for pregnancies with NVP.

After early use of other antipsychotic drugs, there were four twin deliveries (RR = 0.36, 95% CI 0.14-0.96) and after later use one twin delivery (RR = 0.17, 95% CI 0.01-0.94)

The high sex ratio and the low twinning rate could be an effect of the removal from the "other antipsychotics" group of pregnancies where the mother had used dixyrazine or prochlorperazine for NVP. This group will be only a small part of all using dixyrazine or prochlorperazine but a proportionally larger part of the group using other antipsychotic drugs.

Table 50.5. Pregnancy duration and infant birth weight at maternal use of antipsychotic drugs

Variable studied	Drug use in early pregnancy			Drug use later in pregnancy		
	Number	OR/RR	95% CI	Number	OR/RR	95% CI
Dixyrazine or prochlorperazine						
<37 weeks	116	1.05	0.86-1.26	75	1.02	0.80-1.28
<2500g	65	0.94	0.73-1.10	38	0.83	0.60-1.15
≥4500g	93	0.89	0.72-1.10	65	0.93	0.73-1.20
SGA	38	0.83	0.60-1.15	32	1.08	0.76-1.53
LGA	154	0.95	0.81-1.12	92	0.84	0.68-1.04
Other antipsychotic drugs						
<37 weeks	59	1.47	1.11-1.95	27	1.41	0.94-1.10
<2500g	45	1.57	1.14-2.14	18	1.28	0.78-2.10
≥4500g	18	0.69	0.43-1.11	13	0.90	0.52-1.56
SGA	31	1.52	1.05-2.20	15	1.53	0.86-2.53
LGA	33	0.89	0.62-1.29	15	0.67	0.40-1.14

No significant deviations can be seen after maternal use of dixyrazine or prochlorperazine. When other antipsychotic drugs had been used, an increased risk for preterm birth, low birth weight, and SGA is seen, statistically significant only after early use, but OR estimates were increased also after later use.

It has been stated in the literature [8] that term infants born after exposure to second generation antipsychotics (diazepines and oxazepines and "other" antipsychotics (here represented by risperidal) should have a higher birth weight than those exposed to first generation antipsychotics. A study of the present material did not confirm that observation when restricted to singleton term births and after exclusion of dixyrazine and prochlorperazine. The mean birth weight was 3548g after first generation antipsychotics and 3415g after second generation antipsychotics – the weight difference of 33g is not statistically significant (t=0.11).

The rate of preterm births was higher after second generation antipsychotics (OR = 1.96, 95% CI 1.23-3.15) than after first generation antipsychotics (OR = 1.30, 95% CI 0.92-1.84) but this difference may be random. The same was seen for low birth weight and for small-for-gestational age.

Table 50.6. Infant mortality after maternal use of antipsychotics

Variable studied	Drug use in early pregnancy			Drug use later in pregnancy		
	Number	RR	95% CI	Number	RR	95% CI
Dixyrazine or prochlorperazine						
Stillbirth	15	1.98	1.11-3.26	6	1.27	0.47-2.76
Early neonatal death	1	-	-	3	2.38	0.49-6.95
Other antipsychotic drugs						
Stillbirth	6	1.53	0.56-3.34	2	1.27	0.47-2.26
Early neonatal death	3	2.38	0.49-6.95	1	-	-

The only significant deviation is an increased risk for stillbirth after maternal use of dixyrazine or prochlorperazine. This was indicated but not statistically significant in the earlier study [10].

Table 50.7. Neonatal diagnoses after maternal use of antipsychotics

Diagnosis	Drug use in early pregnancy			Drug use later in pregnancy		
	Number	OR/RR	95% CI	Number	OR/RR	95% CI
Dixyrazine or prochlorperazine						
Hypoglycaemia	75	0.90	0.71-1.13	57	1.01	0.77-1.32
Respiratory diagnoses	104	0.92	0.76-1.13	78	1.08	0.86-1.36
Low Apgar score	52	1.26	0.96-1.66	29	1.10	0.76-1.59
CNS diagnoses	15	1.06	0.64-1.77	13	1.32	0.76-2.28
Jaundice	107	1.09	0.90-1.33	70	1.06	0.83-1.36
Other antipsychotic drugs						
Hypoglycaemia	35	1.13	0.79-1.61	18	1.14	0.71-1.85
Respiratory diagnoses	49	1.29	0.96-1.74	32	1.80	1.25-2.59
Low Apgar score	20	1.28	0.81-2.01	12	1.63	0.92-2.89
CNS diagnoses	12	2.34	1.21-4.09#	9	3.03	1.39-5.75#
Jaundice	22	0.67	0.44-1.03	16	0.97	0.58-1.52

#observed over expected number with exact Poisson 95% confidence interval.

After maternal use of dixyrazine or prochlorperazine, no certain deviations from expected numbers are seen but after use of other antipsychotics the odds ratio is increased for respiratory diagnoses after later exposure and for CNS diagnoses both after early and later exposure.

Table 50.8. Congenital malformations in infants whose mothers had used antipsychotic drugs in early pregnancy

Congenital malformation	Dixyrazine or prochlorperazine			Other antipsychotics		
	Number	OR	95% CI	Number	OR	95%CI
All malformations	101	0.89	0.73-1.09	54	1.70	1.27-2.28
Relatively severe malformations	62	0.86	0.67-1.10	44	2.08	1.51-2.82
Chromosome anomalies	7	1.42	0.57-2.93#	2	1.37	0.17-4.95#
Without chromosome anomalies						
Any CNS malformation	0	-	-	3	3.65	0.75-10.7#
Any cardiovascular defect	25	0.97	0.65-1.44	10	1.40	0.67-2.58#
VSD and/or ASD	14	0.99	0.59-1.62	7	2.01	0.81-4.13#
Hypospadias	5	0.70	0.23-1.63#	6	2.78	1.02-6.05#
Pes equinovarus	1	-	-	3	2.94	0.61-8.60#
Hip (sub)luxation, unstable hip	18	1.21	0.76-1.93	4	0.80	0.22-2.06#

#observed over expected number with exact Poisson 95% confidence interval.

There is thus a statistically significant over-risk for congenital malformations and for relatively severe malformations after maternal use of other antipsychotics than dixyrazine or prochlorperazine. The only specific malformation which reaches statistical significance is hypospadias.

An analysis was made of the risk for a relatively severe malformation after exposure for individual drugs when the number of exposed infants was at least 50 (Table 50.9).

Table 50.9. Relatively severe malformations in infants whose mothers used specific antipsychotics

Drug	Number of infants		OR/RR	95% CI
	malformed	total		
Dixyrazine	61	2311	0.87	0.67-1.12
Prochlorperazine	6	255	0.76	0.28-1.65#
Levomepromazine	2	50	1.23	0.15-4.43#
Perphenazine	1	90	0.42	0.01-2.35#
Haloperidol	5	76	2.22	0.72-5.19#
Flupentixol	11	114	2.54	1.27-4.55#
Zuclopenthixol	8	70	3.49	1.51-6.88#
Olanzapine	5	91	1.56	0.51-3.65#
Risperidone	4	58	2.03	0.55-5.20#
Lithium	6	81	2.02	0.74-4.40#

#observed over expected number with exact Poisson 95% confidence interval.

For many of the individual drugs among "other antipsychotics", odds ratios around 2-3 are seen but only for two is statistical significance reached. The eleven malformed infants after flupentixol showed no specific type of malformation. Among the eight infants exposed to zuclopenthixol, three had malformations of the upper alimentary tract, two had pylorostenosis and the third an unspecified malformation (the last one was also exposed to olanzapine). Among the six infants exposed to lithium, three had cardiovascular defects: one had tricuspid and mitral anomalies, one had patent ductus arteriosus in a term infants, and one had a ventricular septum defect.

Summary

Dixyrazine or prochlorperazine seems mainly to have been used for NVP and no major deviations in pregnancy or neonatal outcome is apparent with one exception: an increased risk for stillbirth. No increase in malformation ratE is seen. After use of other antipsychotics, clear-cut effects on pregnancy and neonatal outcomes are seen. There is an increased risk for "relatively severe malformations" but due to low numbers they are difficult to locate to a specific malformation type or a specific antipsychotic drug but statistical significances are reached after two of the thioxanthene derivate drugs. Among the 81 infants exposed to lithium, three had a cardiac defect (4%).

References

[1] Rumeau-Rouqette C, Goujard J, Huel G. Possible teratogenic effect of phenothiazines in human beings. *Teratology* 1977; 15: 57-64.

[2] Heinonen OP, Slone D, Shapiro S. *Birth Defects and Drugs in Pregnancy.* Publishing Sciences Group, Inc. Littleton, MA. 1977.

[3] Diav-Citrin O, Schechtman S, Ornoy S, Arnon J, Schaefer C, Garbis H, Clementi M, Ornoy A. Safety of haloperidol and penfluridol in pregnancy: a multicenter, prospective, controlled study. *I Clin Psychopharm* 2005; 66: 317-322.

[4] Ernst CL, Goldberg JF. The reproductive safety profile of mood stabilizers, atypical antipsychotics, and broad-spectrum psychotropics. *J Clin Psychiatry* 2002; 63 (Suppl. 4): 42-55.

[5] McKenna, Koren G, Tetelbaum M, Wilton L, Shakir S, Diav-Citrin O, Levinson A, Zipursky RB, Einarson A. Pregnancy outcome of women using atypical antipsychotic drugs: a prospective comparative study. *J Clin Psychiatry* 2005; 66:444-449.

[6] Yeshayahu Y. The use of olanzapine in pregnancy and congenital cardiac and musculoskeletal abnormalities. *Amer J Psychiatry* 2007; 164: 1759-1760.

[7] Coppola D, Russo LJ, Kwarta RF Jr, Varughese R, Schmider J. Evaluating the postmarketing experience of risperidone use during pregnancy: pregnancy and neonatal outcomes. *Drug Saf* 2007; 30: 247-264.

[8] Newharn JJ, Thomas SH, MacRitchie K, McElhatton PR, McAllister-Willians, RH. Birth weight of infants after maternal exposure to typical and atypical antipsychotics: prospective comparative study. *B J Psych* 2008; 192: 333-337.

[9] Gentile S. Antipsychotic therapy during early and late pregnancy. A systematic review. Schizophrenia Bull 2008: *E-publ, Doi:10.1093/schul/sbn107.*

[10] Reis M, Källén B. Maternal use of antipsycotics in early pregnancy and delivery outcome. *J Clin Pharmacology* 2008; 28: 279-288.

[11] Moore JA. An assessment of lithum using the IEHR Evaluative Process for Assessing Human Developmental and Reproductive Toxicity of Agents. IEHR Expert Scientific Committee. *Reprod Toxicol* 1999; 9: 175-210.

[12] Schou M, Goldfield MD,Weinstein MR, Villeneuve A. Lithium and pregnancy. I. Report from the Register of Lithium Babies. *BMJ* 1973;ii: 135-136.

[13] Källén B, Tandberg A. Lithium and pregnancy. A cohort study on manic-depressive women. *Acta psych Scand* 1983; 68: 134-139.

[14] Yacobi S, Ornoy A. Is lithium a real teratogen? What can we conclude from the prospective versus retrospective studies? A review. *Isr J Psychiatry Relat Sci* 2008; 45: 95-106.

Chapter 51

SEDATIVES AND HYPNOTICS

Sedatives and hypnotics are often used at various maternal morbidity and the increased rate of pregnancy and neonatal diagnoses seems mainly to be a result of co-morbidity and not a drug effect. No certain signs of teratogenicity have been shown but some specific relationships may occur which are difficult to prove. These drugs should be avoided during pregnancy and when used late in pregnancy may affect the newborn but it is not known if long-term damage can occur. If used in early pregnancy there is no reason to discuss a termination of the pregnancy because of fear for teratogenicity. Further data on the hypnotic benzodiazepine receptor agonists and on specific benzodiazepines including alprazolam are needed.

Use of sedatives and hypnotics, notably benzodiazepines, in late pregnancy may cause withdrawal symptoms and Floppy Infant Syndrome [1,2]. The teratogenic potential of benzodiazepines is uncertain [3]. Most studies which suggest the presence of such an effect are retrospective case-control studies. High doses of benzodiazepines were associated with an increased risk of anomalies and neurodevelopmental disturbances [4,5]. An association between maternal use of lorazepam and infant anal atresia has been suggested [6]. More modern hypnotics, acting as benzodiazepine receptor agonists (HBRA), have been little studied during pregnancy [7]. In a recent study based on the Swedish Medical Birth Register for the years 1995-2004 of benzodiazepines and HBRAs, no certain teratogenic effect could be seen but a suggested increased risk for two specific conditions, pylorostenosis and small bowel atresia [8,9]. An increased risk for preterm birth and low birth weight was also seen.

Table 51.1. Number of women identified using sedatives or hypnotics

Total	5390
Reported use in early pregnancy	4186
Got prescription later in pregnancy	1914
Both early and later use	710

Type of drug	ATC code	Early use	Later use
Sedatives			
Benzodiazepines	N05BA	1408	482
Diazepam	N05BA01	582	171
Chlordiazepoxide	N05BA02	2	0
Oxazepam	N05BA04	517	192
Lorazepam	N05BA06	31	13
Clobazam	N05BA09	15	12
Alprazolam	N05BA12	283	110
Diphenylmetane derivates	N05BB	641	338
Hydroxyzine	N05BB01	641	338
Carbamates	N05BC	1	1
Meprobamate	N05BC01	1	1
Axaspirodecanedione derivates	N05BE	112	48
Buspirone	N05BE01	112	48
Hypnotics			
Barbiturates	N05CA	2	1
Pentobarbital	N05CA01	2	1
Benzodiazepines	N05CD	265	74
Nitrazepam	N05CD02	76	32
Flunitrazepam	N05CD03	170	40
Triazolam	N02CD05	6	2
Midazolam	N05CD08	14	1
Cyclopyrolones (HBRA)	N05CF	1167	326
Zoplicone	N05CF01	612	159
Zolpidem	N05CF02	539	165
Zoleplon	N05CF03	18	3
Other	N05CM	1173	927
Clomethiazole	N05CM02	2	34
Propriomazine	N05CM06	1076	870
Scopolamine	N05CM05	0	1
Valerian	N05CM09	98	23
Unspecified	N05C	27	0

HBRA = Hypnotic benzodiazepine receptor agonists.

Characteristics of Women using Sedatives or Hypnotics

Based on women reporting drug use in early pregnancy (n= 4186). Each variable is adjusted for all other variables and year of delivery. Comparison with all women who gave birth during the period and with information from the first antenatal care (n=967 742). The odds ratios for maternal age, parity, smoking in early pregnancy, number of previous miscarriages, BMI, subfertility, and country of birth are adjusted for all other variables and are shown in Figure 51.1.

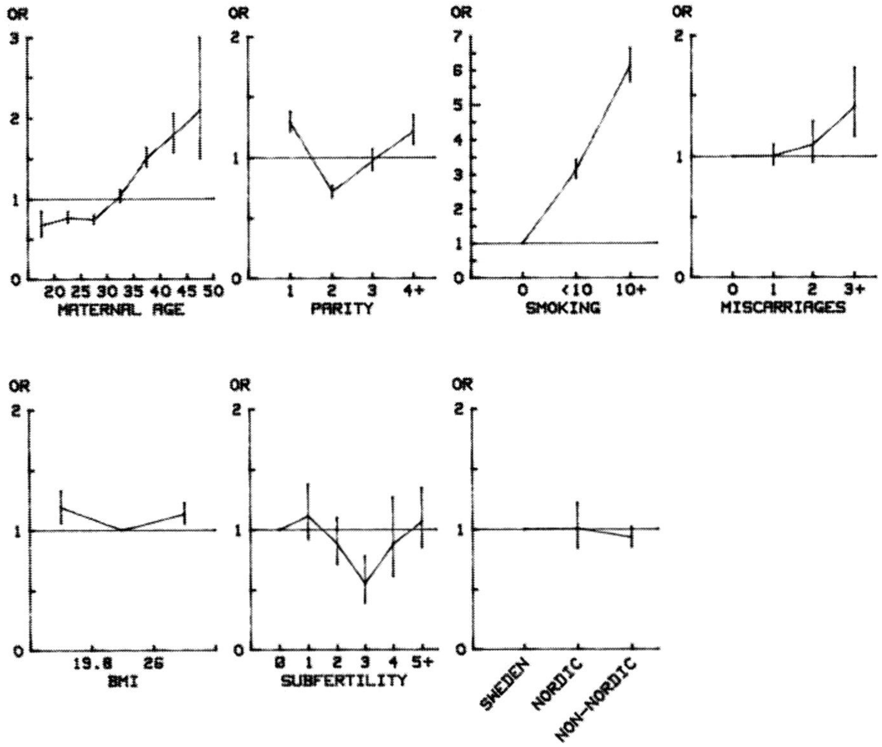

Figure 51.1. Odds ratios for seven maternal characteristics. The odds ratios (OR) for each variable are adjusted for the other variables and year of delivery. Vertical lines mark 95% confidence intervals. For maternal age and parity, each class is compared with all other classes. Unbroken graphs refer to women who used dixyrazine or prochlorperazine, dashed graphs to women using other antipsychotics.

Some further maternal characteristics were analyzed, adjusting for year of delivery, maternal age, parity, smoking, and BMI (Table 51.2).

Table 51.2. Some further characteristics of women using sedatives or hypnotics in early pregnancy

Variable studied	Number	OR	95% CI
Education (1996-2001, 1 974 women with drugs, 526 695 in population)			
Unknown	73		
<12 years	472	1.75	1.56-1.96
12 years	944	1.00	reference
13-14 years	61	0.67	0.52-0.87
≥14 years	424	0.86	0.76-0.98
Family situation			
Unknown	96	-	-
Co-habiting	3326	1.00	reference
Living alone	414	2.92	2.61-3.26
Other family situation	308	2.60	2.28-2.97
Work outside home			
Unknown	775	-	
Full time	1235	1.00	reference
Part time	783	1.38	1.24-1.52
None	1351	2.91	2.67-3.18

Women using sedatives/hypnotics in early pregnancy are thus older than expected. The lowest use is at parity 2 with a high use at first parity and at parity 4 or more. There is a strong association with smoking, an increased use after three or more previous miscarriages and at both low and high BMI. There is little association with subfertility, actually a lower than expected use after three years of unwanted childlessness. Low maternal education increases and high education decreases the use of these drugs. The women are less often than expected cohabiting and are less often than expected working full time.

Table 51.3. Concomitant drug use (early pregnancy)

Drug group	Number	OR/RR	95% CI
Drugs for stomach ulcer and reflux	158	3.87	3.33-4.50
Drugs for inflammatory bowel disease	14	1.25	0.73-2.16
Insulin	14	0.85	0.50-1.46
Multivitamins	151	0.73	0.62-0.85
Folic acid	167	0.89	0.71-1.04
Oral contraceptives	28	2.02	1.40-2.92
Progestogens	12	0.57	0.33-1.00
Gonadotropins	8	0.82	0.35-1.61#
Systemic corticosteroids	44	2.75	2.07-3.67
Thyroid drugs	96	1.65	1.35-2.02
Antibiotics	181	1.38	1.19-1.61
NSAIDs	181	2.01	1.73-2.33
Opioids	256	9.03	8.07-10.1
Minor analgesics	618	1.79	1.64-1.95
Anticonvulsants	42	3.25	2.42-4.36
Antidepressants	1262	25.9	24.6-27.3
Drugs for rhinitis	97	1.77	1.45-2.21
Antiasthmatics	266	1.95	1.72-2.21
Antihistamines	616	3.10	2.86-3.37

#observed over expected number with exact Poisson 95% confidence interval.

Table 51.4. Some maternal diagnoses associated with the use of sedatives and hypnotics

Diagnosis	Drug use in early pregnancy			Drug use later in pregnancy		
	Number	OR	95% CI	Number	OR	95% CI
Pre-existing diabetes	87	1.35	1.08-1.67	44	1.35	0.99-1.84
Chronic hypertension	82	1.40	1.12-1.75	45	1.51	1.12-2.04
Gestational diabetes	68	1.51	1.18-1.93	34	1.53	1.09-2.15
Preeclampsia	247	1.27	1.11-1.45	124	1.37	1.13-1.65
Hyperemesis gravidarum	70	1.46	1.15-1.86	39	1.59	1.15-2.18
Placenta previa	80	1.43	1.14-1.79	39	1.39	1.01-1.91
Abruptio placentae	88	1.39	1.12-1.72	45	1.48	1.04-1.89
Antepartum bleeding	82	1.22	0.98-1.53	45	1.41	1.05-1.90
Intrapartum bleeding	127	1.30	1.08-1.55	74	1.43	1.13-1.81
Postpartum bleeding	254	1.07	0.94-1.22	132	1.26	1.05-1.50
Delivery induction	614	1.37	1.25-1.50	365	1.87	1.66-2.11
Caesarean section	1012	1.49	1.38-1.60	523	1.71	1.54-1.90

There is thus a marked association between the use of sedatives/hypnotics and many other drug groups, notably with antidepressants and opiates, but also drugs for stomach ulcer and reflux, oral contraceptives, systemic corticosteroids, thyroid drugs, antibiotics, NSAIDs and minor analgesics, anticonvulsants, drugs for rhinitis and asthma, and antihistamines. There appears to be a complex co-morbidity.

There are thus signs of an increased pre-existing and gestational morbidity. The risk estimates are of the same magnitude after early and later exposure but some conditions appear to be more strongly associated with use of the drug later in pregnancy.

Outcome after Maternal use of Sedatives and Hypnotics

Infant Sex

After the use of sedatives or hypnotics in early pregnancy there were 2 207 male and 2 032 female infants (three had unknown sex), sex ratio 1.09 (95% CI 1.02-1.15), and after later use there were 1034 male and 913 female infants (one had unknown sex), sex ratio 1.13 (95% CI 1.04-1.24), Both sex ratios are thus somewhat high, but the normal sex ratio (1.06) is contained in the confidence intervals.

Multiple Births

After early use of sedatives or hypnotics there were 54 twin deliveries (OR = 0.80, 95% CI 0.61-1.06). After later use there were 31 twin deliveries (OR =1.00, 95% CI 0.70-1.44). No higher order multiples were born.

Table 51.5. Pregnancy duration and infant birth weight at maternal use of sedatives or hypnotics

Variable studied	Drug use in early pregnancy			Drug use later in pregnancy		
	Number	OR	95% CI	Number	OR	95% CI
<37 weeks	340	1.49	1.33-1.67	191	2.01	1.72-2.33
<2500g	236	1.46	1.29-1.67	114	1.71	1.41-2.07
≥4500g	145	0.93	0.79-1.11	54	0.69	0.53-0.91
SGA	147	1.25	1.06-1.49	69	1.45	1.13-1.85
LGA	234	1.01	0.88-1.16	119	0.99	0.82-1.20

There was thus an increased risk of preterm birth, low birth weight, and SGA both after early and later use of sedatives or hypnotics. After removal of infants which were also exposed in early pregnancy to antihypertensive drugs, corticosteroids, thyroid drugs, NSAIDs, analgesics, antipsychotic drugs, antidepressant, antiasthmatics or antihistamines, all ORs decreased to 0.87-1.16, none of them statistically significant. This procedure removed about ¾ of all cases and it is likely that the remaining ones were less exposed than those removed.

Table 51.6. Infant mortality after maternal use of sedatives or hypnotics

Variable studied	Drug use in early pregnancy			Drug use later in pregnancy		
	Number	OR/RR	95% CI	Number	OR/RR	95% CI
Stillbirth	18	0.96	0.59-1.94	8	1.03	0.45-2.04#
Early neonatal death	3	0.40	0.07-1.17#	3	0.95	0.30-2.77#

#observed over expected number with exact Poisson 95% confidence interval.

No significant perinatal mortality risk is thus indicated.

Table 51.7. Neonatal diagnoses after maternal use of sedatives/hypnotics

Diagnosis	Drug use in early pregnancy			Drug use later in pregnancy		
	Number	OR	95% CI	Number	OR	95% CI
Hypoglycaemia	232	1.36	1.19-1.56	101	1.30	1.06-1.59
Respiratory diagnoses	271	1.22	1.07-1.38	138	1.45	1.22-1.74
Low Apgar score	114	1.29	1.07-1.56	59	1.61	1.24-2.09
CNS diagnoses	40	1.28	0.92-1.79	20	1.45	0.92-2.29
Jaundice	223	1.24	1.08-1.42	114	1.40	1.15-1.70

All studied neonatal diagnoses thus occur more often than expected even though the odds ratios for CNS diagnoses do not reach statistical significance. These effects disappear after removal of infants also exposed to antihypertensive drugs, corticosteroids, thyroid drugs, NSAIDs, analgesics, antipsychotic drugs, antidepressant, antiasthmatics or antihistamines in early pregnancy. The remaining ORs vary between 0.71 and 1.17, none of them statistically significant.

Table 51.8. Congenital malformations in infants whose mothers had used sedatives or hypnotics in early pregnancy

Congenital malformation	Number	OR/RR	95% CI
All malformation	221	1.08	0.94-1.24
Relatively severe malformation	163	1.15	0.95-1.35
Chromosome anomalies	16	1.64	1.00-2.68
Without chromosome anomalies			
Any CNS malformation	5	0.99	0.32-2.31#
Eye malformations	5	1.38	0,45-3.22#
Ear malformations	8	0.86	0.37-1.70#
Orofacial clefts	4	0.53	0.14-1.35#
Any cardiovascular defects	38	0.80	0.58-1.11
VSD and/or ASD	22	0.89	0.58-1.36
Pylorostenosis	10	2.58	1.24-4.74#
Oesophageal, small bowel or anal atresia	6	1.54	0.57-3.36#
Hypospadias	22	1.84	1.21-2.80
Serious kidney malformations	3	1.36	0.28-3.99#
Pes equinovarus	8	1.04	0.45-2.06#
Polydactyly/syndactyly	3	0.35	0.07-1.02#
Limb reduction defects	5	1.59	0.52-3.70#
Hip (su)luxation, unstable hip	14	0.56	0.33-0.84
Craniostenosis	5	1.93	0.63-4.51#

#observed over expected number with exact Poisson 95% confidence interval.

Two conditions occur more often than expected: pylorostenosis and hypospadias. Among the 10 cases of pylorostenosis, three were exposed to alprazolam, two to flunitrazepam, two to zolpidem, two to propiomazine, and one to diazepam.

Among the 22 hypospadias cases, nine were exposed to benzodiazepines, five to HBRA, four to propiomazine, and three to hydroxyine. The remaining one was exposed to buspirone.

Among the drugs which were associated with use of sedatives and hypnotics, anticonvulsants are known teratogens. Among 77 infants exposed to sedatives/hypnotics and anticonvulsants, only three had a congenital malformation (2.8 expected): one with pylorostenosis, one with a ventricular septum defect, and one with syndactyly.

Table 51.9. Distribution of "relatively severe" malformations according to type of sedative or hypnotic used

Sedative or hypnotic	Number of infants with malformations	Total number of infants	OR/RR	95% CI
Benzodiazepines, sedatives	65	1429	1.39	1.08-1.80
Diazepam	20	593	1.00	0.63-1.57
Oxazepam	17	525	0.97	0.59-1.61
Lorazepam	3	32	2.86	0.59-8.35#
Alprazolam	24	284	2.58	1.65-3.84#
Diphenylmethane derivates	23	652	1.03	0.67-1.59
Azaspirodecanedione derivates	5	112	1.29	0.42-3.01#
Benzodiazepines,hypnotics	8	269	0.82	0.36-1.63#
Cyclopyrrolones	33	1169	0.86	0.60-1.20
Zoplicone	20	623	0.99	0.63-1.55
Zolpidem	13	550	0.69	0.39-1.20
Other	42	1183	1.08	0.79-1.48
Propiomazine	37	1086	1.05	0.75-1.47
Valerian	5	98	1.31	0.43-3.05#

#observed over expected number with exact Poisson 95% confidence interval.

Lorazepam and alprazolam thus show high ORs but it is statistically significant only for alprazolam.

Table 51.10. Specfication of malformations in infants exposed to alprazolam

Malformation	Number	Note
Spina bifida with hydromyelia	1	
VSD	4	
ASD + tricuspidal malformation	1	
VSD+ASD	2	One with hydronephrosis
Pulmonary valve stenosis	2	
Hypospadias	2	
Hydronephrosis	1	
Pylorostenosis	3	One with a face/neck anomaly
Megacolon	1	
Malrotation of the guts	1	
Anal/rectal fistula	1	
Bilateral pes equinovarus	1	
Neurofibromatosis	1	
Down syndrome	3	

Nine of the infants thus had cardiac defects, RR = 2.63 (95% CI 1.20-5.00), but these do not explain the total excess risk.

Summary

Maternal use of sedatives and hypnotics is associated with widespread other pathology, apparent also as many associations with other types of drugs, mainly psychoactive drugs. There is an excess risk for pregnancy complications and neonatal pathology which, however, seems to be mainly explained by co-morbidity. There is no general increase in the risk for congenital malformations but it is indicated for benzodiazepine sedatives and then apparently explained by an effect of alprazolam and possibly lorazepam. The putative teratogenic effect of alprazolam appears unspecific as many different malformations occurred. It is unlikely due to confounding as there is no visible effect of related drugs. Either there is causality or the finding is an expression of mass significance.

References

[1] Rementia JL, Bhatt K. Withdrawal symptoms in neonates from intrauterine exposure to diazepam. *J Pediatr* 1977; 90: 123-126.

[2] Gillberg G. "Floppy infant syndrom" and maternal diazepam. *Lancet* 1977; ii: 244.

[3] Dolovich LR, Addis A, Vaillancourt JM, Power JD, Koren G, Einarson TR. Benzodiazepine use in pregnancy and major malformations or oral cleft: meta-analysis of cohort and case-control studies. *BMJ* 1998; 317: 839-43.

[4] Laegreid L, Olegård R, Wahlström J, Conradi N. Abnormalities in children exposed to benzodiazepines in utero. *Lancet* 1987;1:108-9.

[5] Laegreid L, Hagberg G, Lundberg A. The effect of benzodiazepines on the fetus and the newborn. *Neuropediatrics* 1992;23:18-23.

[6] Bonnot O, Vollset SE, Godet PF, D'Amato T, Robert E. In utero exposure to benzodiazepine. Is there a risk for anal atresia with lorazepam? *Encephale* 2003; 29: 553-559.

[7] Diav-Citrin O, Oktore B, Lucarelli K, Koren G. Pregnancy outcome following first-trimester exposure to zoplicone: a prospective controlled cohort study. *Am J Perinatol* 1999; 16: 157-160.

[8] Norstedt Wikner B, Stille C-O, Källén B, Asker C. Use of benzodiazepines and benzodiazepine receptor agonists during pregnancy: maternal characteristics. *Pharmacoepidemiol Drug Safety* 2007; 16: 1-7.

[9] Norstedt Wikner B, Stille C-O, Källén B, Asker C. Use of benzodiazepines and benzodiazepine receptor agonists during pregnancy: neonatal outcome and congenital malformations. *Pharmacoepidemiol Drug Safety* 2007; 16: 1203-1210.

Chapter 52

ANTIDEPRESSANTS

The use of antidepresants during pregnancy is associated with some hazards. No general teratogenic effect is certain after early exposure but the use of clomipramine or paroxetine may be associated with an increased risk for mainly relatively mild cardiovascular defects. If possible, these drugs should be avoided in early pregnancy until more data are available. Use of antidepressants during pregnancy is associated with preterm birth and neonatal symptoms. How much underlying maternal pathology contributes is unclear. Most neonatal symptoms resolve a short time after birth. An association has been described between SSRI and a rare but serious symptom, persistent pulmonary hypertension in the newborn (PPHN). Possible long term effects are not demonstrated with certainty but cannot yet be disregarded. Use of antidepressants during pregnancy is often necessary to ensure the health of the mother (and child) but unnecessary exposure should be avoided. Untreated depression may carry a larger risk than that caused by the drugs. There seems to be little difference between the various SSRI drugs with the exception of the possible specific risk of paroxetine, mentioned above. Data on the modern SNRI drugs are still incomplete and it may be wise to avoid them during pregnancy even though the available data seem rather positive, at least for the risk of teratogenesis. Under no circumstances is exposure for antidepressant drugs in early pregnancy a reason to discuss a termination of the pregnancy.

There are many studies published on the possible effect of use of antidepressants on congenital malformations in the infant. The studies are performed with different methodologies which all carry problems in their interpretation. Some early studies were based on relatively small cohorts from TIS organizations and had a low power to detect anything but very strong effects [1,2]. Some large studies are based on redeemed prescriptions [3,4]. A few case-control studies with retrospective information on drug use are available [5,6]. Some previous studies have been published from the Swedish Medical Birth Register [7,8].

Many reviews are available which more or less critically summarize the available literature [9,10]. There is a consensus that use of antidepressants in late pregnancy can affect neonatal symptoms, perhaps as withdrawal symptoms [11,12]. The most serious one among these is PPHN which in two different studies have been linked to maternal use of SSRI even though a recent small study did not find such an association [13-15]. Effects on pregnancy complications and notably an increased risk for preeclampsia has been described [16].

Many of these effects have been ascribed the underlying diseases, e.g., depression, anxiety, and panic disorder [17]. In many of the studies which tried to demonstrate an effect of such pathology, the possible effect of drug use was not eliminated. It is, however, likely that an effect of stress, anxiety and depression on pregnancy outcome exists but it appears to be stronger when antidepressant drugs have been used [4].

After some initial concerns on a possible teratogenic effect of tricyclic antidepressants, the general opinion has been that the teratogenic potential of antidepressants is low. It has been suggested that the teratogenic risk is lower for SSRI than for TCA [9] and an ongoing discussion exists about possible specific effects of some SSRIs (notably paroxetine) on the risk for cardiovascular defects [18-20].

Possible long term effects on infant neuropsychiatric development have been much discussed but only small studies exist with variable results but so far without any with certainty demonstrated deleterious effects [21].

Table 52.1. Number of women identified using antidepressants

Total	12841
Reported use in early pregnancy	11181
Got prescription later in pregnancy	4940
Both early and later use	3280

Type of drug	ATC code	Early use	Later use
Non-selective monamine reuptak inhibitors (TCA)	N06AA	1560	733
Imipramine	N06AA02	9	3
Clomipramine	N06AA04	1164	565
Trimipramine	N06AA06	15	5
Loperamine	N06AA07	6	1
Amitryptyline	N06AA09	330	137
Nortryptyline	N06AA10	29	21
Protryptyline	N06AA11	1	0
Maprotiline	N06AA21	1	0
Selective serotonin reuptake inhibitors (SSRI)	N06AB	8717	3881
Fluoxetine	N06AB03	1290	716
Citalopram	N06AB04	3439	1364
Paroxetine	N06AB05	1100	354
Sertraline	N06AB06	2774	1436
Fluvoxamine	N06AB08	38	14
Escitalopram	N06AB10	140	49
Unspecified SSRI	N06AB	1	0
Monamine oxidase type A inhibitors	N06AG	35	17
Moclobemide	N06AG02	35	17
Other antidepressants (SNRI)	N06AX	1123	444
Mianserin	N06AX03	74	27
Nefazodone	N06AX06	44	7
Mirtazapine	N06AX11	232	115
Amfebutamone	N06AX12	33	9
Venlafaxine	N06AX16	723	287
Reboxetin	N06AX18	23	5
Duloxetine	N06AX21	8	1
Unspecified antidepressants	N06A	10	0

Characteristics of Women using Antidepressant Drugs

Based on women reporting the drug in early pregnancy (n=11180, four missing maternal age). Each variable is adjusted for all other variables and year of delivery. Comparison with all women who gave birth during the period and with information from the first antenatal care (n=967 742). The odds ratios for maternal age, parity, smoking in early pregnancy, number of previous miscarriages, BMI, subfertility, and country of birth are adjusted for all other variables and are shown in Figure 52.1.

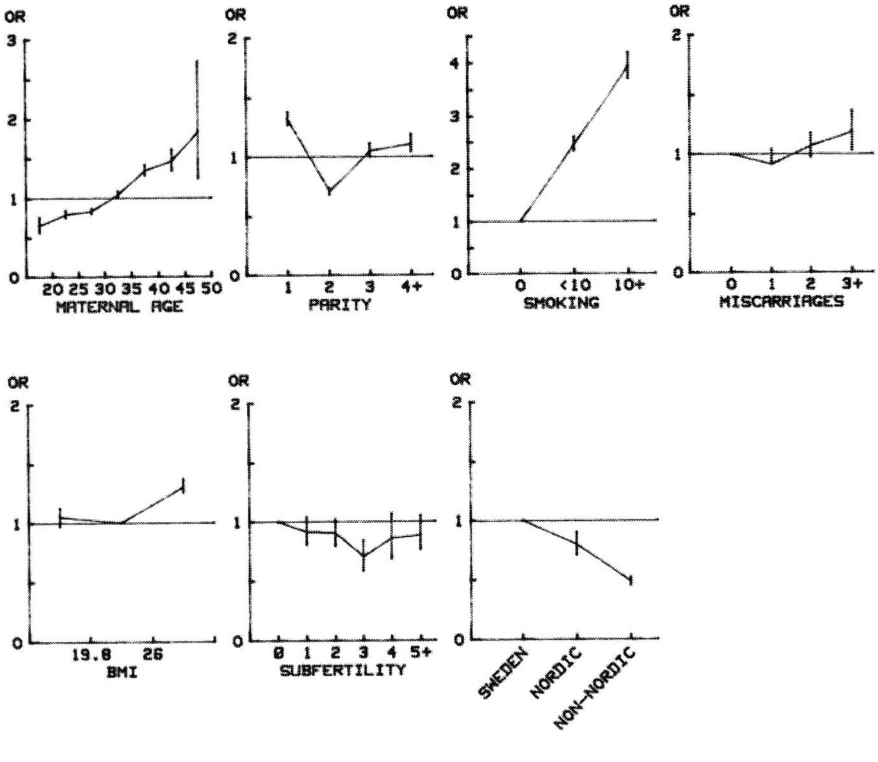

Figure 52.1. Odds ratios for seven maternal characteristics. The odds ratios (OR) for each variable are adjusted for the other variables and year of delivery. Vertical lines mark 95% confidence intervals. For maternal age and parity, each class is compared with all other classes.

Some further maternal characteristics were analyzed, adjusting for year of delivery, maternal age, parity, smoking, and BMI (Table 52.2).

Women using antidepressants are thus older than expected. Usage is lowest at parity 2 and highest at parity 1. There is a strong association with smoking, a slight increase after three or more previous miscarriages, but little association with subfertility. Women born outside Sweden and notably in Non-Nordic countries use less antidepressants than Swedish-born women do. These women are less often than expected co-habiting or working outside home. Their characteristics resemble strongly those of women using sedatives or hypnotics (see Chapter 51).

Table 52.2. Some further characteristics of women using antidepressants in early pregnancy

Variable studied	Number	OR	95% CI
Education (1996-2001, 3891 women with drugs, 526 695 in population)			
Unknown	81	-	-
<12 years	792	1.48	1.35-1.61
12 years	2000	1.00	reference
13-14 years	170	0.85	0.73-1.00
≥14 years	848	0.78	0.72-0.85
Family situation			
Unknown	234	-	
Co-habiting	9437	1.00	reference
Living alone	717	2.34	2.15-2.54
Other family situation	693	2.05	1.87-2.24
Work outside home			
Unknown	1728	-	-
Full time	3716	1.00	reference
Part time	2583	1.48	1.40-1.57
None	3054	2.20	2.07-2.32

Table 52.3. Concomitant drug use (early pregnancy)

Drug group	Number	OR	95% CI
Drugs for stomach ulcer and reflux	316	2.92	2.61-3.26
Drugs for inflammatory bowel disease	41	1.27	0.93-1.73
Insulin	49	1.13	0.85-1.50
Multivitamins	559	0.78	072-0.85
Folic acid	519	0.82	0.75-0.90
Oral contraceptives	160	3.52	3.02-4.11
Progestogens	30	0.56	0.38-0.76
Gonadotropins	22	0.85	0.56-1.28
Systemic corticosteroids	65	1.55	1.21-1.98
Thyroid drugs	317	1.89	1.69-2.11
Antibiotics	321	0.92	082-1.03
NSAIDs	300	1.21	1.08-1.36
Opioids	261	3.48	3.09-3.93
Minor analgesics	835	0.83	0.77-0.89
Anticonvulsants	110	3.17	2.63-3.82
Neuroleptics	283	7.13	6.39-7.97
Sedatives, hypnotics	1202	25.9	24.6-27.3
Drugs for rhinitis	146	0.92	0.78-1.09
Antiasthmatics	533	1.40	1.28-1.53
Antihistamines	1097	1.79	1.68-1.90

There is thus a strong association between the use of antidepressants and opioids, anticonvulsants, neuroleptics, and notably sedatives/hypnotics. Other associations are with oral contraceptives, systemic corticosteroids, thyroid drugs, NSAIDs, antiasthmatics and antihistamines, indicating complex co-morbidity.

Table 52.4. Some maternal diagnoses associated with the use of antidepressants

Diagnosis	Drug use in early pregnancy			Drug use later in pregnancy		
	Number	OR	95% CI	Number	OR	95% CI
Pre-existing diabetes	226	1.27	1.11-1.45	100	1.23	1.00-1.51
Chronic hypertension	212	1.29	1.12-1.49	94	1.25	1.01-1.54
Gestational diabetes	162	1.30	1.00-1.52	63	1.15	0.89-1.48
Preeclampsia	693	1.26	1.16-1.36	338	1.40	1.25-1.57
Hyperemesis gravidarum	189	1.39	1.20-1.61	79	1.28	1.02-1.60
Placenta prevail	207	1.32	1.15-1.52	84	1.19	0.96-1.48
Abruptio placentae	212	1.22	1.06-1.40	80	1.06	0.82-1.28
Antepartum bleeding	218	1.21	1.06-1.39	87	1.11	0.90-1.28
Intrapartum bleeding	362	1.28	1.16-1.44	188	1.42	1.22-1.65
Postpartum bleeding	702	1.11	1.02-1.20	298	1.06	0.94-1.19
Delivery induction	1627	1.30	1.23-1.37	739	1.30	1.21-1.42
Caesarean section	2573	1.37	1.31-1.43	1163	1.35	1.26-1.45

There is thus an excess both of pre-existing and pregnancy morbidity, of the same magnitude after early and later exposure. Both the use of delivery induction and caesarean section is significantly increased with 30-40%.

OUTCOME AFTER MATERNAL USE OF ANTIDEPRESSANTS

Infant Sex

After early use of antidepressants, there were 5 957 male and 5 361 female infants (four with unknown sex) born, sex ratio 1.11 (95% CI 1.07-1.15). After later use, there were 2 606 male and 2 396 female infants (one with unknown sex) born, sex ratio 1.09 (95% CI 1.03-1.15). The former sex ratio is thus somewhat high (normal sex ratio 1.06). It is similar after exposure to tricyclic drugs, SSRI or SNRI drugs.

Multiple Births

After early exposure to antidepressants, there were 141 twin deliveries, OR =0.81 (95% CI 0.68-0.95) and after later exposure there were 62 twin deliveries, OR = 0.82 (95% CI 0.63-1.06). The OR after exposure to TCA was 1.03 (95% CI 0.70-1.50), after SSRI OR = 0.79 (95% CI 0.65-0.96) and after SNRI 0.58 (95% CI 0.31-1.07). There is thus a low twinning rate after SSRI and perhaps after SNRI but not after TCA.

Table 52.5. Pregnancy duration and infant birth weight at maternal use of antidepressants

Variable studied	Drug use in early pregnancy			Drug use later in pregnancy		
	Number	OR	95% CI	Number	OR	95% CI
<37 weeks	832	1.42	1.32-1.53	400	1.60	1.45-1.78
<2500g	476	1.17	1.06-1.29	210	1.23	1.07-1.42
≥4500g	450	1.02	0.93-1.13	175	0.89	0.76-1.04
SGA	283	0.96	0.85-1.09	133	1.08	0.90-1.29
LGA	736	1.16	1.07-1.25	325	1.12	0.99-1.25

There is an increased risk for preterm birth and low birth weight but not for SGA. The OR for preterm birth is higher after later exposure to TCA (2.38, 95% CI 1.89-2.99) than after exposure to SSRI (1.47, 95% CI 1.30-1.66) with the OR intermediate after exposure to SNRI (1.93, 95% CI 1.41-2.63).There are no differences between drug groups with respect to SGA or LGA.

Table 52.6. Infant mortality after maternal use of antidepressants

Variable studied	Drug use in early pregnancy			Drug use later in pregnancy		
	Number	OR	95% CI	Number	OR	95% CI
Stillbirth	41	0.90	0.66-1.23	20	1.11	0.71-1.73
Early neonatal death	14	0.76	0.44-1.29	5	0.67	0.22-1.56#

#observed over expected number with exact Poisson 95% confidence interval

There is thus no increased risk for perinatal mortality.

Table 52.7. Neonatal diagnoses after maternal use of antidepressants

Diagnosis	Drug use in early pregnancy			Drug use later in pregnancy		
	Number	OR	95% CI	Number	OR	95% CI
Hypoglycaemia	584	1.33	1.22-1.45	291	1.47	1.30-1.66
Respiratory diagnoses	793	1.40	1.30-1.51	398	1.69	1.52-1.88
Low Apgar score	332	1.49	1.33-1.66	170	1.83	1.57-2.13
CNS diagnoses	120	1.49	1.24-1.71	69	1.83	1.44-2.33
Jaundice	558	1.14	1.05-1.25	273	1.24	1.09-1.40

All studied neonatal diagnoses thus occur more often than expected and with higher risk estimates after later exposure than after early exposure.

There were differences in risk estimates according to which antidepressant category had been used. Risk estimates are consistently higher for TCA than for SSRI while for SNRI the confidence intervals are relatively wide due to small numbers (Table 52.8).

Table 52.8. Risk estimates for neonatal diagnoses after maternal use of antidepressants in late pregnancy

Outcome	TCA		SSRI		SNRI	
	OR	95% CI	OR	95% CI	OR	95% CI
Hypoglycaemia	1.65	1.23-2.22	1.18	1.02-1.38	1.37	1.06-1.78
Respiratory diagnoses	2.37	1.87-3.00	1.42	1.25-1.61	1.39	0.95-2.02
Low Apgar score	1.83	1.23-2.74	1.35	1.11-1.66	1.38	0.71-2.41
CNS-diagnosis	3.20	1.86-5.13#	1.59	1.19-2.13	1.79	0.66-3.89#
Jaundice	1.51	1.11-2.05	1.11	1.01-1.35	1.47	1.01-2.15

#observed over expected number with exact Poisson 95% confidence interval.

There is thus a slight excess of relatively severe malformations but the only specific malformation which occurs more often than expected is hypospadias.

Table 52.9. Congenital malformations in infants whose mothers had used antidepressants in early pregnancy

Congenital malformation	Number	OR	95% CI
All malformation	519	0.97	0.88-1.06
Relatively severe malformation	408	1.12	1.01-1.24
Chromosome anomalies	22	0.84	0.54-1.29
Without chromosome anomalies			
Any CNS malformation	10	0.82	0.44-1.55
Eye malformations	10	1.05	0.50-1.93#
Ear malformations	22	0.90	0.59-1.38
Orofacial clefts	20	0.99	0.63-1.53
Any cardiovascular defect	144	1.16	0.98-1.37
VSD and/or ASD	78	1.15	0.92-1.45
Unspecified cardiac defects	9	0.88	0.45-1.70
Small bowel atresia	3	0.98	0.20-2.86#
Anal atresia	6	1.20	0.44-2.61#
Pylorostensois	14	1.52	0.83-2.55#
Hypospadias	45	1.40	1.04-1.88
Severe kidney malformations	11	1.56	0.78-2.79#
Pes equinovarus	24	1.31	0.86-1.99
Polydacytly/syndactyly	18	0.82	0.51-1.31
Limb reduction defects	3	0.47	0.10-1.38#
Hip (sub)luxation, unstable hip	28	0.41	0.28-0.59
Body wall defects	5	1.64	0.53-3.83#
Diaphragmatic hernia	2	0.72	0.09-2.59#
Craniostenosis	10	1.45	0.69-2.66#

#observed over expected number with exact Poisson 95% confidence interval.

Table 52.10. Relatively severe malformations and cardiovascular defects according to antidepressant drug used

Drug (group)	"Relatively severe" malformation			Cardiovascular defect		
	Number	OR/RR	95% CI	Number	OR/RR	95%CI
TCA	74	1.38	1.09-1.75	29	1.67	1.15-2.44
Clomipramine	60	1.52	1.17-1.98	26	2.02	1.36-3.01
Amitryptiline	12	1.01	0.56-1.82	3	0.80	0.17-2.24#
SSRI	310	1.10	0.98-1.24	101	1.05	0.86-1.88
Fluoxetine	47	1.16	0.86-1.55	17	1.22	0.76-1.97
Citalopram	124	1.11	0.92-1.33	34	0.90	0.64-1.27
Paroxetine	45	1.20	0.82-1.63	22	1.72	1.12-2.65
Setraline	91	1.05	0.85-1.30	25	0.82	0.55-1.23
SNRI	33	0.91	0.64-1.30	13	1.53	0.82-2.62
Mirtazapine	6	0.85	0.31-1.85#	3	1.15	0.24-3.37#
Venlafaxine	26	1.11	0.74-1.65	13	1.53	0.82-2.67#

#observed over expected number with exact Poisson 95% confidence interval.

Only clomipramine shows a significant increase in the risk for a "relatively severe" malformation. This may be a TCA-specific effect but is not seen for amitryptiline but the confidence interval for that estimate is relatively wide. Both clomipramine and paroxetine show statistically significant risk estimates for any cardiovascular defect. For fluoxetine and for SNRI drugs, an increased odds ratio is seen but they are far from statistically significant.

When the risk for a VSD and/or ASD is analyzed for clomipramine and paroxetine, slightly higher odds ratios are obtained than for any cardiovascular defect. For clomipramine the OR is 2.22 (95% CI 1.21-3.72) and for paroxetine 1.81 (95% CI 1.17-2.82). After removal from the analysis of infants whose mothers had also used drugs for hypertension, anticonvulsants, systemic corticosteroids, thyroid drugs, and drugs for rhinitis (all drugs which were used in excess and which may affect the risk for a cardiac defect) the odds ratios increased slightly to 2.31 and 1.94, respectively.

The risk increase for hypospadias is slightly higher for TCA than for SSRI and SNRI but these differences may be random. There were nine cases of hypospadias among 1 588 infants exposed to TCA, 35 among 8821 exposed to SSRI, and four among 1 133 exposed to SNRI. These rate do not differ significantly (p=0.59).

Summary

Maternal use of antidepressants is associated with an increased risk for pregnancy and neonatal complications, especially after use in late pregnancy. Effects of tricyclic antidepressants and notably clomipramine appear stronger than effects of SSRI. The perinatal death risk seems not to be increased. In general, antidepressants appear not to be associated with teratogenesis but when specific drugs and specific malformations are analyzed, some effects appear. Clomipramine increases the risk for any relatively severe malformation and specifically for cardiovascular defects. No certain general effect is seen for SSRI but among the four SSRIs studied, paroxetine showed a significant effect on cardiovascular defects. The cardiac defects seen are to a large extent VSD or ASD. There is an increased risk for hypospadias, apparently independent of the antidepressant used. – An interesting note is the significantly low occurrence of twin deliveries after maternal use of SSRI and perhaps SNRI but not TCA. This observation has not been supported by independent studies and the mechanism behind it is unknown.

References

[1] Pastuszak A, Schick-Boschetto B, Zuber C, Feldkamp M, Pinelli M, Sihn S, Donnenfeld A, McCormack M, Leen-Mitchell M, Woodland C, Gardner A, Hom M, Koren G. Pregnancy outcome following first-trimester exposure to fluoxetine (Prozac). *JAMA* 1993; 269: 2246-2248.

[2] McElhatton PR, Gaarbis HM, Eléfant E, Vial T, Bellemin B, Mastroiacovo P, Arnon J, Rodrígues-Pinilla E, Schaefer C, Pexieder T, Merlob P, dal Verme S. The outcome of pregnancy in 689 women exposed to therapeutic doses of antidepressants. A collaborative study of the European Network of Teratology Information Services (ENTIS). *Reprod Toxicol* 1996; 10: 285-294.

[3] Simon GE, Cunningham ML, Davis RL. Outcomes of prenatal antidepressant exposure. *Am J Psychiatry* 2002; 159: 2055-2061.

[4] Oberlander TF, Warburton W, Misri S, Aghajanian J, Herzman C. Neonatal outcomes after prenatal exposure to selective seotonin reuptake inhibitor antidepressants and maternal depression using population-based linked health data. *Arch Gen Psychiatry* 2006; 63: 898-906.

[5] Louik C, Lin AE, Werler MM, Hernández-Dáz S, Mitchell A. First-trimester use of selective serotonin-reuptake inhibitors and the risk of birth defects. *New Engl J Med* 2007; 356: 2675-2683.

[6] Alwan S, Reefhuis J, Rasmussen SA, Olney RS, Friedman JM for the National Birth Defets Prevention Study. Use of selective serotonin-reuptake inhibitors in pregnancy and the risk of birth defecs. *New Engl J Med* 2007; 356: 2684-2692.

[7] Ericson A, Källén B, Wiholm B-E. Delivery outcome after the use of antidepressants in early pregnancy. *Eur J Clin Pharmacol* 1999; 55: 503-508.

[8] Källén B, Otterblad Olausson P. Maternal use of selective serotonin re-uptake inhibitors in early pregnancy and infant congenital malformations. *Birth Def Res (A)* 2007; 79: 301-308.

[9] Källén B. The safety of antidepressant drugs during pregnancy. *Exper Opin Drug Saf* 2007; 6: 357-370-

[10] Pearlstein T. Perinatal depression: treatment options and dilemmas. *J Psychiatry Neurosci* 2008; 33: 302-318.

[11] Costei AM, Kozer E, Ho T, Ito S, Koren G. Perinatal outcome following third trimester exposure to paroxetiine. *Arch Pediatr Adolesc Med* 2002; 156: 1129-1132.

[12] Källén B. Neonate charcteristics after maternal use of antidepressants in late pregnancy. *Arch Pediatr Adolesc Med* 2004; 158: 312-316.

[13] Chambers CD, Hernandez-Diaz S, van Marter LJ, Werler MM, Louik C, Jones KL, Mitchell AA. Selective serotonin-reuptake inhibitors and risk of persistent pulmonary hypertension of the newborn. *New Engl J Med* 2006; 354: 579-587.

[14] Källén B, Otterlad Olausson P. Maternal use of selective serotonin re-uptake inhibitors and persistent pulmonary hypertension of the newborn. *Pharmacoepid Drug Safety* 2008; 17: 801-806.

[15] Andrade SE, McPhillips H, Loren D, Raebel MA, Lane K, Livinston J, Boudreau SM,Smith DH, Davis RL, Willy ME, Platt R. Antidepressant medication use and risk of persistent pulmonary hypertension of the newborn. *Pharacoepid Drug Safety* 2009; 18: 246-252.

[16] Toh S, Mitchell AA, Louik C, Werler MM, Chambers CD, Hernánderz-Díaz S. Selective serotonin reuptake inhibitor used and risk of gestational hypertension. *Am J Psychiatry Epub* 2009. DOI 10.1176/appi.ajp.2008.08060817.

[17] Dayan J, Creveuil C, Marks MN, Conroy S, Herlicoviez M, Dreyfus M, Tordjman S. Prenatal depression, prenatal anxiety, and spontaneous preterm birth: a prospective cohort study among women with early and regular care. *Psychosom Med* 2006; 68: 938-946.

[18] Cole JA, Ephross SA, Cosmatos IS, Walker AM. Paroxetine in the first trimester and the prevalence of congenital malformations. *Pharmacoepid Drug Safety* 2007; 16: 1075-1085.

[19] Källén B, Otterblad Olausson P. Antidepressant drugs during pregnancy and infant congenital heart defect. *(Letter) Reprod Toxicol* 2006; 21: 221-222.

[20] Davis RL, Rubanowice D, McPhillips H, Raebel MA, Andrade SA, Smith D, Yood MU, Platt R. For the HMO Research Network Center for Education in Therapeutics. Risks of congenital malformations and perinatal events among infants exposed to antidepressant medications during pregnancy, *Pharmacoepidem Drug Safety* 2007; 16: 1086-1094.

[21] Oberlander TF, Reebye P, Misri S, Papsdorf M, Kim J, Grunau RE. Externalizing and attentional behaviors in children of depressed mothers treated with a selective

reuptake inhibitor antidepressant during pregnancy. *Arch Pediatr Adolesc Med* 2007; 161: 22-29.

Chapter 53

OTHER DRUGS AFFECTING THE NERVOUS SYSTEM

Only small studies exist to clarify possible harmful effects of drugs affecting the nervous system, many of which are used in connexion with maternal dependency which in itself has a negative effect on the offspring. There are mounting evidence that the use of nicotine as an antismoking drug could carry a risk for the infant and it may be wise to avoid it during pregnancy. If nicotine has been used, the effects are uncertain and at most moderate and do not motivate a termination of pregnancy. Other methods of reduction of smoking may be more preferable.

This group of drugs is heterogeneous and has different uses. One group is used at myasthenia gravis, one at vertigo, and one for treating dependencies. Each group is small.

Myasthenia gravis is a serious condition during pregnancy and antibodies transferred to the foetus can affect its movement and lead to paralysis and limb malpositions, including arthrogryposis [1]. Supportive treatment with anticholinesterases and similar drugs can be used to reduce clinical symptoms – their effect on the embryo or foetus is little studied.

The hazards associated with maternal smoking during pregnancy are well known even if the actual component(s) which cause the damage are not fully clarified. One way to smoking cessation is the use of pure nicotine. Its effectiveness in pregnancy has been much debated but relatively little is known on possible ill effects on the newborn. In one study an increased risk for preterm birth and low birth weight was found, larger than those after maternal smoking [2]. Another study found an increased risk for stillbirths [3], and a third an increased risk for congenital malformations, notably "musculoskeletal malformations" [4]. A risk for neurobehavioral disturbances has also been proposed [5].

Maternal alcoholism is a serious hazard for the infant. A few early case reports suggested that disulfiram could have a teratogenic effect but the close association with alcoholism makes conclusions uncertain.

Maternal use and misuse of opioids is associated with withdrawal symptoms in the infant, with preterm birth and low birth weight but not with structural malformations [6] and methadone maintenance during pregnancy is regarded as safe [7].

Table 53.1. Number of women identified using other drugs affecting the nervous system

Total	620
Reported use in early pregnancy	491
Got prescription later in pregnancy	190
Both early and later use	61

Type of drug	ATC code	Early use	Later use
Parasympathomimetic drugs			
Anticholinesterases	N07AA	74	27
Neostigmine	N07AA01	1	1
Pyridostigmine	N07AA02	72	26
Ambenonium	N07AA30	2	4
Choline esters	N07AB	1	0
Carbachol	N07AB01	1	0
Other parasympathomimetics	N07AX	3	1
Pilocarpine	N07AX01	3	1
Antismoking agents	N07BA	187	116
Nicotine	N07BA01	187	116
Drugs for alcohol dependence	N07BB	54	11
Disulfiram	N07BB01	51	10
Acamprosate	N07BB03	3	1
Drugs for opioid dependence	N07BC	44	22
Buprenorphine	N07BC01	5	4
Methadone	N07BC02	39	18
Drugs for vertigo	N07CA	126	4
Cinnarizine	N07CA02	126	4
Other	N07XX	2	0
Tirilazol	N07XX01	1	0
Riluzol	N07XX02	1	0

None of the women used two or more drugs belonging to different groups.

CHARACTERISTICS OF WOMEN USING DRUGS AFFECTING THE NERVOUS SYSTEM

The heterogeneity between drugs belonging to this group and the low number in each subgroup make analysis of maternal characteristics imprecise. Some features can, howere, be pointed out.

The use of anticholinesterases, choline esters, and other parasympathicomimetics shows no association with maternal age, parity, smoking, number of previous miscarriages, or BMI. There is, however, an association with subfertility: the OR for having a period of unwanted childlessness is 2.09 (95% CI 1.06-4.16), based on 10 among the 74 women.

The use of nicotine is associated with an age of 35 or more (OR = 1.64, 95% CI 1.17-2.28), first parity (OR = 2.12, 95% CI 1.59-2.83), smoking (OR = 2.36, 95% CI 1.22-4.55), and previous miscarriage (OR = 1.43, 95% CI 1.03-2.00), but shows no association with BMI or subfertility.

Among women using cinnarizine for vertigo, no significant deviations in maternal characteristics were seen.

Women who used drugs for alcohol or opioid dependence were older than expected: the OR for being 35 or more was 1.92 (95% CI 1.23-3.00), were more often than expected of first parity (OR = 1.72, 95% CI 1.10-2.69), smoked more than expected (OR = 8.76, 95% CI 4.56-16.9) but had a normal BMI distribution and no increase in earlier miscarriages or subfertility.

Table 53.2. Concomittant drug use (early pregnancy)

Drug group	Number	OR/RR	95% CI
Parasympathomimetic drugs			
Antidepressants	33	19.5	12.0-24.5#
Antiasthmatics	5	2.07	0.67-4.82#
Antismoking drugs			
Drugs for stomach ulcer and reflux	5	2.69	0.87-6.27#
Multivitamins	14	1.62	0.79-2.74#
Folic acid	6	0.71	0.26-1.55#
Antibiotics	5	0.87	0.28-2.03#
NSAIDs	7	1.59	0.64-3.28#
Minor analgesics	30	2.00	1.36-2.95
Sedatives, hypnotics	4	3.23	0.86-8.26#
Antidepressants	7	2.36	0.95-4.86#
Drugs for rhinitis	9	3.08	1.41-5.84#
Antiasthmatics	5	0.79	0.26-1.84#
Antihistamines	12	1.13	0.63-2.02
Drugs for alcohol or opioid dependence			
Drugs for stomach ulcer and reflux	4	3.67	1.00-9.40#
Folic acid	6	1.58	0.58-3.45#
Opioids	40	16.5	11.8-22.4#
Minor analgesics	8	0.83	0.36-1.64#
Sedatives, hypnotics	15	8.43	4.72-13.9#
Antidepressants	20	6.69	4.09-10.3#
Antiasthmatics	14	3.20	1.75-5.38#
Antihistamines	9	1.67	0.76-3.18#
Drugs for vertigo (antihistamine)			
NSAIDs	6	4.05	1.49-8.82#
Minor analgesics	25	3.02	1.96-4.49#
Drugs for rhinitis	5	3.04	0-99-7.11#
Antihistamines for NVP	22	4.71	2.95-7.13#

#observed over expected number with exact Poisson 95% confidence interval.

There are thus strong associations between parasympathomimetic drugs (mainly used at myasthenia gravis) and antidepressants, between anti-smoking drugs and minor analgesics and drugs for rhinitis, between drugs for alcohol or opioid dependency and opioids, psychoactive drugs, and antiasthmatics, and between drugs for vertigo and analgesics and antihistamines used for NVP.

Due to low number of exposures for specific subgroups, most matrnal diagnoses during pregnancy occurred so seldom that analysis was relatively useless. If the whole group of drugs was analyzed together, the only statitically significant deviation was in the rate of caesarean sections: OR = 1.20 (95% CI 1.04-1.62). Divided according to subgroup, two showed significantly increased risks for caesarean section: parasympathomimetics (OR = 1.83, 85% CI 1.10-3.05) and drugs used for opioid dependency (OR = 2.22, 95% CI 1.26-4.12), for the remaining groups the OR varied between 1.07 and 1.17, none of them statistically significant.

Outcome after Maternal use of Drugs Affecting the Nervous System

Infant Sex

Numbers were not large enough to show deviations in sex distribution. For the total group, the sex ratio (based on 250 male and 248 female infants) was 1.01 (95% CI 0.85-1.20).

Multiple Births

Among all deliveries, there were seven twin deliveries which is close to the expected number (7.7).

Table 53.3. Pregnancy duration and infant birth weight at maternal use of drugs affecting the nervous system

Variable studied	Drug use in early pregnancy			Drug use later in pregnancy		
	Number	OR/RR	95% CI	Number	OR/RR	95% CI
<37 weeks	31	1.17	0.82-1.69	13	1.28	0.73-2.24
<2500g	17	0.88	0.54-1.43	12	1.44	0.74-2.51
≥4500g	21	1.14	0.73-1.78	5	0.75	0.24-1.75#
SGA	13	0.92	0.53-1.62	11	1.81	0.90-3.24#
LGA	33	1.30	0.91-1.87	7	0.67	0.31-1.48

#observed over expected number with exact Poisson 95% confidence interval.

Table 53.4. Neonatal diagnoses after maternal use of drugs affecting the nervous system

Diagnosis	Drug use in early pregnancy			Drug use later in pregnancy		
	Number	OR/RR	95% CI	Number	OR/RR	95% CI
All drugs						
Hypoglycaemia	27	1.42	0.96-2.08	13	1.71	0.91-2.93#
Respiratory diagnoses	32	1.20	0.84-1.72	16	1.74	1.00-2.84#
Low Apgar score	11	1.03	0.57-1.87	5	1.37	0.44-3.20#
CNS diagnoses	6	1.90	0.70-4.15#	2	1.49	0.18-5.39#
Jaundice	23	1.10	0.72-1.67	6	0.75	0.27-1.62#
Drugs for opioid dependence						
Hypoglycaemia	7	3.26	1.31-6.71#			
Respiratory diagnoses	9	3.73	1.71-7.09#			
Low Apgar score	4	4.65	1.27-11.9#			
CNS diagnoses	4	14.8	4.04-37.9#			
Jaundice	3	1.85	0.38-5.41#			

#observed over expected number with exact Poisson 95% confidence interval.

There is thus no significant deviations in these variables. This is also true for the different subgroups but then numbers are low. There were no perinatal deaths among the exposed infants.

In the total group, the only marginally significant effect was on respiratory diagnoses after later exposure. When the different subgroups were studied no deviations were seen except for drugs used at opioid dependence. Numbers are low but formal statistical significance is reached for four of the diagnoses.

Table 53.5. Congenital malformations in infants whose mothers had used drugs in erly pregnancy affecting the nervous system

Congenital malformation	Number	OR	95% CI
All drugs			
All malformations	28	1.15	0.78-1.71
Relatively severe malformation	20	1.20	0.76-2.90

Table 53.6 specifies the infants with relatively severe malformations.

Table 53.6. Infants with relatively severe malformations after maternal use of drugs affecting the nervous system

Drug group and malformation	Specific drug	Other drugs
Parasympathomimetic drugs		
Choanal atresia	pilocarpine	celecoxib, citalopram, hydroxychloroquine
VSD	pyridostigmin	loratadine, hydroxyzine
VSD+CoA+hypospadias	pyridostigmin	
Pes calcaneovalgus	pyridostigmin	
Antismoking drugs		
TGV+ atresia of pulmonary artery	nicotine	Xylomatazoline
VSD	nicotine	phenylpropanolamine
VSD	nicotine	citalopram, terfenadine
ASD	nicotine	ASA, lactulose
ASD+pulmonary and aortic stenosis	nicotine	-
Hand redution and syndactyly	nicotine	-
Polydactyly	nicotine	azithromycine, salbutamol
Hydronephrosis	nicotine	-
Hydronephrosis	nicotine	multivitamiins, ASA
Drugs for alcohol dependency		
Congenital ptosis	disulfiram	Paracetamol
Pulmonary malformation	disulfiram	risperidon, budesonide, terbutalin
Down syndrome	acamprosate	thyroxine, diazepam, escitalopram
Drugs for vertigo		
Unspecified facial defecct	cinnerazine	-
Malrotation of the gut	cinnerazine	-
Unspecifed cardiac defect	cinnerazine	-
Chromosomal deletion	cinnerazine	-

After use of nicotine as an antismoking agent, there are thus nine malformed infants among 188 exposed infants: RR = 1.44 (95% CI 0.54-5.07). Five of these had cardiovascular defects (RR = 2.27, 95% CI 0.74-5.30), an increased risk which obviously can be random. For the other groups there are no signs of a teratogenic risk but numbers are small.

Summary

Clear effects on neonatal symptoms were present only after maternal use of drugs for opioid dependency. No certain effects on congenital malformations could be seen, but infants born after maternal use of nicotine as an antismoking drug had a tendency to have an increased rate of malformations, notably cardiovascular defects, but numbers were small and confidence intervals wide.

References

[1] Polizzi A, Huson SM, Vincent A. Teratogen update: maternal myasthenia gravis as a cause of congenital arthrogryposis. *Teratology* 2000; 62: 332.341.

[2] Gaither KH, Brunner Huber LR, Thomson ME, Huet-Hudson YM. Does the use of nicotine replacement therapy during pregnancy affect pregnancy outcomes? *Matern Child Health J E-publ* 2008. DOI 10.1007/s10995-008-0361-1.

[3] Strandberg-Larsen K, Tinggaard M, Nybo Andersen A-M, Olsen J, Grønbaek M. Use of nicotine replacement therapy during pregnancy and stillbirth: a cohort study. *BJOG* 2008; E-publ 2008: DOI10.1111/j.1471-0528.01867x.

[4] Morales-Suárez-Varela MM, Bille C, Christensen K, Olsen J. Smoking habits, nicotine use, and congenital malformations. *Obstet Gynecol* 2006; 107: 51-57.

[5] Pauly JR, Slotkin TA. Maternal tobacco smoking, nicotine replacement and neurobehavioural development. *Acta Paediatrica* 2008; 97: 1331-1337.

[6] Rayburn WF, Bogenschutz MP. Pharmacotherapy for pregnant women with addictions. *Amer J Obst Gynecol* 2004; 191: 1885-1897.

[7] McCarthy JJ, Leamon MH, Stenson G, Biles LA. Outcomes of neonates conceived on methadone maintenance therapy. *J Subst Abuse Treatm* 2008; 35: 202-206.

Chapter 54

ANTIMALARIALS

Use of antimalarial drugs as malaria prophylaxis is important for women living in or travelling to countries with endemic malaria. There is no certain ill effects on the embryo or foetus. The choice of antimalarial drug should mainly be decided according to the pattern of plasmoidum resistence but if pyrimethamine can be avoided, this is recommended. High doses of aminoquinolines at rheumatic diseases or SLE appears to carry no major risk for foetal damage. If exposure has occurred in early pregnancy, there is no reason to discuss a termination of the pregnancy.

Antimalarials are used in Sweden as prophylactic treatment during travel in countries with malaria, and some of them also in the treatment of rheumatoid arthritis or SLE.

Use of chloroquine has not been associated with teratogenicity. Use of hydrocychloroquine for connective tissue diseases during pregnancy was not associated with an increased risk for infant congenital malformations [1] but this study was based on only 177 livebirths, three of them malformed. Previous studies were still smaller, and so was a later study [2] where a high rate of preterm births was found, perhaps due to underlying maternal disease. A scare for ototoxicity exists after the use of quinine or chloroquine but this seems at least not to be a common effect even though many case descriptions are available [3]. When used at lower doses for malaria prophylaxis, no risks seem to exist with these drugs.

Mefloquine during pregnancy has been studied repeatedly. An increased risk for stillbirth has been described [4]. A post-marketing study performed by the producer found no evidence for teratogenicity. Among 476 infants born after first trimester exposure, there were 24 with congenital malformations (5%) [5].

The general opinion [6,7] is that antimalarial drugs in pregnancy can be used for malaria prophylaxis without risk and is definitely to be recommended if the pregnant woman will be exposed to malaria which is a very serious disease in pregnancy.

Pyrimethamine has a folic-acid antagonistic effect and it has been suggested that such drugs could be teratogenic even though the evidence is weak [8].

Table 54.1. Number of women identified using antimalarias

Total	772
Reported use in early pregnancy	698
Got prescription later in pregnancy	120
Both early and later use	46

Type of drug	ATC code	Early use	Later use
Aminoquinolines	P01BA	567	98
Chloroquine	P01BA01	405	51
Hydroxychloroquine	P01BA02	62	34
Mefloquine	P01BA05	105	13
Biguanides	P01BB	153	51
Proguanil	P01BB01	128	20
Proguanil+atovaquone	P01BB51	25	11
Quinine alkaloids	P01BC	13	2
Quinine	P01BC01	13	2
Diaminopyrimidines	P01BD	6	1
Pyrimethamine	P01BD01	3	0
Pyrimethamine+sulfadioxine	P01BD51	3	1
Unspecified antimalarials	P01B	67	2

The most common drug combination was an aminoquinoline and a biguanide (154 early and 31 later exposures). One of the former also had a diaminopyramidine drug. One early exposure was for a combination of an aminoquinoline and a quinine alkaloid, and two were for a combination of a biguanide and quinine.

Characteristics of Women using Antimalarial Drugs

Based on women reporting the drug in early pregnancy (n=698). Each variable is adjusted for all other variables and year of delivery. Comparison with all women who gave birth during the period and with information from the first antenatal care (n=967 742). The odds ratios for maternal age, parity, smoking in early pregnancy, number of previous miscarriages, BMI, subfertility, and country of birth are adjusted for all other variables (Table 54.2).

Some further maternal characteristics were analyzed, adjusting for year of delivery, maternal age, parity, smoking, and BMI (Table 54.3).

Women using antimalarials were thus older than the average and had fewer deliveries among women <25 years. They were much more often than expected of parity one while previous miscarriages or subfertility occurred less often than expected. They had more often than expected a high education.

The very strong association with corticosteroids is limited to aminoquinolines which are used at rheumatoid arthritis and SLE. This may also explain the association with NSAIDs. There is also a strong association with drugs used at immunological bowel disease, also that with aminoquinolines. An association with anticonvulsants is more difficult to understand but is based on only six cases.

The only statistically significant deviation is an increased risk for delivery induction. For many conditions, the odds ratio estimates are low.

Table 54.2. Characteristics of women using antimalarials in early pregnancy

Variable studied	Number	OR	95% CI
Maternal age			
<25 years	75	0.45	0.35-0.56
25-34 years	513	1.00	reference
≥35 years	110	1.23	0.99-1.52
Parity			
1	509	3.87	3.29-4.56
≥2	189	1.00	reference
Smoking			
Unknown	15		
No	626	1.00	reference
Yes	57	0.83	0.46-1.52
Previous miscarriage			
No	620	1.00	reference
Yes	78	0.58	0.46-0.73
BMI			
Unknown	64	-	-
<19.8	77	1.27	0.99-1.61
19.8-25.9	446	1.00	reference
≥26	111	0.68	0.55-0.84
Unwanted childlessness			
No	669	1.00	reference
Yes	29	0.38	0.27-0.55
Country of birth			
Unknown	13	1	-
Sweden	575	1.00	reference
Other Nordic country	16	1.00	0.61-1.65
Non-Nordic country	94	0.97	0.77-1.22

Table 54.3. Some further characteristics of women using antimalarials in early pregnancy

Variable studied	Number	OR	95% CI
Education (1996-2001,437 women with drugs, 526 695 in population)			
Unknown	9		
<12 years	24	0.87	0.55-1.37
12 years	163	1.00	reference
≥13 years	251	2.08	1.68-2.57
Family situation			
Unknown	19	-	
Co-habiting	632	1.00	reference
Living alone	21	1.15	0.71-1.84
Other family situation	19	1.48	0.87-2.52
Work outside home			
Unknown	96	-	
Full time	416	1.00	reference
Part time	77	0.63	0.48-0.82
None	102	1.02	0.78-1.32

Table 54.4. Concomitant drug use (early pregnancy)

Drug group	Number	OR/RR	95% CI
Drugs for stomach ulcer and reflux	9	1.50	0.69.2,85#
Drugs for inflammatory bowel disease	15	7.98	4.47-13.2#
Multivitamins	20	0.81	0.51-1.30
Folic acid	13	0.54	0.31-0.94
Oral contraceptives	7	3.07	1.23-6.33#
Progestogens	4	0.90	0.25-2.32#
Systemic corticosteroids	30	9.90	6.68-14.1#
Thyroid drugs	9	1.17	0.54-2.22#
Antibiotics	26	1.25	0.84-1.85
NSAIDs	41	3.30	2.44-4.47
Opioids	4	1.41	0.39-3.62#
Minor analgesics	41	0.72	0.53-0.99
Anticonvulsants	6	3.26	1.20-2.10#
Sedatives, hypnotics	8	2.74	1.18-5.40#
Antidepressants	9	1.16	0.53-2.20#
Drugs for rhinitis	9	0.87	0.45-1.68
Antiasthmatics	19	0.86	0.55-1.36
Antihistamines	35	0.86	0.62-1.21

#observed over expected number with exact Poisson 95% confidence interval.

Table 54.5. Some maternal diagnoses associated with the use of antimalarials

Diagnosis	Drug use in early pregnancy			Drug use later in pregnancy		
	Number	OR/RR	95% CI	Number	OR/RR	95% CI
Pre-existing diabetes	4	0.52	0.14-1.34#	2	1.23	0.15-4.43#
Chronic hypertension	5	0.74	0.24-1.72#	3	1.96	0.40-5.73#
Gestational diabetes	3	0.57	0.12-1.66#	2	1.85	0.22-6.69#
Preeclampsia	38	1.07	0.77-1.49	8	1.37	0.59-2.70#
Hyperemesis gravidarum	3	0.54	0.11-1.58#	2	1.59	0.19-5.73#
Placenta previa	4	0.62	0.17-1.59#	2	1.44	0.17-5.20#
Abruptio placentae	2	0.28	0.03-1.00#	2	1.29	0.16-4.66#
Antepartum bleeding	3	0.34	0.07-0.98#	2	1.20	0.15-4.35#
Intrapartum bleeding	9	0.70	0.36-1.35	2	0.68	0.08-2.49#
Postpartum bleeding	35	0.80	0.57-1.13	8	1.13	0.49-2.24#
Delivery induction	92	1.27	1.01-1.58	22	1.70	1.06-2.95
Caesarean section	114	0.96	0.79-1.18	27	1.28	0.83-1.97

#observed over expected number with exact Poisson 95% confidence interval.

Outcome after Maternal use of Antimalarials

Infant Sex

After early use, there were 350 male and 348 female infants born, sex ratio 1.03 (95% CI 0.89-1.19) and after later use there were 60 males and 60 females, sex ratio 1.00 (95% CI 0.70-1.44). The normal sex ratio (1.06) is thus contained within both confidence intervals.

Multiple Births

After early use of antimalarials, there were eight twin deliveries (OR = 0.76, 95% CI 0.38-1.52). After later exposure, there were no twin deliveries.

Table 54.6. Pregnancy duration and infant birth weight at maternal use of antimalarials

Variable studied	Drug use in early pregnancy			Drug use later in pregnancy		
	Number	OR/RR	95% CI	Number	OR/RR	95% CI
<37 weeks	33	0.88	0.62-1.25	10	1.61	0.77-2.96#
<2500g	26	1.03	0.70-1.53	6	1.46	0.53-3.17#
≥4500g	14	0.63	0.37-1.07	0	-	-
SGA	28	1.41	0.97-2.06	7	2.14	0.86-4.41#
LGA	19	0.74	0.47-1.18	2	0.34	0.04-1.22#

#observed over expected number with exact Poisson 95% confidence interval.

The only markedly increased odds ratio was for SGA but it did not reach statistical significance.

Table 54.7. Infant mortality after maternal use of antimalarials

Variable studied	Drug use in early pregnancy			Drug use later in pregnancy		
	Number	OR/RR	95% CI	Number	OR/RR	95% CI
Stillbirth	5	1.95	0.63-4.54#	2	4.31	0.52-15.6#
Early neonatal death	1	-	-	0	-	-

#observed over expected number with exact Poisson 95% confidence interval.

The increased stillbirth rate may well be random.

Table 54.8. Neonatal diagnoses after maternal use of antimalarials

Diagnosis	Drug use in early pregnancy			Drug use later in pregnancy		
	Number	OR/RR	95% CI	Number	OR/RR	95% CI
Hypoglycaemia	19	0.68	0.43-1.07	7	1.49	0.60-3.06#
Respiratory diagnoses	22	0.50	0.33-0.76	2	0.34	0.04-1.22#
Low Apgar score	8	0.45	0.23-0.89	0	-	-
CNS diagnoses	2	0.40	0.05-1.43#	0	-	-
Jaundice	20	0.61	0.40-0.95	5	0.93	0.30-2.18#

#observed over expected number with exact Poisson 95% confidence interval.

There are thus no signs of an increased neonatal morbidity, on the contrary some of the odds ratios are significantly lower than 1.

There were 22 infants with relatively severe malformations among 574 infants after exposure to aminoquinolines (OR = 1.13, 95% CI 0.74-1.73), five among 155 infants exposed to proguanil (RR = 0.92, 95% CI 0.30-2.14), and one among 14 infants exposed to quinine. None of the six infants exposed to pyrimethamine had a malformation diagnosis. One of the 67 infants exposed to an unspecified antimalarial had a malformation. Four of the malformed infants exposed to proguanil were also exposed to aminoquinolines. The malformations are specified in Table 54.10.

Table 54.9. Congenital malformations in infants whose mothers had used antimalarials in early pregnancy

Congenital malformation	Number	OR	95% CI
All malformation	32	0.87	0.61-1.24
Relatively severe malformation	25	1.03	0.69-1.53
Chromosome anomalies	2	1.40	0.17-5.05#
Without chromosome anomalies			
Any cardiovascular defect	10	1.31	0.63-2.40#

#observed over expected number with exact Poisson 95% confidence interval.

Table 54.10. Specification of malformations in infants whose mothers used antimalarials in early pregnancy

Drug group and malformation	Number
Amnioquinolines	
Choanal atresia	1
Tracheomalacia + unstable hip	1
Ventricular septum defect	2
Endocardial cushion defect	1
Aorta stenosis	1
Unspecified cardiac defect	1
Duplication and malposition of ureter	1
Hypospadias	1
Pes equinovarus	2
Pes calcaneovalgus	2
Polydactyly thumb	1
Arthrogryposis with pulmonary hypoplasia and pulmonary artery atresia	1
Diaphragmatic hernia + hypospadias	1
Syndrome with cleft palate and laryngeal malformation	1
Down syndrome	1
Trisomy 13	1
Amnioquinoline with proguanil	
Ventricular septum defect	1
Pes equinovarus	1
Polydactyly	1
Proguanil	
Congenital cardiac block	1
Quinine	
Ventricular septum defect	1

There are no signs of a teratogenic effect even though the number of exposed infants is low and a moderate increase can well be hidden.

Summary

In the present material, no ill effects were seen from maternal use of antimalarials. It should be stressed that a drug which has been suspected of teratogenicity because of its anti-folic acid effect, pyrimethamine, was rarely used and only six exposed infants were included in the study.

REFERENCES

[1] Costedoat-Chalumeau N, Amoura Z, Duhaut P. Huong DLT, Sebbough D, Wechslaer B, Vauthier D, Denjoy I, Lupoglazoff J-M, Piette J-C. Safety of hydroxychloroquine in pregnant patients with connective tissue diseases. *Arthritis Rheumatism* 2003; 48: 3207-3211.

[2] Motta M, Tincani A, Faden D, Zinzini E, Lojacono A, Marchesi A, Frassi M, Biasini C, Zatti S, Chirico G. Follow-up of infants exposed to hydroxychloroquine given to mothers during pregnancy and lactation. *J Perinatol* 2005; 25: 86-89.

[3] Borba EF, Turrini-Filho JR, Kuruma KA, Bertola C, Pedalini ME, Lorenzi MC, Bonfá E. Chloroquine gestational use in systemic lupus erythematosus: assessing the risk of child ototoxicity by pure tone audiometry. *Lupus* 2004; 13: 223-227.

[4] Nosten F, Vincenti M, Simpson J, Yei P, Thwai KL, de Vries A, Chongsuphajaisiddhi T, White NJ. The effects of mefloquine treatment in pregnancy. *Clin Infect Dis* 1999; 28: 808-815.

[5] Vanhauwere B, Maradit H, Kerr L. Post-marketing surveillance of prophylactic mefloquine (Lariam®) use in pregnancy. *Am J Trop Med* 1998; 58: 17-21.

[6] Phillips-Howard PA, Steffen R, Kerr L, Vanhauwere B, Schildknecht J, Fuchs E, Edwards R. Safety of mefloquine and other antimalarial agents in the first trimester of pregnancy. *J Travel Med* 1998; 5: 121-126.

[7] Newman RD, Parise ME, Slutsker L, Nahlen B, Steketee RW. Safety, efficacy and determinants of effectiveness of antimalarial drugs during pregnancy: implications for prevention programmes in Plasmodium falciparum-endemic sub-Saharan Africa. *Trop Med Int Health* 2003; 8: 488-56.

[8] Hernandez-Diaz S, Werler MM, Walker AM, Mitchell AA. Folic acid antagonists during pregnancy and the risk of birth defects. *N Engl J Med* 2000; 343: 1608-1614.

Chapter 55

ANTHELMINTICS

Anthelmintic treatment of pregnant women in areas with endemic infections can be of benefit but if possible should first trimester treatment be avoided. Treatment of threadworm appears to be without any risk also during the first trimester. There are no signs of teratogenicity of mebendazole or pyrvinium when used as single dose therapies but the available evidence is based on limited data. There is no reason to discuss a termination of the pregnancy if exposure has occurred in early pregnancy.

Anthelmintic use in Sweden is dominated by threadworm therapy, usually consisting of one treatment only and perhaps easily forgotten because reporting and recording of these drugs are low and probably very incomplete.

One paper suggested a possible teratogenic effect of mebendazole but the slightly increased risk was not statistically significant [1]. Two other studies, also of small size, have not been able to find signs of teratogenicity of this drug [2,3]. Few data exist on the use of pyrvinium during pregnancy. The use of anthelmintics in areas with significant helmintic problems offers many advantages for the pregnant woman but first trimester exposures should be avoided [4,5].

Table 55.1. Number of women identified using anthelmintics

Total	579
Reported use in early pregnancy	458
Got prescription later in pregnancy	130
Both early and later use	9

Type of drug	ATC code	Early use	Later use
Antinematodal agents	P02C	441	121
Mebendazole	P02CA01	116	12
Pyrvinium	P02CX01	327	111
Anticetodals	P02D	0	1
Niclosamide	P02DA01	0	1
Unspecified	P02	17	8

Two women reported both mebendazole and pyrvinium in early pregnancy and later in pregnancy.

CHARACTERISTICS OF WOMEN USING ANTHELMINTICS

Based on women reporting the drug in early pregnancy (n=457, one missing maternal age). Each variable is adjusted for all other variables and year of delivery. Comparison with all women who gave birth during the period and with information from the first antenatal care (n=967 742) (Table 55.2).

Table 55.2. Characteristics of women using anthelmintics in early pregnancy

Variable studied	Number	OR	95% CI
Maternal age			
<25 years	36	0.78	0.54-1.12
25-34 years	314	1.00	reference
≥35 years	107	0.95	0.75-1.19
Parity			
1	83	0.30	0.24-0.39
≥2	374	1.00	reference
Smoking			
Unknown	9	-	-
No	411	1.00	reference
Yes	37	0.68	0.37-1.26
Previous miscarriage			
No	358	1.00	reference
Yes	99	0.84	0.67-1.05
BMI			
Unknown	44	-	-
<19.8	28	0.87	0.67-1.05
19.8-25.9	278	1.00	reference
≥26	107	0.82	0.66-1.03
Unwanted childlessness			
No	429	1.00	reference
Yes	28	1.24	0.84-1.83
Country of birth			
Unknown	1	-	-
Sweden	396	1.00	reference
Other Nordic country	13	1.02	0.58-1.77
Non-Nordic country	47	0.58	0.43-0.78

Some further maternal characteristics were analyzed, adjusting for year of delivery, maternal age, parity, smoking, and BMI (Table 55.3).

The most obvious deviation in the characteristics of women using anthelmintics is the increased usage in parity 2 or higher – a reasonable explanation is infection from previous children. There is a weak effect of education with an increased use at higher education, a lower use among women born outside the Nordic countries and among women who do not work outside home.

The only significantly increased use concerns minor analgesics.

Table 55.3. Some further characteristics of women using anthelmintics in early pregnancy

Variable studied	Number	OR	95% CI
Education (1996-2001, 289 women with drugs, 526 695 in population)			
Unknown	6	-	-
<12 years	22	0.64	0.41-1.01
12 years	140	1.00	reference
≥13 years	121	1.32	1.03-1.71
Family situation			
Unknown	4	-	-
Co-habiting	430	1.00	reference
Living alone	12	0.98	0.53-1.82
Other family situation	6	0.75	0.32-1.79
Work outside home			
Unknown	61	-	-
Full time	192	1.00	reference
Part time	140	0.96	0.76-1.22
None	59	0.70	0.50-0.98

Table 55.4. Concomitant drug use (early pregnancy)

Drug group	Number	OR/RR	95% CI
Multivitamins	12	0.64	0.42-0.98
Folic acid	14	0.88	0.52-1.48
Thyroid drugs	6	0.96	0.35-2.10#
Antibiotics	20	1.32	0.84-2.07
Naiads	10	1.30	0.62-2.38#
Minor analgesics	52	1.44	1.08-1.92
Antidepressants	5	0.91	0.30-2.12#
Drugs for rhinitis	5	0.80	0.26-1.88#
Antiasthmatics	8	0.58	0.29-1.15
Antihistamines	28	1.02	0.70-1.50

#observed over expected number with exact Poisson 95% confidence interval.

Table 55.5. Some maternal diagnoses associated with the use of anthelmintics in early pregnancy

Diagnosis	Drug use in early pregnancy		
	Number	OR/RR	95% CI
Pre-existing diabetes	5	0.85	0.27-1.97#
Chronic hypertension	5	0.92	0.30-2.15#
Gestational diabetes	5	1.08	0.35-2.51#
Preeclampsia	10	0.57	0.31-1.07
Hyperemesis gravidarum	5	1.07	0.35-2.50#
Placenta previa	5	0.95	0.31-2.23#
Abruptio placentae	5	0.89	0.29-2.08#
Antepartum bleeding	7	1.08	0.43-2.22#
Intrapartum bleeding	6	0.69	0.25-1.54#
Postpartum bleeding	26	1.04	0.70-1.55
Delivery induction	48	0.95	0.70-1.29
Caesarean section	46	0.68	0.50-0.92

#observed over expected number with exact Poisson 95% confidence interval.

No deviations from expected values were thus seen after early exposure to anthelmintics. After later exposure, numbers are low. There were four women with preeclampsia (RR = 0.64, 95% CI 0.17-1.64), 11 women with postpartum bleeding (RR = 1.55, 95% CI 0.77-2.78), 18 with delivery inductions (OR 1.18, 95% CI 0.77-2.78), and 21 with caesarean section (OR = 1.01, 95% CI 0.64-1.62). There are thus no signs of an increased pregnancy complication rate.

Outcome after Maternal use of Anthelmintics

Infant sex

After early use, there were 231 male and 231 female infants (one with unknown sex). The sex ratio is thus 1.00 (95% CI 0.83-1.20). After later exposure there were 60 male and 72 female infants, sex ratio 0.83 (95% CI 0.59-1.17). The normal sex ratio (1.06) is contained in both confidence intervals.

Multiple births

After early use, there were four twin deliveries (RR = 0.53, 95% CI 0.14-1.35) and after later use two (RR = 1.00, 95% CI 0.12-3.61).

Table 55.6. Pregnancy duration and infant birth weight at maternal use of anthelmintics

Variable studied	Drug use in early pregnancy			Drug use later in pregnancy		
	Number	OR/RR	95% CI	Number	OR/RR	95% CI
<37 weeks	13	0.67	0.38-1.16	0	-	-
<2500g	10	0.88	0.46-1.68	0	-	-
≥4500g	29	1.27	0.87-1.86	7	1.18	0.47-2.43#
SGA	9	1.35	0.62-2.56#	3	1.28	0.20-3.75#
LGA	44	1.18	0.86-1.63	11	1.15	0.57-2.05#

#observed over expected number with exact Poisson 95% confidence interval.

No significant deviations were found. There was one stillbirth after early exposure.

Table 55.7. Neonatal diagnoses after maternal use of anthelmintics in early pregnancy

Diagnosis	Number	OR/RR	95% CI
Hypoglycaemia	13	0.90	0.81-1.57
Respiratory diagnoses	16	0.74	0.45-1.22
Low Apgar score	3	0.37	0.08-1.09#
CNS diagnoses	1	-	-
Jaundice	14	0.88	0.51-1.50

#observed over expected number with exact Poisson 95% confidence interval.

The only diagnosis present in more than two infants after later exposure was respiratory diagnoses: three cases (RR = 0.50, 95% CI 0.10-1.45). There were thus no ill effects seen on the newborns.

Table 55.8. Congenital malformations in infants whose mothers had used anthelmintics in early pregnancy

Congenital malformation	Number	OR/RR	95% CI
All malformations	13	0.60	0.35-1.03
Relatively severe malformation	10	0.66	0.30-1.23
Chromosome anomalies	0	-	-
Without chromosome anomalies			
Any cardiovascular defect	3	0.60	0.12-1.77#

#observed over expected number with exact Poisson 95% confidence interval.

Among the infants with a relatively severe malformation, six were exposed to pyrvinium, three to mebendazole, and one to an unspecified anthelmintic.

Table 55.9. Specification of congenital malformations after maternal use of anthelmintics in early pregnancy

Malformation	Number	Anthelmintic
Laryngeal hypoplasia	1	pyrvinium
Ventricular septum defect	2	mebendazole; pyrvinium
Coarctatio aortae and aortic stenosis	1	mebendazole
Unspecified cardiac defect	1	pyrvinium
Hypospadias	1	unspecified
Hydronephrosis	1	pyrvinium
Vesico-uretro-renal reflux	1	pyrvinium
Polydactyly	2	mebendazole; pyrvinium

No signs of teratogenicity can be seen but the number of exposures is low.

Summary

In Sweden, the dominant anthelmintic therapy concerns threadworm. Most likely, anthelmintic use is heavily underreported. There are no signs of an ill effect of either of the two drugs used, mebendazole or pyrvinium.

References

[1] de Silva NR, Sirisena JL, Gunasekera DP, Ismail MM, de Silva HJ. Effect of mebendazole therapy during pregnancy and birth outcome. *Lancet* 1999; 353: 1145-1149.

[2] Diav-Citrin O, Schechtman S, Arnon J, Lubart I, Ornoy A. Pregnancy outcome after gestational exposure to mebendazole: a prospective controlled cohort study. *Am J Obstet Gynecol* 2003; 188: 282-285.

[3] Ács N, Bánhidy F, Puhó E, Czeizel A. Population-based case-control study of mebendazole in pregnant women for birth outcomes. *Cong Anomalies* 2005; 45: 85-88.

[4] Christian P, Khatry S, West KP. Antenatal anthelmintic treatment, birthweight, and infant survival in rural Nepal. *Lancet* 2004; 364: 981-983.

[5] Savioli L, Crompton DWT, Neira M. Use of anthelminthic drugs during pregnancy. *Am J Obstet Gynecol* 2003; 188: 5-6.

Chapter 56

DRUGS FOR ECTOPARASITES

Insectisides may have unwanted effects on pregnancy but a topical use is probably not associated with any risk even though only few data are available. If possible, use during the first trimester should be avoided but if exposure has occurred there is no reason to discuss a termination of the pregnancy.

Exposure to insecticides can occur in different ways: as occupational exposure, environmental exposure (e.g., after aerial spraying, local indoor use or at gardening), from residues in food etc. Therapeutic use of parmethrin [1,2] or benzyl benzoate [2] during pregnancy seemed not to be associated with any foetal risk. In Sweden the main therapeutic use is local treatment of head lice, mainly among school children and exposure of pregnant women will be rare.

Table 56.1. Number of women identified using drugs for ectoparasites

Total	28
Reported use in early pregnancy	19
Got prescription later in pregnancy	9
Both early and later use	0

Type of drug	ATC code	Early use	Later use
Disulfiram with benzylbenzoate	P03AA54	8	4
Malathion	P03AX03	11	5

The very low number of exposures makes a detailed analysis of pregnancy or neonatal complications meaningless. A short summary of the data will only be given.

OUTCOME AFTER MATERNAL USE OF DRUGS FOR ECTOPARASITES

There were five male and 14 female infants born after early exposure. The sex ratio is thus low. The exact 95% CI for being male is 9-51%, that is, just below the expected male percentage of 51.5. There were no twin deliveries. One infant was born preterm and had a low birth weight: gestational duration 31 weeks, birth weight 1980g. The baby was not small for gestational age. No infant died perinatally. Two were malformed; both had been exposed to malathion. One infant had a mild anomaly, preauricular appendix, the other had a knee deformity.

SUMMARY

The small material of women who reported the use of drugs for ectoparasites showed no aberrations but the power of the analysis is very low.

REFERENCES

[1] Kennedy D, Hurst V, Konradsdottir E, Einarson A. Pregnancy outcome following exposure to permethrin and use of teratogen information. *Am J Perinatol* 2005; 22: 87-90.

[2] Mytton OT, McGready R, Lee SJ, Roberts CH, Ashley EA, Carrara VI, Thwai KL, Jay MP, Wiangambun T, Singhasivanon P, Nosten F. Safety of benzyl benzoate lotion and permethrin in pregnancy: a retrospective matched cohort study. *BJOG* 2007; 114:582-587.

Chapter 57

NASAL DECONGESTANT PREPARATIONS

No certain ill effects of the use of topical nasal decongestans have been demonstrated, including the use of nose drops containing corticosteroids. The use of oral decongestants is more doubtful even though the postulated associations with some specific malformations are uncertain and based on possibly biased retrospective information. It may be wise to avoid such drugs in early pregnancy but if exposure has occurred there is no reason to discuss a termination of pregnancy. Use of these drugs later in pregnancy may increase the risk for preeclampsia and should be avoided. The risk increase is small, however.

Nasal decongestant preparations are used at upper respiratory tract infections, notably common cold, at allergic rhinitis, and at pregnancy rhinitis. A possible association was described with clubfoot, eye and ear malformations and maternal use of sympathicomimetic drugs [1]. A number of retrospective case-control studies found an association between the use of oral nasal decongestants and certain specific malformations: gastroschisis, small bowel atresia, and hemifacial microsomia [2], all based on small numbers of malformed and exposed infants. Recently an association also with transverse limb reductions has been suggested [3]. The idea has been that these – and some other malformations – are due to vascular disruption, a popular idea for which there is little evidence, notably with respect to gastroschisis [4].

A previous study [5] of the use of oral decongestants during pregnancy showed no significant teratogenic effect but fewer than expected preterm birth, probably a positive effect of the underlying condition of pregnancy rhinitis.

Table 57.1. Number of women identified using nasal decongestant preparations

Total	19226
Reported use in early pregnancy	12981
Got prescription later in pregnancy	7698
Both early and later use	1433

Type of drug	ATC code	Early use	Later use
Sympathicomimetics	R01AA	3024	1468
Oxymethazoline	R01AA05	2458	1177
Xylomethazoline	R01AA07	605	300
Antiallergic agents, not corticosteroids	R01AC	2047	1004
Cromoglicic acid	R01AC01	1420	776
Levocabastine	R01AC02	683	257
Azelastine	R01AC03	3	2
Corticosteroids	R01AD	5068	2801
Beclometasone	R01AD01	171	46
Flunisolide	R01AD04	4	1
Budesonide	R01AD05	3541	1746
Fluticasone	R01AD08	582	339
Mometasone	R01AD09	712	646
Triamcinolone	01AD11	50	26
Other	R01AX	4	1
Ipatropium	R01AX03	4	1
Peroral decongestants	R01B	3655	3186
Phenylpropanolamine	R01BA01	3490	3113
Phenylpropanolamine+cinnarizine	R01BA51	15	82
Pseudoephedrine+dexbrompheniramine	R01BA52	28	3

In early pregnancy, 475 women used both local and peroral decongestants, in later pregnancy 989 did.

Characteristics of Women using Nasal Decongestants in Early Pregnancy

Based on women reporting the drug in early pregnancy (n=7913, one missing maternal age). Each variable is adjusted for all other variables and year of delivery. Comparison with all women who gave birth during the period and with information from the first antenatal care (n=967 742). The odds ratios for maternal age, parity, smoking in early pregnancy, number of previous miscarriages, BMI, subfertility, and country of birth are adjusted for all other variables and are shown in Figure 57.1.

Some further maternal characteristics were analyzed, adjusting for year of delivery, maternal age, parity, smoking, and BMI (Table 57.2).

The maternal age distribution shows fewer than expected young women and the use of these drugs declines with parity. The women smoke less than expected. There is an increase in use with BMI and a higher use among Swedish-born women than other women. A long education, co-habitation, and work outside home are associated with an increased use of the drugs.

There are a number of associations. Some indicate the presence of allergy and asthma, other the presence of respiratory infections (e.g., antibiotics, cough medicines, minor analgesics and NSAIDs). Associations with drugs for NVP and drugs for stomach ulcer and reflux may mirror an association between pregnancy rhinitis and NVP.

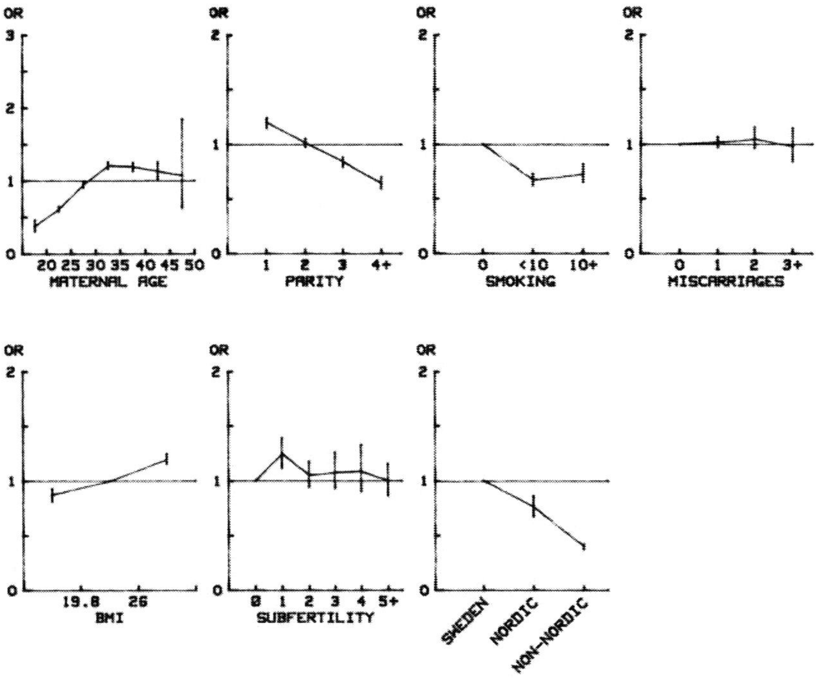

Figure 57.1. Odds ratios for seven maternal characteristics. The odds ratios (OR) for each variable are adjusted for the other variables and year of delivery. Vertical lines mark 95% confidence intervals. For maternal age and parity, each class is compared with all other classes.

Table 57.2. Some further characteristics of women who nasal decongestants in early pregnancy

Variable studied	Number	OR	95% CI
Education (1996-2001, 6626 women with drugs, 526 695 in population)			
Unknown	57		
<12 years	429	0.66	0.60-0.74
12 years	3322	1.00	reference
13-14 years	423	1.09	0.98-1.20
≥14 years	2395	1.14	1.07-1.19
Family situation			
Unknown	202	-	-
Co-habiting	12264	1.00	reference
Living alone	190	0.70	0.61-0.81
Other family situation	212	0.80	0.68-0.92
Work outside home			
Unknown	1323	-	-
Full time	6693	1.00	reference
Part time	3368	1.06	1.01-1.12
None	1484	0.72	0.67-0.77

Table 57.3. Concomitant drug use (early pregnancy)

Drug group	Number	OR/RR	95% CI
Drugs for stomach ulcer and reflux	172	1.50	1.29-1.75
Drugs for inflammatory bowel disease	41	1.08	0.79-1.47
Insulin	21	0.43	0.28-0.65
Multivitamins	789	1.01	0.94-1.08
Folic acid	547	0.83	0.76-0.91
Antihypertensives	38	0.76	0.55-1.04
Oral contraceptives	42	1.15	0.84-1.55
Progestogens	57	0.84	0.65-1.09
Gonadotropins	21	0.58	0.38-0.88
Systemic corticosteroids	137	3.17	2.72-3.70
Thyroid drugs	174	0.93	0.80-1.08
Antibiotics	1543	4.21	4.00-4.43
NSAIDs	397	1.70	1.53-1.88
Opioids	89	1.39	1.13-1.72
Minor analgesics	2370	2.63	2.51-2.74
Drugs for migraine	65	1.64	1.29-2.10
Anticonvulsants	23	0.60	0.40-0.90
Sedatives, hypnotics	97	1.79	1.46-2.19
Antidepressants	145	0.92	0.78-1.09
Antiasthmatics	2895	9.51	9.17-9.80
Cough medicines	540	8.55	7.92-9.24
Antihistamines	2775	4.45	4.28-4.63
For NVP	1122	2.02	1.90-2.14
For allergy	1771	10.6	10.2-11.1

Table 57.4. Some maternal diagnoses associated with the use of nasal decongestant preparations

Diagnosis	Drug use in early pregnancy			Drug use later in pregnancy		
	Number	OR/RR	95% CI	Number	OR/RR	95% CI
Pre-existing diabetes	147	0.82	0.69-0.97	88	0.78	0.63-0.97
Chronic hypertension	169	1.03	0.89-1.21	111	1.07	0.89-1.30
Gestational diabetes	131	1.04	0.88-1.25	70	0.92	0.72-1.16
Preeclampsia	673	1.06	0.98-1.15	440	1.20	1.09-1.33
Hyperemesis gravidarum	132	0.98	0.81-1.15	83	0.95	0.77-1.19
Placenta previa	154	1.00	0.85-1.18	81	0.83	0.66-1.02
Abruptio placentae	172	1.04	0.89-1.21	97	0.92	0.75-1.13
Antepartum bleeding	188	1.03	0.89-1.19	100	0.92	0.75-1.12
Intrapartum bleeding	304	1.05	0.94-1.18	190	1.01	0.88-1.17
Postpartum bleeding	780	1.04	0.96-1.12	453	1.05	0.96-1.16
Delivery induction	1494	1.05	1.00-1.11	932	1.09	1.02-1.17
Caesarean section	2281	1.06	1.02-1.12	1389	1.07	1.01-1.14

The only deviation concerns the occurrence of preeclampsia which is significantly increased after exposure during late pregnancy. This effect is most marked after the use of peroral decongestants which are sympathicomimetics. There were 185 cases of preeclampsia among 3186 women using such drugs, OR = 1.30 (95% CI 1.11-1.51). The dominating oral decongestant drug used in late pregnancy was phenylpropanolamine. No such effect was seen after local use of sympathicomimetics: OR = 1.05 (95% CI 0.82-1.33).

Outcome after Maternal use of Nasal Decongestant Preparations

Infant Sex

After early use there were 6 788 male and 6 378 female infants (3 with unknown sex), sex ratio 1.06 (95% CI 1.03-1.10). After later use there were 3 996 male and 3 832 female infants, sex ratio 1.04 (95% CI 1.00-1.09). The normal sex ratio (1.06) was thus included in both confidence intervals.

Multiple Births

After early use there were 205 twin deliveries (OR = 1.01, 95% CI 0.88-1.16) and one triplet delivery. After later use there were 130 twin deliveries (OR = 1.11, 95% CI 0.93-1.32).

Table 57.5. Pregnancy duration and infant birth weight at maternal use of nasal decongestant preparations

Variable studied	Drug use in early pregnancy			Drug use later in pregnancy		
	Number	OR/RR	95% CI	Number	OR/RR	95% CI
<37 weeks	586	0.94	0.87-1.03	322	0.90	0.81-1.01
<2500g	374	0.97	0.87-1.08	190	0.87	0.74-1.00
≥4500g	556	1.00	0.92-1.09	371	1.10	0.99-1.22
SGA	257	0.96	0.85-1.09	139	0.96	0.81-1.13
LGA	801	0.99	0.92-1.07	576	1.14	1.04-1.24

The only indicated deviation was an increased rate of LGA infants after later exposure. This is formally statistical significant but could be random nevertheless. It could also be associated with the presence of pregnancy rhinitis which (like NVP) has been associated with a better than expected intrauterine growth.

Table 57.6. Infant mortality after maternal use of nasal decongestants

Variable studied	Drug use in early pregnancy			Drug use later in pregnancy		
	Number	OR/RR	95% CI	Number	OR/RR	95% CI
Stillbirth	31	0.69	0.49-0.99	19	0.75	0.48-1.18
Early neonatal death	14	0.70	0.42-1.19	6	0.52	0.19-1.14#

#observed over expected number with exact Poisson 95% confidence interval.

The perinatal death risk is thus if anything lower than expected.

The only indicated deviations represent statistically significant low rates of low Apgar score.

Table 57.7. Neonatal diagnoses after maternal use of decongestants

Diagnosis	Drug use in early pregnancy			Drug use later in pregnancy		
	Number	OR/RR	95% CI	Number	OR/RR	95% CI
Hypoglycaemia	473	0.98	0.39-1.08	285	1.02	0.91-1.15
Respiratory diagnoses	659	0.98	0.91-1.07	351	0.96	0.86-1.07
Low Apgar score	208	0.79	0.69-0.91	105	0.76	0.63-0.92
CNS diagnoses	86	1.02	0.82-1.27	55	1.08	0.83-1.41
Jaundice	566	1.05	0.96-1.14	311	0.99	0.88-1.11

Table 57.8. Congenital malformations in infants whose mothers had used nasal decongestants in early pregnancy

Congenital malformation	Number	OR	95% CI
All malformation	616	0.98	0.90-1.06
Relatively severe malformation	422	0.99	0.90-1.09
Chromosome anomalies	25	0.95	0.63-1.41
Without chromosome anomalies			
Any CNS malformation	17	1.08	0.67-1.75
Neural tube defects	8	1.61	0.69-3.17#
Any cardiovascular defect	157	1.11	0.95-1.31
VSD and/or ASD	90	1.21	0.98-1.49
Unspecified cardiac defects	26	1.88	1.26-2.80
Oesophageal atresia	1	0.26	0.01-1.44#
Small bowel atresia	3	0.96	0.20-2.79#
Anal atresia	7	1.42	0.57-2.93#
Pylorostenosis	13	1.38	0.93-2.35#
Abdominal wall defects	1	0.30	0.01-1.67#
Diaphragmatic hernia	2	0.64	0.08-2.31#
Hypospadias	30	0.79	0.55-1.13
Severe kidney malformation	4	0.51	0.14-2.30#
Pes equinovarus	4	0.84	0.23-2.14#
Poly/syndctyly	38	1.42	1.03-1.96
Limb reduction defects	4	0.53	0.14-1.36#
Hip (sub)luxation, unstable hip	89	1.02	0.82-1.26
Craniostenosis	5	0.65	0.21-1.53#

#observed over expected number with exact Poisson 95% confidence interval.

Table 57.9. Relatively severe malformations and cardiovascular defects according to group of nasal decongestant used

Drug group	Number of infants		OR	95% CI
	malformed	total		
Relatively severe malformation				
Sympathicomimetic, local	100	3074	1.03	0.84-1.26
Antiallergics, except corticosteroids, local	58	2075	0.86	0.66-1.12
Corticosteroids, local	168	5150	1.00	0.86-1.17
Peroral decongestants	123	3711	1.02	0.85-1.22
Any cardiovascular defect				
Sympathicomimetic, local	36	3074	1.12	0.81-1.56
Antiallergics, except corticosteroids, local	18	2075	0.83	0.52-1.32
Corticosteroids, local	65	5150	1.18	0.92-1.51
Peroral decongestants	49	3711	1.21	0.90-1.61

The risk of a relatively severe malformation or a cardiac defect is similar in the different groups of decongestants.

Use of peroral decongestants has been associated with some specific malformations, notably gastroschisis, small bowel atresia, and transverse limb reduction defects. In the present material, there were only two infants, exposed to peroral decongestants, with any of these malformations (expected number 3.0): one had gastroschisis (expected number 0.9) and one had an upper limb reduction malformation of unclear nature, combined with hand polydactyly and therefore probably not of transverse reduction type.

SUMMARY

The only adverse effect of the use of nasal decongestants is an indicated increased risk for preeclampsia after exposure to peroral sympathicomimetic drugs during late pregnancy,. No signs of any teratogenic effects were seen

REFERENCES

[1] Heinonen OP. Slone D, Shapiro S. *Birth Defects and Drugs in Pregnancy*. Littleton (MA): Publishing Sciences Group, Inc; 1977.

[2] Werler MM. Teratogen update: Pseudoephedrine. *Birth Def Res (Part A)* 2006; 76:445-452.

[3] Werler MM, Bosco JL, Shapira SK, National Birth Defects Prevention Study. Maternal vasoactive exposure, amniotic band, and terminal transverse limb defects. *Birth Def Res (Part A)* 2009; 85: 52-57.

[4] Feldkamp ML, Carey JC, Sadler TW. Development of gastroschisis: Review of hypotheses, a novel hypothesis, and implications for research. *Amer J Med Genet (Part A)* 2007; 143A: 639-652.

[5] Källén B, Otterblad Olausson P. Use of oral decongestants during pregnancy and delivery outcome. *Am J Obst Gynecol* 2006; 194: 480-485.

Chapter 58

ANTIASTHMATIC DRUGS

Maternal asthma could affect pregnancy and neonatal conditions and adequate treatment is needed to optimize the outcome. There are very little evidence that maternal antiasthmatic drugs can negatively affect pregnancy or neonatal outcome. Most of the alleged associations with congenital malformations are uncertain and scare for such effects should not prevent adequate asthma therapy during pregnancy. Exposure to antiasthmatic drugs in early pregnancy is no reason to discuss a termination of pregnancy.

Asthma is relatively common among pregnant women and many studies have been published on the outcome after asthma or use of antiasthmatic drugs. Relatively recent reviews are available [1-4]. Some anomalies in pregnancy and neonatal outcomes are observable but it is uncertain to what extent they are due to asthma or antiasthmatic drugs. A recent study [5] suggested that treatment of asthma did not increase the risk for a congenital malformation compared with non-treated asthma but found a possible teratogenic effect of "other anti-inflammatory medication" (cromoglicate, nedocromil, montelukast, or zafirlukast) but this statement was based on only nine cases. A small TIS study [6] found no certain risk increase for a congenital malformation after maternal use of leucotrine receptor antagonists based on five infants with malformations among 96 exposed infants. Use of inhaled corticosteroids was not found to increase the risk for congenital malformations [7] but the study did not specifically discuss orofacial clefts, which are probably associated with systemic corticosteroid use. A retrospective case-control study of infants with gastroschisis found an association with maternal use of bronchodilators [8]. The estimated odd ratio after use of anti-inflammatory drugs was of the same magnitude but did not reach statistical significance.

Previous analyses of data from the Swedish Medical Birth Register are available [9-11]. Those studies described an increased risk for various pregnancy complications including preterm birth and an increased risk for neonatal complications including respiratory problems and hypoglycaemia. A slight teratogenic effect could be seen, observable for cardiovascular defects, median cleft palate, and anal atresia.

Table 58.1. Number of women identified using antiasthmatic drug

Total	36250
Reported use in early pregnancy	29160
Got prescription later in pregnancy	5643
Both early and later use	36250

Type of drug	ATC code	Early use	Later use
Adrenergics	R03AA/R03AC/R03CA/R03CC	24752	10651
Epinephrine	R03AA01	92	14
Ephedrine	R03CA02	23	8
Salbutamol	R03AC02/R03CC02	5723	2128
Terbutaline	R03AC03/R03CC03	18430	8254
Fenoterol	R03AC04	35	0
Salmeterol	R03AC12	1567	543
Formoterol	R03AC13	932	509
Formoterol+budesonide	R03AK07	974	714
Bambuterol	R03CC12	14	2
Clenbuterol	R03CC13	1	1
Unspecified	R03CA	1	0
Adrenergics and glucocorticosteroids	R03AK	1769	1252
Salbutamol+ipratropium	R03AK04	12	20
Salmeterol+fluticasone	R03AK06	789	527
Formoterol+budesonide	R03AK07	974	714
Inhaled glucocorticosteroids	R03BA	12753	5167
Beclometasone	R03BA01	596	135
Budesonide	R03BA02	11542	4659
Betamethasone	R03BA04	0	1
Fluticasone	R03BA05	675	401
Mometasone	R03BA07	16	13
Unspecified	R03BA	6	1
Anticholinergics	R03BB	183	76
Ipratropium	R03BB01	181	73
Thiotropium	R03BB04	2	3
Antiallergic, not corticosteroids	R03BC	1453	477
Cromoglicic acid	R03BC01	1453	477
Nedocromat	R03BC03	0	1
Xanthines	R03DA	183	59
Choline theophyllinate	R03DA02	35	13
Theophylline	R03DA04	145	46
Aminophylline	R03DA05	5	0
Leucotrine receptor antagonists	R03DC	190	102
Montelukast	R03DC03	190	102
Unspecified	R03	36	2

Number of different categories of antiasthmatic drugs

One	16789	7468
Two	10951	4374
Three	1209	751
Four	161	123
Five	18	15

The most common combination was between an adrenergic and an inhaled glucocorticosteroid (early exposure 11 863, later exposure 5 100 women) but nearly all possible combinations occurred.

Characteristics of Women using Antiasthmatic Drugs

Based on women reporting the drug in early pregnancy (n= 29 157, three missing maternal age). Each variable is adjusted for all other variables and year of delivery. Comparison with all women who gave birth during the period and with information from the first antenatal care (n=967 742). The odds ratios for maternal age, parity, smoking in early pregnancy, number of previous miscarriages, BMI, subfertility, and country of birth are adjusted for all other variables and are shown in Figure 58.1.

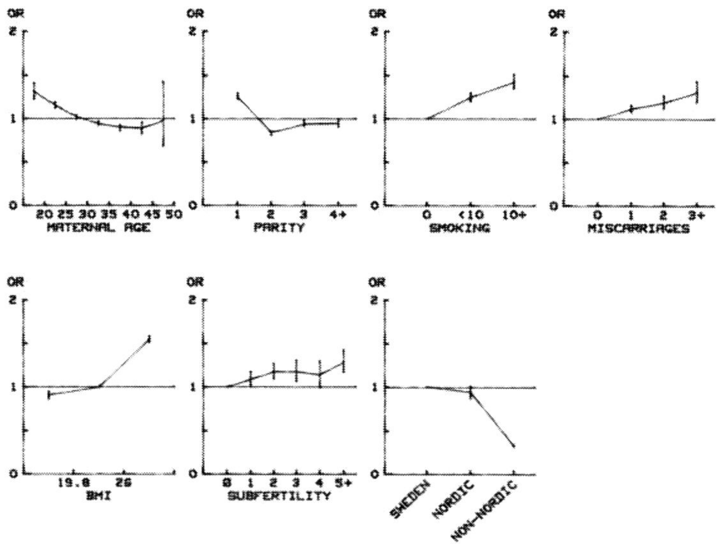

Figure 58.1. Odds ratios for seven maternal characteristics. The odds ratios (OR) for each variable are adjusted for the other variables and year of delivery. Vertical lines mark 95% confidence intervals. For maternal age and parity, each class is compared with all other classes.

Table 58.2. Some further characteristics of women using antiasthma tics in early pregnancy

Variable studied	Number	OR	95% CI
Education (1996-2001, 14 708 women with drugs, 526 695 in population)			
Unknown	187	-	-
<12 years	1934	0.96	0.91-1.02
12 years	7976	1.00	reference
13-14 years	763	0.93	0.86-1.00
≥14 years	3848	0.90	0.87-0.94
Family situation			
Unknown	557	-	-
Co-habiting	26426	1.00	reference
Living alone	688	1.25	1.16-1.33
Other family situation	1749	1.13	1.05-1.22
Work outside home			
Unknown	4184	-	
Full time	13768	1.00	reference
Part time	6566	0.99	0.95-1.02
None	4420	0.85	0.81-0.88

Some further maternal characteristics were analyzed, adjusting for year of delivery, maternal age, parity, smoking, and BMI (Table 58.2).

Antiasthmatic drugs are more often used by young than by older women, at first parity, and among smokers. There is a slightly increased use after previous miscarriage or a period of subfertility. Women with a high education use such drugs less often than women with a low education and women born in the Nordic countries use more such drugs than women born outside the Nordic countries. Women using antiasthmatics are overrepresented among non-cohabiting women but they worked outside home more often than other women.

Table 58.3. Concomitant drug use (early pregnancy)

Drug group	Number	OR/RR	95% CI
Drugs for stomach ulcer and reflux	407	1.59	1.44-1.76
Drugs for inflammatory bowel disease	107	1.43	1.18-1.94
Insulin	92	0.85	0.69-1.04
Multivitamins	1194	0.75	0.71-0.79
Folic acid	1063	0.80	0.75-0.85
Oral contraceptives	103	1.16	0.97-1.40
Progestogens	83	0.64	0.51-0.79
Gonadotropins	58	0.80	0.62-1.04
Systemic corticosteroids	697	7.82	7.27-8.40
Thyroid drugs	516	1.38	1.26-1.51
Antibiotics	1148	1.25	1.17-1.32
NSAIDs	442	0.76	0.69-0.84
Opioids	283	1.81	1.61-2.04
Minor analgesics	2120	0.86	0.82-0.90
Drugs for migraine	143	1.69	1.43-2.00
Anticonvulsants	93	1.06	0.86-1.31
Neuroleptics	108	1.07	0.88-1.30
Sedatives, hypnotics	266	1.95	1.72-2.21
Antidepressants	533	1.40	1.28-1.53
Drugs for rhinitis	2870	9.50	9.16-9.85
Cough medicines	513	3.56	3.27-3.89
Antihistamines	4914	3.43	3.33-3.53
For NVP	1921	1.51	1.44-1.59
For allergy	3191	9.24	8.93-3.89

There is a strong association with systemic corticosteroids and cough medicines, also used at asthma, and with drugs for allergy including rhinitis. Weaker but statistically significant associations are seen for instance with drugs for inflammatory bowel disease and for stomach ulcer and reflux, for thyroid drugs, antibiotics, opioids, drugs for migraine, sedatives and hypnotics, and antidepressants. Some of these drugs are used for asthma complications, e.g., antibiotics, other may indicate co-morbidity (e.g., drugs for inflammatory bowel disease and thyroid drugs). Other drugs are used less often than expected, e.g., vitamins, NSAIDs, and analgesics.

There is thus an indicated increased risk for some pregnancy complications and for delivery induction and caesarean section. The odds ratio for preeclampsia and for caesarean section after late use of antiasthmatic drugs varied with the number of different asthma drug categories used as an estimate of the severity of the asthma (Table 58.5).

Table 58.4. Some maternal diagnoses associated with the use of antiasthmatic drugs

Diagnosis	Drug use in early pregnancy			Drug use later in pregnancy		
	Number	OR/RR	95% CI	Number	OR/RR	95% CI
Pre-existing diabetes	391	0.96	0.87-1.07	205	1.05	0.92-1.22
Chronic hypertension	393	1.09	0.98-1.20	201	1.14	0.98-1.31
Gestational diabetes	308	1.08	0.97-1.22	154	1.16	0.98-1.36
Preeclampsia	1670	1.15	1.09-1.21	758	1.20	1.11-1.29
Hyperemesis gravidarum	356	1.15	1.03-1.28	182	1.21	1.04-1.41
Placenta previa	358	1.05	0.94-1.17	183	1.10	0.95-1.27
Abruptio placentae	413	1.08	0.98-1.20	220	1.20	1.05-1.38
Antepartum bleeding	436	1.05	0.95-1.16	215	1.14	0.99-1.30
Intrapartum bleeding	686	1.10	1.02-1.19	387	1.24	1.12-1.38
Postpartum bleeding	1746	1.04	0.99-1.10	772	1.08	1.01-1.17
Delivery induction	3695	1.17	1.13-1.22	1748	1.22	1.16-1.29
Caesarean section	5548	1.22	1.18-1.25	2590	1.24	1.19-1.30

Table 58.5. Two pregnancy complications according to number of antiasthmatic drugs used

Number of drug groups	Number	OR	95% CI
Preeclampsia			
One	402	1.12	1.01-1.24
Two	284	1.26	1.11-1.42
Three or more	71	1.49	1.17-1.91
Caesarean section			
One	1444	1.20	1.14-1.28
Two	930	1.25	1.16-1.35
Three or more	214	1.44	1.23-1.69

Outcome after Maternal use of Antiasthmatics

Infant Sex

After early use of antiasthmatics there were 15 273 male and 14 332 female infants, sex ratio 1.07 (95% CI 1.04-1.09). After later use, there were 6 655 male and 6 336 female infants and one infant with unknown sex, sex ratio 1.05 (95% CI 1.01-1.09). Both estimates are thus close to the normal sex ratio (1.06)

Multiple Births

After early use there were 448 twin deliveries (OR = 1.05, 95%. CI 0.96-1.16) and eight triplet deliveries. After later use, there were 257 twin deliveries (OR = 1.40, 95% CI 1.23-1.58) and two triplet deliveries. The increased multiple birth rate is reasonably explained by the use of certain antiasthmatic drugs for threatened preterm delivery which is common at multiple births.

Table 58.6. Pregnancy duration and infant birth weight at maternal use of antiasthmatics

Variable studied	Drug use in early pregnancy			Drug use later in pregnancy		
	Number	OR/RR	95% CI	Number	OR/RR	95% CI
<37 weeks	1625	1.11	1.06-1.17	861	1.41	1.31-1.51
<2500g	1099	1.18	1.11-1.26	502	1.26	1.15-1.38
≥4500g	1223	1.02	0.96-1.08	479	0.89	0.81-0.98
SGA	765	1.16	1.08-1.25	302	1.10	0.98-1.24
LGA	1772	1.03	0.98-1.09	761	0.96	0.89-1.04

The excess risk for preterm birth after early use is smaller after the use of only one antiasthmatic drug group (OR = 1.08, 95% CI 1.00-1.17) than after the use of two different antiasthmatic groups (OR = 1.16, 95% CI 1.05-1.29) which indicates that this effect can be the result of asthma severity. The excess risk after later exposure is confounded by the use of some antiasthmatic drugs (e.g., terbutaline) for threatened preterm delivery. When only such adrenergic drugs had been used, the OR for preterm birth was 1.35 (95% CI 1.12-1.56) – when only other antiasthmatic drugs had been used, no increase in the OR was seen: after the use of only inhaled corticosteroids, for example, the OR = 0.95, 95% CI 0.73-1.25.

Table 58.7. Infant mortality after maternal use of anatiasthmatic drugs

Variable studied	Drug use in early pregnancy			Drug use later in pregnancy		
	Number	OR/RR	95% CI	Number	OR/RR	95% CI
Stillbirth	90	0.86	0.70-1.06	52	1.14	0.86-1.51
Early neonatal death	47	1.02	0.76-1.36	19	1.01	0.64-1.61

No increased perinatal mortality can thus be seen.

Table 58.8. Neonatal diagnoses after maternal use of antiasthmatics

Diagnosis	Drug use in early pregnancy			Drug use later in pregnancy		
	Number	OR/RR	95% CI	Number	OR/RR	95% CI
Hypoglycaemia	1161	1.05	0.99-1.11	581	1.19	1-09-1.29
Respiratory diagnoses	1607	1.05	1.00-1.10	726	1.18	1.09-1.27
Low Apgar score	554	0.91	0.83-0.99	279	1.17	1.04-1.32
CNS diagnoses	206	1.07	0.93-1.23	108	1.18	0.97-1.44
Jaundice	1378	1.11	1.05-1.17	683	1.25	1.16-1.35

The increased risk for neonatal complications after later use of antiasthmatics could be due to the increased risk for preterm birth but when the analysis was restricted to term infants, the statistically significant risk increases remained. For hypoglycaemia the OR was 1.20 (95% CI 1.08-1.32), for respiratory diagnoses 1.13 (95% CI 1.03-1.25), for low Apgar score 1.19 (95% CI 1.03-1.37), for CNS diagnoses 1.29 (95% CI 1.04-1.60), and for jaundice 1.17 (95% CI 1.04-1.30).

Table 58.9. Congenital malformations in infants whose mothers had used antiasthmatics in early pregnancy

Congenital malformation	Number	OR	95% CI
All malformations	1503	1.06	1.01-1.12
Relatively severe malformations	1024	1.05	0.99-1.12
Chromosome anomalies	56	1.01	0.77-1.32
Without chromosome anomalies			
Any CNS malformations	33	0.87	0.62-1.24
Neural tube defects	12	1.00	0.56-1.78
Eye malformations	30	0.99	0.68-1.43
Ear malformations	76	1.07	0.85-1.35
Orofacial clefts	60	1.09	0.84-1.42
Any cardiovascular defect	350	1.10	0.99-1.23
VSD and/or ASD	195	1.17	1.01-1.36
Unspecified cardiac defects	29	0.88	0.61-1.28
Oesophageal atresia	6	0.67	0.25-1.46#
Small bowel atresia	11	1.49	0.74-2.66#
Anal atresia	14	1.17	0.68-2.01
Pylorostenosis	32	1.48	1.04-2.12
Abdominal wall defect	8	0.93	0.40-1.83#
Diaphragmatic hernia	8	1.14	0.49-2.24#
Hypospadias	83	0.95	0.76-1.18
Severe kidney malformations	16	0.83	0.51-1.37
Pes equinovarus	48	1.10	0.82-1.47
Poly/syndactyly	70	1.21	0.95-1.53
Limb reduction defect	21	1.16	0.75-1.81
Hip (sub)luxation, unstable hip	165	0.89	0.76-1.04
Craniostenosis	13	0.75	0.43-1.30

#observed over expected number with exact Poisson 95% confidence interval.

There is thus a weak increase in the risk of a relatively severe malformation and specifically for VSD/ASD and pylorostenosis. No significantly increased risk for anal atresia was found in this study.

The risk increase for a relatively severe malformation is increased for infants exposed to three groups of antiasthmatics (OR = 1.35, 95% CI 0.93-1.99) or for more than three drug groups (OR = 1.55, 95% I 0.57-4.22), but none of the two estimates are thus statistically significant.

For VSD/ASD, the OR is 1.20 (95% CI 0.99-1.96) after exposure to one drug group, 1.17 (95% CI 1.01-1.36) after exposure to two drug groups, and the RR is 1.67 (95% CI 0.72-3.28) after exposure to three or more groups. The suggested higher risk among the latter can thus be random.

Specific types of antiasthmatics or (when numbers were enough) specific antiasthmatics were analyzed for relatively severe malformations, for any cardiovascular defect, for VSD/ASD, and for pylorostenosis, that is, the conditions which showed a possible overrisk.

Table 58.10. Groups of malformations after different groups of antiasthmatics and specific antiasthmatics

Malformation Drug (group)	Number of infants		OR	95% CI
	malformed	total		
Relatively severe malformations				
Adrenergics	879	25142	1.06	0.99-1.14
Salbutamol	209	5809	1.10	0.95-1.26
Terbutaline	651	16869	1.06	0.98-1.15
Salmeterol	63	1601	1.17	0.91-1.51
Formoterol	22	944	0.72	0.47-1.09
Adrenergic+inhaled glucocorticosteroids	53	1794	0.98	0.75-1.30
Salmeterol+fluticasone	27	802	1.13	0.86-1.67
Formoterol+budesonide	26	988	0.87	0.59-1.29
Inhaled glucocorticosteroids	439	12938	1.03	0.94-1.14
Beclometasone	24	604	1.13	0.75-1.71
Budesonide	395	11710	1.03	0.93-1.14
Fluticasone	21	684	0.93	0.60-1.85
Anticholinergics	6	188	0.79	0.29-1.72#
Antiallergic, non-steroid	52	1480	1.04	0.79-1.38
Xanthines	7	187	1.04	0.42-2.14#
Leucotrine receptor antagonists	6	192	1.04	0.38-2.26#
Any cardiovascular defect				
Adrenergics	304	25142	1.13	1.00-1.27
Adrenergic+inhaled glucocorticosteroids	24	1794	1.22	0.81-1.84
Inhaled glucocorticosteroids	144	12938	1.04	0.88-1.23
Antiallergic, non-steroid	17	1480	1.09	0.67-1.26
VSD/ASD				
Adrenergics	165	25142	1.17	1.00-1.37
Adrenergic+inhaled glucocorticosteroids	18	1794	1.59	0.99-2.56
Inhaled glucocorticosteroids	82	12938	1.12	0.90-1.40
Antiallergic, non-steroid	12	1480	1.53	0.79-2.68#
Pylorostenosis				
Adrenergics	24	25142	1.29	0.85-1.95
Adrenergic+inhaled glucocorticosteroids	0	1794		-
Inhaled glucocorticosteroids	11	12938	1.17	0.58-2.09#
Antiallergic, non-steroid	5	1480	4.85	1.58-11.3#

There are thus no certain differences in risk according to the type of antiasthmatic (or specific antiasthmatic) used. The only unusual finding is the strong association between cromoglicic acid and pylorostenosis but this is based on only five cases and may be random in spite of formal statistical significance.

There were thus seven malformed infants which had been exposed to xanthines. One had a ventricular septum defect, one had pulmonary valve stenosis, one pulmonary artery stenosis, one pylorostenosis and pes equinovarus, one omphalocele, one ureter duplication with vesico-uretero-renal reflux, and one a malformation syndrome.

There were six malformed infants who had been exposed to montelukast: two with ventricular septum defect, one with a laryngeal malformation, two with polydactyly, and one with a malformation of the thumb.

A concern has been raised that inhaled glucocorticoids could increase the risk for orofacial clefts. There were 14 587 infants exposed in early pregnancy to inhaled glucocorticoids – either alone or in combination with other antiasthmatic drugs. Among them, 32 had orofacial clefts (OR = 1.18, 95% CI 0.83-1.09). If the cases were divided into isolated cleft palate and cleft lip with or without cleft palate, the OR for the former ones was 1.59 (95% CI 0.96-2.65), for the latter 0.94 (95% CI 0.57-1.55). None of the 16 infants with isolated cleft palate was exposed to systemic corticosteroids. There is thus a suggested association with isolated cleft palate but statistical significance is not reached.

SUMMARY

There are relatively slight deviations in pregnancy and neonatal outcome, including congenital malformations, after use of antiasthmatic drugs. Asthma disease may be an important confounder and could explain some of the deviations. For some variables, the risks increased with the number of antiasthmatic drugs used which may mirror disease severity. Little difference between different categories of drugs is seen. There is a suggested association between use of inhaled glucocorticoids and cleft palate.

REFERENCES

[1] Tan KS, Thomson NO. Asthma in pregnancy. *Am J Med* 2000; 109: 727-733.

[2] Chambers C. Safety of asthma and allergic medications in pregnancy. *Immunol Allergy Clin North Amer* 2006; 26: 13-28.

[3] Murphy VE, Clifton VL, Gibson PG. Asthma exacerbations during pregnancy: incidence and association with pregnancy outcome. *Thorax* 2006; 61: 169-176.

[4] Källén B. The safety of asthma medications during pregnancy. *Expert Opinion Drug Saf* 2007; 6: 15-26.

[5] Tata LJ, Lewis SA, McKeever TM, Smith CJP, Doyle P, Smeeth L, Gibson JE, Hubbard RB. Effect of maternal asthma, exacerbations and asthma medication use on congenital malformations in offspring; a UK population-based study. *Thorax* 2008; 63: 981-987.

[6] Bakhireva L, Jones KL, Schatz M, Klonoff-Cohen HS, Johnson D, Slymen DJ, Chambers CD; Organization of Teratology Information Specialists Collaborative Research Group. Asthma control during pregnancy and the risk for preterm delivery or impaired fetal growth. *J Allergy Clin Immunol* 2007; 119: 618-625.

[7] Blais L, Beauchesne M-F, Rey É, Malo J-L, Forget A. Use of inhaled corticosteroids during the first trimester of prgnancy and the risk of congenital malformations among women with asthma. *Thorax* 2007; 62: 320-328.

[8] Lin S, Munsie JPW, Hardt-Losavio ML, Bell E, Druschel C, Romitti PA, Oley R and the National Birth Defects Prevention Study. Maternal asthma mediation use and the risk of gastroschisis. *Am J Epidemiol* 2008; 168: 73-79.

[9] Källén B, Otterblad Olausson P. Use of anti-asthmatic drugs during pregnancy. 1. Maternal characteristics, pregnancy and delivery complications. *Europ J Pharmacol* 2007; 63: 363-373.

[10] Källén B, Otterblad Olausson P. Use of anti-asthmatic drugs during pregnancy. 2. Infants characteristics excluding congenital malformations. *Europ J Pharmacol* 2007; 63: 375-381.

[11] Källén B, Otterblad Olausson P. Use of anti-asthmatic drugs during pregnancy. 3. Congenital malformations in the infants. *Europ J Pharmacol* 2007; 63: 383-388.

Chapter 59

COUGH MEDICINES

There is very little evidence that the use of cough medicines during pregnancy can have a negative influence on pregnancy or neonatal outcomes and no effects on the risk for congenital malformations. Exposure in early pregnancy carries no detectable risk for the embryo and there is no reason to discuss a termination of the pregnancy.

Table 59.1. Number of women identified using cough medicines

Total	7275
Reported use in early pregnancy	4697
Got prescription later in pregnancy	2786
Both early and later use	208

Type of drug	ATC code	Early use	Later use
Expectorants	R05CA	21	12
Guaifenesin	R05CA01	21	12
Mucolytics	R05CB	2262	1478
Acetylcysteine	R05CB01	392	166
Bromhexine	R05CB02	643	270
Bromhexine+ephedrine	R05CB10	1282	1075
Ambroxol	R05CB06	1	0
Cough suppressants, opioid derivates	R05DA	1052	455
Ethylmorphine	R05DA01	5	2
Ethylmorphine+ephedrine	R05DA20	240	160
Codeine	R05DA04	34	22
Noscapine	R05DA07	771	271
Dextromethorphan	R05DA09	6	3
Other cough suppressants	R05DB	121	120
Pentoxyverine	R05DB05	116	120
Dfenhydramine	R05DB20	5	0
Combinations with opioids	R05FA	1456	931
Ethylmorphine+coccilana+senega	R05FA02	1456	931
Other	R05FB02	138	49[a]
Unspecified	R05	65	3

[a]Two different drugs with the same ATC code are included: difenhydramine with ammonium chloride and quillaja and ammonium chloride.

Cough medicines have their foremost use in connection with upper respiratory tract infections, including common cold. Some chronic conditions like asthma are also associated with the use of cough medicines. Relatively little is known in the literature on pregnancy outcome after maternal use of cough medicines. In the Collaborative Perinatal Project [1] no certain increase in congenital malformation risk was seen among 948 mother-child pairs after use of cough medicines in early pregnancy. Concern was raised concerning one antitussive drug, dextromorphan, but one case-control study [2] and one small prospective study [3] could not verify its teratogenicity. The possibility that the use of common cold and cough medicines could be associated with an increased risk for ventricular septum defects [4] was identified in a retrospective case-control study and the authors linked the observed risk increase to sympathicomimetic components in cough medicines.

Various combinations of cough medicines of different categories were common.

Characteristics of Women using Cough Medicines

Based on women reporting the drug in early pregnancy (n=4697). Each variable is adjusted for all other variables and year of delivery. Comparison with all women who gave birth during the period and with information from the first antenatal care (n=967 742). The odds ratios for maternal age, parity, smoking in early pregnancy, number of previous miscarriages, BMI, subfertility, and country of birth are adjusted for all other variables and are shown in Figure 59.1.

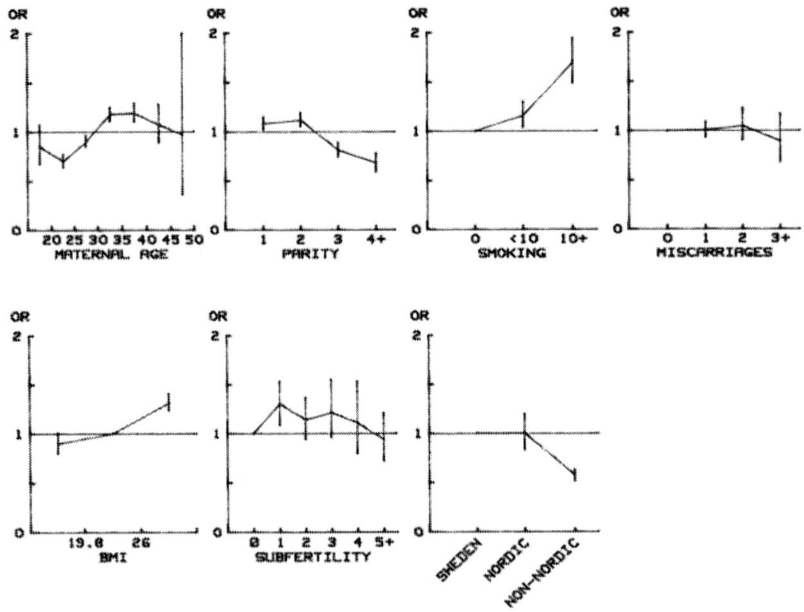

Figure 59.1. Odds ratios for seven maternal characteristics. The odds ratios (OR) for each variable are adjusted for the other variables and year of delivery. Vertical lines mark 95% confidence intervals. For maternal age and parity, each class is compared with all other classes.

Some further maternal characteristics were analyzed, adjusting for year of delivery, maternal age, parity, smoking, and BMI (Table 59.2).

Table 59.2. Some further characteristics of women using cough medicines in early pregnancy

Variable studied	Number	OR	95% CI
Education (1996-2001, 2463 women with drugs, 526 695 in population)			
Unknown	48		
<12 years	194	0.68	0.58-0.80
12 years	1254	1.00	reference
13-14 years	149	1.08	0.91-1.29
≥14 years	818	1.12	1.02-1-24
Family situation			
Unknown	55	-	
Co-habiting	4360	1.00	reference
Living alone	122	0.99	0.82-1.10
Other family situation	121	1.04	0.84-1.28
Work outside home			
Unknown	516	-	-
Full time	2364	1.00	reference
Part time	1189	1.03	0.95-1.11
None	589	0.69	0.62-0.77

Table 59.3. Concomitant drug use (early pregnancy)

Drug group	Number	OR/RR	95% CI
Drugs for stomach ulcer and reflux	65	1.53	1.18-1.92
Drugs for inflammatory bowel disease	14	1.08	0.64-1.83
Insulin	7	0.40	0.19-0.82
Multivitamins	271	0.93	0.84-1.04
Folic acid	186	0.78	0.68-0.91
Antihypertensives	10	0.55	0.30-1.02
Oral contraceptives	17	1.15	0.72-1.85
Progestogens	20	0.85	0.55-1.31
Gonadotropins	11	0.87	0.48-1.58
Systemic corticosteroids	35	1.87	1.35-2.60
Thyroid drugs	40	0.59	0.43-0.81
Antibiotics	1012	8.30	7.82-8.81
NSAIDs	188	2.22	1.92-2.56
Opioids	45	1.78	1.33-2.39
Minor analgesics	1325	4.45	4.19-4.72
Drugs for migraine	7	0.45	0.21-0.95
Anticonvulsants	14	0.97	0.57-1.64
Neuroleptics	10	0.58	0.32-1.07
Sedatives, hypnotics	24	1.03	0.69-1.55
Antidepressants	44	0.72	0.53-0.97
Drugs for rhinitis	542	8.56	7.92-9.24
Antiasthmatics	513	3.56	3.27-3.89
Antihistamines	401	1.46	1.32-1.61
For NVP	267	1.27	1.12-1.43
For allergy	144	1.85	1.57-2.18

Women using cough medicines are thus on average a little older than other women, have low parity, smoke, and have a high BMI. There is a slight association with previous childlessness and women born outside the Nordic countries use less cough medicines than women born within the Nordic countries. Use increases with education while family situation plays little role. Women not working outside home use less such medicines than other women.

There is a strong association with other drugs used at upper respiratory tract infections like antibiotics, drugs for rhinitis, analgesics, and NSAIDs. There is also a strong association with asthma and allergy medicines including systemic corticosteroids. Drugs for stomach ulcer and reflux are also used more often than expected.

Table 59.4.Some maternal diagnoses associated with the use of cough medicines

Diagnosis	Drug use in early pregnancy			Drug use later in pregnancy		
	Number	OR	95% CI	Number	OR	95% CI
Pre-existing diabetes	49	0.75	0.56-0.99	28	0.62	0.43-0.90
Chronic hypertension	53	0.89	0.68-1.17	35	0.85	0.61-1.18
Gestational diabetes	48	1.04	0.78-1.39	26	0.83	0.56-1.23
Preeclampsia	250	1.11	0.97-1.26	149	1.10	0.93-1.31
Hyperemesis gravidarum	49	0.97	0.73-1.30	32	0.92	0.65-1.30
Placenta previa	50	0.89	0.67-1.17	36	0.92	0.66-1.28
Abruptio placentae	67	1.08	0.85-1.38	37	0.86	0.62-1.18
Antepartum bleeding	67	1,03	0.81-1.31	36	0.83	0.60-1.15
Intrapartum bleeding	111	1.06	0.87-1.28	76	1.08	0.86-1.36
Postpartum bleeding	282	1.06	0.94-1.19	159	1.02	0.87-1.20
Delivery induction	515	1.00	0.91-1.10	330	1.03	0.91-1.16
Caesarean section	828	1.07	0.99-1.16	511	1.08	0.97-1.19

No pregnancy complication thus occurred more often than expected.

Outcome after Maternal use of Cough Medicines

Infant Sex

After early exposure there were 2 472 male and 2 289 female infants (one with unknown sex), sex ratio = 1.08 (95% CI 1.02-1.14). After later exposure there were 1 410 male and 1 419 female infants, sex ratio 0.99 (95% CI 0.92-1.07). The normal sex ratio (1.06) in thus contained in both confidence intervals.

Multiple Births

After early exposure there were 70 twin deliveries, OR = 0.97 (95% CI 0.76-1.23) and after later exposure 45 twin deliveries, OR = 1.03 (95% CI 0.76-1.39).

No statistically significant deviations from expected values are thus seen.

No increased risk for perinatal mortality is thus seen.

Only one diagnosis appears in excess, jaundice after early exposure.

Individual cough medicines (irrespective of other components) showed no certain increased risk for any relatively severe malformation (Table 59.9).

Table 59.5. Pregnancy duration and infant birth weight at maternal use of cough medicines

Variable studied	Drug use in early pregnancy			Drug use later in pregnancy		
	Number	OR	95% CI	Number	OR	95% CI
<37 weeks	244	1.07	0.94-1.22	124	0.93	0.77-1.11
<2500g	147	1.01	0.85-1.19	75	0.89	0.71-1.12
≥4500g	182	0.91	0.78-1.06	127	1.01	0.84-1.20
SGA	102	1.02	0.83-1.24	42	0.77	0.57-1.05
LGA	288	0.98	0.87-1.11	201	1.03	0.89-1.19

Table 59.6. Infant mortality after maternal use of cough medicines

Variable studied	Drug use in early pregnancy			Drug use later in pregnancy		
	Number	OR/RR	95% CI	Number	OR/RR	95% CI
Stillbirth	20	1.19	0.76-1.85	8	0.82	0.35-1.62#
Early neonatal death	5	0.71	0.23-1.67#	3	0.70	0.14-2.04#

#observed over expected number with exact Poisson 95% confidence interval.

Table 59.7. Neonatal diagnoses after maternal use of cough medicines

Diagnosis	Drug use in early pregnancy			Drug use later in pregnancy		
	Number	OR	95% CI	Number	OR/RR	95% CI
Hypoglycaemia	154	0.88	0.74-1.03	82	0.77	0.62-0.97
Respiratory diagnoses	228	0.98	0.83-1.08	129	0.96	0.80-1.14
Low Apgar score	73	0.78	0.62-0.98	38	0.74	0.54-1.03
CNS diagnoses	25	0.83	0.56-1.23	12	0.65	0.36-1.16
Jaundice	226	1.18	1.03-1.35	122	1.08	0.90-1.30

Table 59.8. Congenital malformations in infants whose mothers had used cough medicines in early pregnancy

Congenital malformation	Number	OR	95% CI
All malformations	207	0.91	0.79-1.05
Relatively severe malformations	138	0.89	0.85-1.06
Chromosome anomalies	4	0.40	0.11-1.04#
Without chromosome anomalies			
Ear malformations	13	1.17	0.68-2.01
Orofacial clefts	11	1.25	0.62-2.23#
Any cardiovascular defect	50	0.99	0.75-1.31
VSD and/or ASD	28	1.05	0.72-1.52
Unspecified cardiac defects	8	1.62	0.70-3.20#
Hypospadias	14	1.03	0.60-1.74
Pes equinovarus	6	0.85	0.31-1.85#
Poly/syndactyly	7	0.75	0.30-1.54#
Hip (sub)luxation, unstable hip	32	1.05	0.74-1.49

#observed over expected number with exact Poisson 95% confidence interval.

Table 59.9. Relative severe congenital malformations and some specific cough medicines

Drug	Number malformed	Number total	OR/RR	95% CI
Acetylcysteine	14	395	1.01	0.59-1.72
Bromhexine	62	1929	1.00	0.78-1.30
Noscapine	31	782	1.26	0.88-1.81
Ethylmorphine	37	1706	0.66	0.48-0.92
Pentoxyvirine	6	116	1.56	0.53-3.40#

#observed over expected number with exact Poisson 95% confidence interval.

There is thus a non-statistically significant excess of malformations after noscapine. Among them there were five infants with hypospadias (RR = 2.23, 95% CI 0.72-5.71). Among the six malformed infants, exposed to pentoxyvirine, one had VSD and aortic valve insufficiency, one had ASD, one had pulmonary valve stenosis and median cleft palate, and one had penoscrotal hypospadias, one hydronephrosis, and one pes equinovarus.

Summary

There is no evidence in the present material that use of cough medicines has any ill effect on pregnancy or neonatal outcome. This observation also throws doubt on the idea that common cold can act as a teratogenic factor, usually demonstrable in retrospective case-control studies with risks for recall bias.

References

[1] Heinonen OP, Slone D, Shapiro S. *Birth Defects and Drugs in Pregnancy*. Publishing Scineces Group, Inc. Littleton (MA). 1977.

[2] Martínez-Frás M-L, Rodrígues-Pinilla E. Epidemiologic analysis of prenatal exposure to cough medicines containing dextramethorphan: no evidence of human teratogenicity. *Teratology* 2001; 63: 38-41.

[3] Einarson A, Lyszkiewicz D, Koren G. The safety of dextromethorphan in pregnancy. *Chest* 2001; 119: 466-469.

[4] Bateman DN, McElhatton PR, Dickinson D, Wren C, Matthews JNS, O´Keeffe M, Thomas SHL. A case control study to examine the pharmacological factors underlying ventricular septal defects in the North of England. *Eur J Clin Pharmacol* 2004; 60: 635-641.

Chapter 60

ANTIHISTAMINES

Use of antihistamine drugs in early pregnancy has not been shown to be associated with any increased risk for pregnancy or neonatal complications, including congenital malformations. Actually, use of most antihistamines for nausea and vomiting in pregnancy is associated with a lower than expected risk of many outcomes including malformations, probably due to an association between the underlying condition and a favourable pregnancy outcome. – Antihistamines for allergy have no certain teratogenic effect and an increased risk of some pregnancy and neonatal complications may be related to underlying pathology. Use of antihistamines in early pregnancy is no reason to discuss a termination of the pregnancy.

Antihistamines are generally regarded as safe to use during pregnancy [1,2]. Some concerns were raised about a drug used for NVP called Bendectin® but detailed study could not detect any teratogenic effect [3]. More recently, a concern was raised about loratadine and a possible association with the origin of hypospadias [4] but further studies showed that this alarm with all probability was false [5]. One relatively small study of cetirizine [6] found no evidence of teratogenicity.

Antihistamines used for NVP have been associated with a better than expected pregnancy outcome [1,7-8]. It has been postulated that the explanation could be better placental function and hormonal status which might increase the intensity of NVP and therefore result in an association with use of antiemetic drugs [8].

Table 60.1. Number of women identified using antihistamines

Total	68910
Reported use in early pregnancy	53991
Got prescription later in pregnancy	24065
Both early and later use	9146

Type of drug	ATC code	Early use	Later use
Aminoalkyl esters	R06AA	4837	4844
Diphenylhydramine	R06AA02	220	88
Clemastine	R06AA04	4620	4758
Substituted alkylamines	R06AB	529	387
Dexchlorpheniramine	R06AB02	529	387
Phenothiazine derivates	R06AD	10604	7315
Alimemazine	R06AD01	108	49
Promethazine	R06AD02	4714	3415
Promethazine+caffeine+ephedrine	R06AD52	5744	3914
Thietylperazine	R06AD03	314	186
Piperazine derivates	R06AE	34585	12040
Cyclizine	R06AE03	2078	1224
Chlorcyclizine	R06AE04	0	2
Meclozine	R06AE05	29774	10012
Meclozine+hydroxzine+nicotinic acid	R06AE55	3	5
Cetirizine	R06AE07	3470	964
Combination of antihistamines	R06AK06	3	0
Other antihistamines	R06AX	7176	1201
Cyproheptadine	R06AX02	13	13
Terfenadine	R06AX12	1180	65
Loratadine	R06AX13	5031	735
Acrivastine	R06AX18	54	12
Ebastine	R06AX22	494	253
Mizolastine	R06AX25	2	1
Fexofenadine	R06AX27	185	41
Unspecified	R06	73	6

Drugs of different categories were often combined (Table 60.2).

Table 60.2. Use of two antihistamines belonging to different groups

	Substituted alkylamines	Phenothiazine derivates	Piperazine derivates	Other
Early use				
Aminoalkyl esters	11	110	383	240
Substituted alkylamines	-	5	12	33
Phenothiazine derivates	-	-	2530	42
Piperazine derivates	-	-	-	287
Later use				
Aminoalkylesters	12	190	230	98
Substituted alkylamines	-	12	11	5
Phenothiazine derivates	-	-	1011	11
Piperazine derivates	-	-	-	58

A combination of three different antihistamine groups in early pregnancy was reported by 54 women and in later pregnancy by 13. The most common combination was aminoalkyl ester + phenothiazine derivate + piperazine derivate (32 women, early pregnancy).

Among the different antihistamines, some were mainly used for NVP (diphenhydramine, promethazine, cyclizine, meclozine) and the remaining ones were mainly used as antiallergics. In early pregnancy 39 188 women reported the use of antihstamines for NVP and 15 605 antihistamines for allergy, in 817 instances both types were reported. In later pregnancy the corresponding numbers were 17 324, 7 303, and 568. Thus about 70% of usage was related to NVP.

CHARACTERISTICS OF WOMEN USING DRUGS FOR ANTIHISTAMINES

Characteristics are given separately for women who used antihistamines for NVP (n=39 182, six missing maternal age, unbroken graphs) and for women using antihistamines for allergy (n=15 605, dashed graphs). Each variable is adjusted for all other variables and year of delivery. Comparison with all women who gave birth during the period and with information from the first antenatal care (n=967 742). The odds ratios for maternal age, parity, smoking in early pregnancy, number of previous miscarriages, BMI, subfertility, and country of birth are adjusted for all other variables and are shown in Figure 60.1.

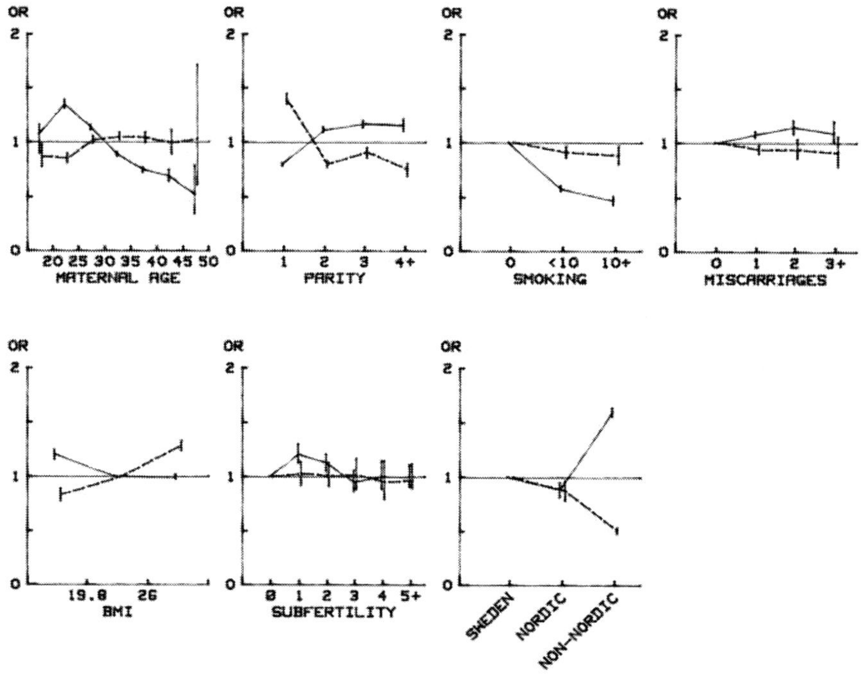

Figure 60.1. Odds ratios for seven maternal characteristics. The odds ratios (OR) for each variable are adjusted for the other variables and year of delivery. Vertical lines mark 95% confidence intervals. For maternal age and parity, each class is compared with all other classes. Unbroken graphs show data for antihistamines mainly used for NVP, dashed graphs for antihistamines mainly used for allergy.

Some further maternal characteristics were analyzed, adjusting for year of delivery, maternal age, parity, smoking, and BMI (Table 60.3).

Table 60.3. Some further characteristics of women using antihistamines in early pregnancy

Variable studied	Antihistmines for NPV			Antihistamines for allergy		
	Number	OR	95% CI	Number	OR	95% CI
Education (1996-2001, 18 931 women with drugs for NVP, 7 722 women with drugs for allergy, 526 695 in population)						
Unknown	638	-	-	92	-	-
<12 years	2596	1.29	1.23-1.36	606	0.77	0.70-0.84
12 years	9607	1.00	reference	3907	1.00	reference
13-14 years	885	0.96	0.93-1.00	506	1.16	1.06-1.28
≥14 years	5205	0.95	0.92-0.98	2551	1.11	1.05-1.17
Family situation						
Unknown	399	-	-	256	-	-
Co-habiting	29142	1.00	reference	14463	1.00	reference
Living alone	671	0.88	0.81-0.95	428	1.17	1.06-1.30
Other family situation	8970	1.60	1.56-1.64	458	1.16	1.05-1.30
Work outside home						
Unknown	5339	-	-	1866	-	-
Full time	16265	1.00	reference	8122	1.00	reference
Part time	9443	1.07	1.03-1.10	3578	0.99	0.93-1.01
None	8135	1.30	1.27-1.35	2039	0.76	0.72-0.80

Table 60.4. Concomitant drug use (early pregnancy)

Drug group	Anthihistamines for NVP			Antihistamines for allergy		
	Number	OR	95% CI	Number	OR	95% CI
Drugs for stomach ulcer and reflux	887	2.93	2.74-3.14	244	1.88	1.65-2.13
Drugs for inflammatory bowel disease	48	0.43	0.33-0.57	45	1.10	0.82-1.48
Insulin	46	0.34	0.25-0.44	34	0.61	0.44-0.85
Multivitamins	1756	0.82	0.78-0.86	634	0.72	0.66-0.77
Folic acid	1914	1.07	1.02-1.12	527	0.73	0.67-0.80
Antihypertensives	101	0.80	0.66-0.98	54	0.99	0.76-1.30
Oral contraceptives	94	0.67	0.55-0.83	36	1.57	1.25-1.97
Progest.ogens	141	0.90	0.76-1.07	43	0.59	0.44-0.80
Gonadotropins	68	0.75	0.59-0.95	21	0.53	0.35-0.89
Systemic corticosteroids	110	0.74	0.61-0.90	533	11.2	10.4-12.1
Thyroid drugs	369	0.72	0.65-0.79	212	1.06	0.93-1.22
Antibiotics	1242	0.98	0.93-1.04	601	1.29	1.19-1.40
NSAIDs	763	1.07	0.99-1.15	316	1.10	0.98-1.23
Opioids	335	1.81	1.62-2.02	114	1.51	1.26-1.82
Minor analgesics	5151	1.78	1.73-1.84	1162	0.95	0.90-1.01
Drugs for migraine	112	1.00	0.83-1.21	76	1.68	1.34-2.10
Anticonvulsants	70	0.62	0.49-0.78	29	0.65	0.45-0.94
Neuroleptics	924	9.20	8.62-9.82	48	0.93	0.70-1.24
Sedatives, hypnotics	415	2.86	2.59-3.16	201	3.18	2.77-3.65
Antidepressants	842	1.91	1.78-2.05	255	1.40	1.24-1.59
Drugs for rhinitis	608	1.09	1.00-1.19	1346	13.5	12.9-14.0
Antiasthmatics	1021	0.81	0.86-0.76	1194	11.9	11.6-12.3
Cough medicine	256	1.29	1.13-1.46	181	1.81	1.53-2.13

Maternal characteristics for the two groups of antihistamines thus differ markedly in many aspects.

Use of antihistamines for NVP is strongly associated with use of psychopharmaca, notably neuroleptics, a group which contains at least two drugs also used for NVP (dixyrazine an prochlorperazine). An association with some other drug groups is also seen.

Use of antihistamines for allergy is as expected associated with systemic corticosteroids and drugs for rhinitis and asthma but also with sedatives/hypnotics and some other drug categories.

There seems to be an overlapping between the associations with the two groups of antihistamines – some women who used antihistamines for NVP also used antihistamines for allergy and this occurred more often than among other women (OR = 5.54, 95% CI 5.33-5.76).

Table 60.5. Some maternal diagnoses associated with the use of antihistamines

Diagnosis	Drug use in early pregnancy			Drug use later in pregnancy		
	Number	OR	95% CI	Number	OR	95% CI
Antihistamines for NVP						
Pre-existing diabetes	383	0.78	0.70-0.86	244	1.04	0.91-1.18
Chronic hypertension	406	0.94	0.85-1.04	250	1.20	1.05-1.36
Gestational diabetes	349	1.02	0.92-1.14	205	1.30	1.13-1.49
Preeclampsia	1657	0.96	0.91-1.01	860	1.12	1.04-1.20
Hyperemesis gravidarum	706	1.85	1.72-2.00	419	2.30	2.08-2.53
Placenta previa	422	1.00	0.91-1.11	251	1.24	1.10-1.41
Abruptio placentae	475	1.02	0.93-1.12	271	1.22	1.08-1.38
Antepartum bleeding	502	0.98	0.90-1.08	282	1.23	1.09-1.39
Intrapartum bleeding	835	1.07	1.00-1.15	471	1.28	1.17-1.41
Postpartum bleeding	2124	0.99	0.94-1.03	995	1.08	1.01-1.15
Delivery induction	4472	1.11	1.08-1.15	2266	1.24	1.18-1.29
Caesarean section	6298	1.09	1.05-1.12	3043	1.14	1.10-1.19
Antihistamines for allergy						
Pre-existing diabetes	204	0.95	0.82-1.09	114	1.04	0.86-1.26
Chronic hypertension	209	1.08	0.94-1.24	113	1.13	0.94-1.37
Gestational diabetes	173	1.16	0.99-1.15	86	1.17	0.94-1.45
Preeclampsia	836	1.07	0.99-1.15	449	1.22	1.11-1.34
Hyperemesis gravidarum	189	1.16	1.00-1.34	103	1.22	1.00-1.49
Placenta previa	200	1.11	0.96-1.28	100	1.07	0.88-1.31
Abruptio placentae	213	1.07	0.93-1.23	109	1.07	0.88-1.30
Antepartum bleeding	229	1.04	0.91-1.19	113	1.06	0.88-1.39
Intrapartum bleeding	366	1.08	0.97-1.20	192	1.07	0.92-1.24
Postpartum bleeding	928	1.02	0.96-1.10	482	1.18	1.07-1.29
Delivery induction	1863	1.09	1.04-1.15	1151	1.43	1.34-1.52
Caesarean section	2756	1.08	1.04-1.13	1365	1.10	1.03-1.16

After early use of antihistmines for NVP, the only pregnancy complications which are significantly increased are hyperemesis gravidarum and intrapartum bleeding but both delivery inductions and caesarean sections occur more often than expected. After later use, the association with hypremesis is still stronger but now a number of different pregnancy complications occur more often than expected and all odds ratios are higher than after early use. Long-standing NVP or hyperemesis gravidarum is apparently associated with a moderately increased risk for various pregnancy complications.

After early use of antihistamines for allergy, a moderately increased risk for hyperemesis gravidarum is seen, again indicating the association between the two groups of antihistamines. The occurrence of delivery induction and caesarean section is increased also for this group of antihistamines. After later use, an association is seen with preeclampsia, hyperemesis, and postpartum bleeding and delivery induction and caesarean section occur more often than expected.

OUTCOME AFTER MATERNAL USE OF ANTIHISTAMINES

Infant Sex

After early use of antihistamines for NVP, there were 19 160 male and 20 898 female infants born (11 with unknown sex), sex ratio 0.92 (95% CI 0.90-0.93) and after later use there were 8 595 male and 9 104 female infants (eight with unknown sex), sex ratio 0.94 (95% CI 0.92-0.97). The low sex ratio (the normal sex ratio is 1.06) is typical for infants born after intense NVP or hyperemesis gravidarum.

After early use of antihistamines for allergy, there were 8 184 male and 7 650 female infants (5 with unknown sex), sex ratio 1.07 (95% CI 1.04-1.10), and after later use 3 812 male and 3 664 female infants (three with unknown sex), sex ratio 1.04 (95% CI 0.99-1.09). The normal sex ratio is thus contained within both confidence intervals.

Multiple Births

After early use of antihistamines for NVP, there were 875 twin deliveries (OR =1.56, 95% CI 1.46-1.68) and nine triplet deliveries. After later use, there were 373 twin deliveries (OR 1.60, 95% CI 1.44-1.77) and five triplet deliveries. A high rate of multiple birth is a well-known factor in the origin of NVP and hyperemesis gravidarum.

Table 60.6. Pregnancy duration and infant birth weight at maternal use of antihistamines

Variable studied	Drug use in early pregnancy			Drug use later in pregnancy		
	Number	OR	95% CI	Number	OR	95% CI
Antihistamines for NVP						
<37 weeks	1680	0.95	0.89-0.98	842	1.05	0.98-1.13
<2500g	975	0.88	0.82-0.94	525	1.05	0.96-1.15
≥4500g	1692	1.04	0.99-1.09	719	1.01	0.93-1.09
SGA	676	0.91	0.84-0.98	335	0.99	0.88-1.10
LGA	2637	1.08	1.04-1.12	1110	1.03	0.96-1.09
Antihistamines for allergy						
<37 weeks	781	1.01	0.94-1.09	365	1.02	0.92-1.14
<2500g	498	1.02	0.93-1.12	213	0.95	0.83-1.09
≥4500g	636	0.99	0.91-1.07	302	0.98	0.87-1.10
SGA	363	1.04	0.93-1.15	151	0.97	0.82-1.14
LGA	980	1.03	0.96-1.10	463	1.05	0.95-1.15

After early use of antihistamines for allergy, there were 238 twin deliveries (OR = 1.01, 95% CI 0.88-1.15) and two triplet deliveries. After later use, there were 174 twin deliveries (OR = 1.64, 95% CI 1.41-1.91). The high rate of twin deliveries after later use explains some of the increased risks for pregnancy complications (see above).

The risks for preterm birth, low birth weight, and SGA are thus slightly but significantly reduced and the risk for LGA slightly increased after early use of antihistamines for NVP while no certain effects are seen after later use of antihistamines for NVP or use of antihistamines for allergy.

Table 60.7. Infant mortality after maternal use of antihistamines

Variable studied	Drug use in early pregnancy			Drug use later in pregnancy		
	Number	OR	95% CI	Number	OR	95% CI
Antihistamines for NVP						
Stillbirth	124	1.02	0.85-1.22	46	0.89	0.66-1.19
Early neonatal death	48	0.83	0.62-1.00	19	0.80	0.35-1.25
Antihistamines for allergy						
Stillbirth	45	0.80	0.60-1.08	26	1.00	0.68-1.47
Early neonatal death	25	1.10	0.74-1.64	8	0.80	0.35-1.58#

#observed over expected number with exact Poisson 95% confidence interval.

The risk for early neonatal death is thus reduced after early and later use of antihistamines for NVP but statistical significance is not reached.

Table 60.8. Neonatal diagnoses after maternal use of antihistamines

Diagnosis	Drug use in early pregnancy			Drug use later in pregnancy		
	Number	OR	95% CI	Number	OR	95% CI
Antihistamines for NVP						
Hypoglycaemia	1204	0.90	0.84-0.95	657	1.07	0.99-1.16
Respiratory diagnoses	1766	0.93	0.89-0.98	775	0.98	0.91-1.05
Low Apgar score	626	0.87	0.80-0.94	328	1.11	0.99-1.24
CNS diagnoses	222	0.96	0.84-1.10	134	1.20	1.01-1.42
Jaundice	1667	1.07	1.02-1.13	813	1.14	1.06-1.23
Antihistamines for allergy						
Hypoglycaemia	572	0.96	0.89-1.05	313	1.13	1.01-1.27
Respiratory diagnoses	826	1.01	0.94-1.08	375	1.05	0.93-1.14
Low Apgar score	290	0.90	0.80-1.01	147	1.05	0.89-1.24
CNS diagnoses	117	1.19	0.99-1.43	54	1.10	0.84-1.44
Jaundice	692	1.10	1.02-1.19	312	1.07	0.95-1.20

After early use of antihistamines against NVP, neonatal outcome (with the exception of jaundice) is better than expected while a tendency towards the opposite is seen after later use even though only the odds ratios for CNS diagnoses and jaundice reach statistical significance. Early use of antihistamines against allergy gives an increased risk for jaundice and after later use the risk for hypoglycaemia is increased.

After exposure to antihistamines used for NVP, the total malformation rate is thus slightly but significantly low and the same is seen for some malformations: orofacial clefts, any cardiovascular malformation, pylorostenosis, hypospadias, and cystic kidney. Among individual such drugs, a significantly low malformation rate is seen only for meclozine but the estimates are low also for diphenhydramine and cyclizine, but not for the two relatively large materials after exposure to promethazine. Promethazine is used also for other purposes than as an antiemetic which could explain the difference, but the sex ratio after exposure to this drug is 0.92 (95% CI 0.88-0.95) which is the same as for all antihistamines used at NVP. This indicates that promethazine actually carries a higher risk than the other similar drugs (notably meclozine) which makes the low risk associated with NVP to disappear.

Table 60.9. Congenital malformations in infants whose mothers had used antihistamines in early pregnancy

Congenital malformation	Antihistamines for NVP			Antihistamines for allergy		
	Number	OR	95% CI	Number	OR	95%CI
All malformations	1722	0.93	0.89-0.98	743	0.98	0.91-1.06
Relatively severe malformations	1153	0.91	0.86-0.97	518	1.01	0.92-1.10
Chromosome anomalies	66	0.90	0.70-1.15	29	0.94	0.65-1.36
Without chromosome anomalies						
Any CNS malformations	37	0.78	0.56-1.08	21	1.08	0.70-1.67
Neural tube defects	8	0.53	0.27-1.07	6	0.86	0.32-1.08#
Eye malformations	41	1.05	0.76-1.43	16	1.03	0.63-1.70
Ear malformations	89	0.98	0.79-1.21	42	1.12	0.82-1.52
Orofacial clefts	54	0.75	0.57-0.98	35	1.21	0.87-1.70
Any cardiovascular defect	372	0.90	0.81-0.98	182	1.08	0.93-1.26
VSD and/or ASD	196	0.88	0.77-1.02	97	1.07	0.88-1.32
Unspecified cardiac defects	40	1.00	0.73-1.38	13	0.80	0.46-1.38
Oesophageal atresia	10	0.90	0.48-1.69	2	0.40	0.05-1.45#
Small bowel atresia	4	0.40	0.11-1.03	2	0.67	0.08-2.42#
Anal atresia	18	1.18	0.73-1.90	6	0.91	0.34-1.99#
Pylorostenosis	30	0.81	0.61-0.99	14	1.21	0.71-2.07
Abdominal wall defects	11	1.15	0.57-2.05#	4	0.92	0.25-2.35#
Diaphragmatic hernias	10	1.16	0.56-2.13#	1	0.27	0.01-1.52#
Hypospadias	93	0.81	0.66-0.99	44	0.93	0.69-1.25
Kidney a/dysgenesis	6	0.52	0.24-1.17	3	0.66	0.14-1.94#
Cystic kidney	7	0.45	0.22-0.94	3	0.51	0.10-1.48#
Pes equinovarus	53	1.00	0.76-1.31	19	0.84	0.53-1.33
Poly/syndactyly	74	0.91	0.72-1.15	29	0.92	0.64-1.34
Limb reduction defect	18	0.81	0.50-1.30	9	0.98	0.44-1.86#
Hip (sub)luxation, unstable hip	225	0.93	0.81-1.06	70	0.68	0.53-0.86
Craniostenosis	22	0.97	0.63-1.49	10	1.04	0.50-1.92#

#observed over expected number with exact Poisson 95% confidence interval.

Among antihistamines used for allergy, no certain effect on the malformation risk is seen. The only indicated increased risk is after dexchlorpheniramine but it does not quite reach statitical significance.

The relatively severe malformations observed after exposure to dexchlorpheniramine are shown in Table 60.11.

Among the 25 malformed infants, eight had cardiac defects (RR = 1.40, 95% CI 0.60-2.76). There seemed to be no specific pattern of other malformations even though some were serious. This supports the idea that the finding was random but further data are needed.

Table 60.10. The relatively severe malformations according to antihistamines used

Drug or drug group	Number malformed	Number total	OR	95% CI
Drug group				
Aminoalkyl esters	164	4949	1.04	0.89-1.32
Substituted alkylamines	25	537	1.45	0.97-2.17
Phenothiazine derivates	334	10895	0.99	0.89-1.11
Piperazine derivates	1024	35285	0.91	0.87-0.97
Other antihistamines	223	7269	0.93	0.81-1.06
Specific drugs				
Diphenhydramine	3	226	0.42	0.09-1.23#
Clemastine	161	4706	1.07	0.92-1.26
Dexchlorpheniramine	25	537	1.45	0.97-2.17
Alimemazine	3	109	0.90	0.19-2.64#
Promethazine	150	4830	1.00	0.85-1.18
Promethazine+caffeine+ephedrine	184	5923	1.01	0.87-1.17
Thietylperazine	5	321	0.59	0.27-1.31
Cyclizine	58	2128	0.87	0.67-1.13
Meclozine	868	30393	0.90	0.84-0.96
Cetirizine	120	3516	1.06	0.88-1.27
Terfenadine	35	1201	0.80	0.57-1.12
Loratadine	162	5095	0.97	0.83-1.14
Acrivastine	1	56	0.54	0.01-3.01#
Ebastine	13	496	0.83	0.48-1.45
Fexofenadine	10	305	1.05	0.50-1.93
Desloratadine	2	187	0.35	0.04-1.28#

#observed over expected number with exact Poisson 95% confidence interval.

Table 60.11. Specification of malformations observed after exposure to dexchlorpheniramine in early pregnancy

Congenital malformations	Number
Anophthalmia+holoprosencepahly+nose malformation+cleft lip/palate	1[a]
Lacrimal duct stenosis	1
Cleft lip/palate	1
Median cleft palate	1
Ventricular septum defect	1
Atrium septum defect	1
Ventricular and atrium septum defect	2
Endocardial cushion defect	1
Unspecified cardiac defect	1
Tracheomalacia	1
Pylorostenosis	1
Omphalocele+ ventricular septum defect	1
Hypospadias	1
Unspecified genital malformation	1
Ureter duplication and ureter obstruction	1
Hydronephrosis	2
Craniostenosis	2
Chondrodystrophy+lens luxation+atrium septum defect+unstable hip	1
Unspecified musculoskeletal malformation	1
Down syndrome	3

[a]This infant appeares to have trisomy 13 but had no such diagnosis.

Summary

Antihistamines used for NVP is associated with a better pregnancy outcome than expected, including a lower than expected risk for a congenital malformation. There seems to be a difference between promethazine and other such drugs but this must be verified. It should be stressed that NVP usually does not appear until a few weeks into pregnancy and a possible effect on the formation of malformations originating very early (e.g., neural tube defects) cannot be evaluated from the present or similar studies.

Antihistamines used for allergy seem to be associated with some pregnancy complications but otherwise no certain ill effects are noted. An increased risk for hypoglycaemia may well be random or due to underlying pathology and notably gestational diabetes. No certain teratogeni effect is seen – the only indicated and statistically non-significant increase is seen after exposure to dexchlorpheniramine but this observation must be further explored.

Reference

[1] Seto A, Einarson T, Gideon K. Pregnancy outcome following first trimester exposure to antihistamines: meta-analysis. *Am J Perinatol* 1997; 14: 119-124.

[2] Källén B. Use of antihistamine drugs in early pregnancy and delivery outcome. *J Maternal-Foetal Neonat Med* 2002; 11: 146-152.

[3] Brent BL. Bendectin: review of the medical literature of a comprehensively studied human nonteratogen and the most prevalent tortogen-litigen. *Reprod Toxicol* 1995; 9: 337-349.

[4] Källén B, Otterblad Olausson P. Monitoring of maternal drug use and infant congenital malformations. Does loratadine cause hypospadias? *Int J Risk Safety Med* 2001; 14: 115-119.

[5] Källén B, Otterblad Olausson P. No increased risk of infant hypospadias after maternal use of loratadine in early pregnancy. *Int J Med Sci* 2006; 3: 106-107.

[6] Webet-Schoendorfer C, Schaefer C.The safety of cetirizine during pregnancy. A prospective observational cohort study. *Reprod Toxicol* 2008; 26: 19-23.

[7] Källén B, Mottet I. Delivery outcome after the use of meclozine in early pregnancy. *Europ J Epidemiol* 2003; 18: 665-669.

[8] Asker C, Norstedt Wikner B, Källén B. Use of antiemetic drugs during pregnancy in Sweden. *Eur J Clin Pharmacol* 2005; 61: 899-906.

Chapter 61

OPHTHALMOLOGICALS

It is unlikely that drugs applied locally in the eye could be absorbed to a degree which could represent a hazard for the embryo or foetus. No certain deviations in pregnancy or neonatal outcome were seen with two exceptions. One was an increase of the rate of infants with cystic kidney which appeared to be a random occurrence, the other an increased risk of severe eye malformations. If a link exists is seem more likely that it consists of a genetic link than it is a drug effect.

Locally applied ophthalmologicals may be absorbed but the amounts are unlikely to cause any damage to the embryo or foetus, even if many of the drugs are pharmacologically potent. Early studies in mice indicated that corticosteroids, applied locally in the eye, could increase the risk for cleft palate in the offspring [1] but as far as I know there are no systematic studies on this issue in humans.

Table 61.1. Number of women identified using ophthalmologicals

Total	2949
Reported use in early pregnancy	2008
Got prescription later in pregnancy	1202
Both early and later use	261

Type of drug	ATC code	Early use	Later use
Antiinfectives	S01A	92	89
Chloramphenicol	S01AA01	40	30
Gentamicin	S01AA11	0	1
Tobramycin	S01AA12	1	0
Fusidic acid	S01AA13	26	23
Antibiotic unspecified	S01AA20	0	1
Aciclovir	S01AD03	17	32
Bibrocathol	S01AX05	2	3
Ciprofloxacin	S01AX13	0	1
Unspecified antiinfective	S01A	2	0
Antiinflammatory agents	S01B	111	77
Dexamethasone	S01BA01	40	29
Hydrocortisone	S01BA02	27	16
Rimexolone	S01BA13	3	1
Diclofenac	S01BC03	7	14
Unspecified antiinflammatory agent	S01B	2	0

Table 61.1 (Continued)

Type of drug	ATC code	Early use	Later use
Antiinflammatory agents+antiinfectives	S01C	1	2
Prednisolone+sulfa+metaoxedrin	S01C02	1	2
Antiglaucoma preparations, miotics	S01E	83	60
Epinephrine	S01EA01	6	1
Dipevifrine	S01AE02	1	1
Brimonidine	S01AE05	5	5
Pilocarpine	S01EB01	7	3
Pilocarpine+physostigmine	S01EB51	1	0
Acetazolamide	S01EC01	18	14
Diclofenamide	S01EC02	1	0
Dorzolamide	S01EC03	3	3
Brinzolamide	S01EC04	5	5
Timolol	S01ED01	29	18
Timolol+dorzolamide/pilocarpine/latanoprost	S01ED51	9	5
Betaxolol	S01ED02	1	1
Latanoprost	S01EE01	15	14
Travoprost	S01EE04	0	1
Unspecified antiglaucoma preparation	S01EX00	0	9
Mydriatics and cycloplegics	S01F	35	19
Atropine	S01FA01	22	11
Cyclopentolate	S01FA04	7	3
Homatropine	S01FA05	1	1
Tropicamide	S01FA06	5	4
Decongestants and antiallergics	S01G	1632	936
Naphazoline	S01GA01	1	1
Naphazoline+antazoline	S01GA51	152	63
Phenylephrine+zinc sulphate	S01GA55	5	2
Cromoglicid acid	S01GX01	1385	802
Levocabastine	S01GX02	19	18
Nedocromil	S01GX04	63	34
Emedastine	S01GX06	19	22
Olopatadine	S01GX09	1	0
Unspecified decongestant/antiallergic	S01G	2	0
Local anestethics	S01H	23	2
Oxybuprocaine	S01HA02	6	0
Tetracaine	S01HA03	17	2
Diagnostics	S01J	12	8
Fluorescein	S01JA01	7	4
Hyaluronic acid	S01KA	5	4
Other ophthalmologicals	S01X	24	29
Artifical tears	S01XA	20	27
Other	S01X	4	2

The largest group is thus decongestants and antiallergics (notably cromoglicid acid), followed by antinflammatory drugs, antiinfective drugs, and drugs for glaucoma.

CHARACTERISTICS OF WOMEN USING OPHTHALMOLOGICALS

Based on women reporting the drug in early pregnancy (n=2 008). Each variable is adjusted for all other variables and year of delivery. Comparison with all women who gave birth during the period and with information from the first antenatal care (n=967 742). The odds ratios for maternal age, parity, smoking in early pregnancy, number of previous miscarriages, BMI, subfertility, and country of birth are adjusted for all other variables and are shown in Figure 61.1.

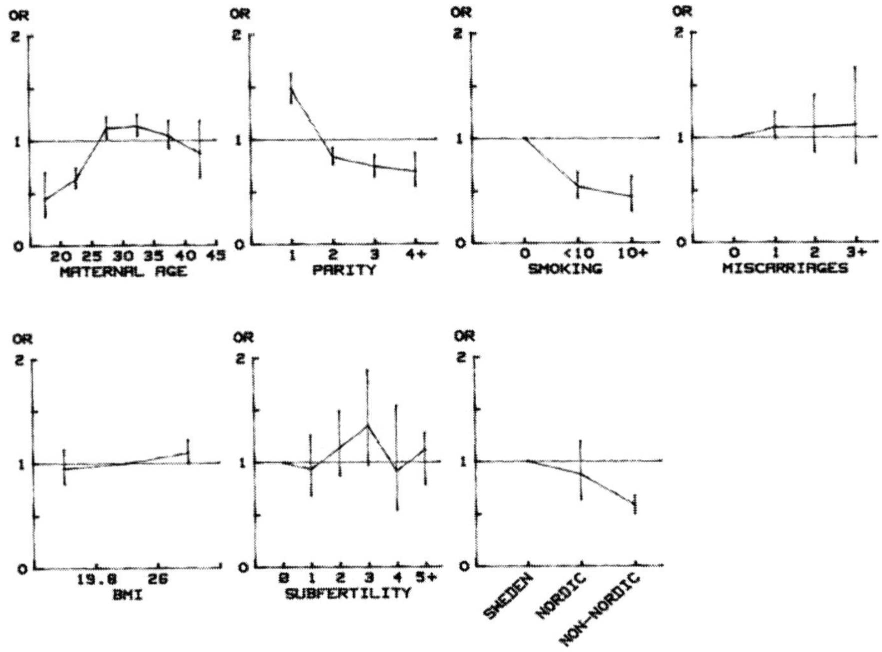

Figure 61.1. Odds ratios for seven maternal characteristics. The odds ratios (OR) for each variable are adjusted for the other variables and year of delivery. Vertical lines mark 95% confidence intervals. For maternal age and parity, each class is compared with all other classes.

Some further maternal characteristics were analyzed, adjusting for year of delivery, maternal age, parity, smoking, and BMI (Table 61.2).

Young women thus used ophthalmologicals less often than expected, first parity was associated with a high use, women using these drugs smoked less than expected and were under-represented among women born outside the Nordic countries. They had a higher education than expected and were more often than expected cohabiting and worked outside home.

There was thus a strong association with drugs used for allergy, rhinitis, and asthma including systemic corticosteroids. Other associations are with opioids, drugs for inflammatory bowel disease, and antihistamines for NVP.

Table 61.2. Some further characteristics of women using ophthalmologicals in early pregnancy

Variable studied	Number	OR	95% CI
Education (1996-2001, 876 women with drugs, 526 695 in population)			
Unknown	13	-	-
<12 years	51	0.63	0.47-0.86
12 years	415	1.00	reference
13-14 years	51	1.40	1.21-1.63
>14 years	146	1.35	1.17-1.56
Family situation			
Unknown	26	-	-
Co-habiting	1912	1.00	reference
Living alone	30	0.98	0.54-1.14
Other family situation	28	0.53	0.34-0.83
Work outside home			
Unknown	207	-	-
Full time	1082	1.00	reference
Part time	452	1.00	0.88-1.13
None	255	0.76	0.65-0.90

Table 61.3. Concomitant drug use (early pregnancy)

Drug group	Number	OR/RR	95% CI
Drugs for stomach ulcer and reflux	22	1.27	0.84-1.94
Drugs for inflammatory bowel disease	15	2.46	1.38-4.06#
Insulin	10	1.40	0.67-2.58#
Multivitamins	135	0.94	0.79-1.12
Folic acid	94	0.82	0.66-1.01
Oral contraceptives	1	0.17	0.04-0.97#
Progestogens	8	0.72	0.37-1.40
Gonadotrophines	3	0.51	0.10-1.48#
Systemic corticosteroids	37	7.14	5.41-9.25#
Thyroid drugs	34	1.20	0.85-1.68
Antibiotics	73	1.19	0.94-1.50
NSAIDs	38	1.03	0.75-1.63
Opioids	18	1.89	1.20-2.99
Minor analgesics	149	0.94	0.80-1.12
Drugs for migraine	11	1.77	0.88-3.10#
Anticonvulsants	8	1.38	0.60-2.72#
Neuroleptics	7	1.01	0.41-2.08#
Sedatives, hypnotics	10	1.27	0.68-2.34#
Antidepressants	18	0.72	0.45-1.14
Drugs for rhinitis	945	61.9	58.8-65.1
Antiasthmatics	555	11.9	11.0-12.8
Cough medicine	27	2.61	1.81-3.77
Antihistamines	713	8.78	8.12-9.48
For NVP	221	2.58	2.25-2.96
For allergy	525	22.1	20.6-23.7

#observed over expected number with exact Poisson 95% confidence interval.

Table 61.4. Some maternal diagnoses associated with the use of ophthalmologicals

Diagnosis	Drug use in early pregnancy			Drug use later in pregnancy		
	Number	OR	95% CI	Number	OR	95% CI
Pre-existing diabetes	27	1.04	0.71-1.53	15	0.90	0.54-1.51
Chronic hypertension	26	1.10	0.74-1.62	18	1.18	0.74-1.18
Gestational diabetes	20	1.13	0.72-1.75	12	1.08	0.61-1.92
Preeclampsia	94	0.94	0.76-1.16	52	0.87	0.66-1.15
Hyperemesis gravidarum	19	0.96	0.61-1.51	15	1.16	0.69-1.94
Placenta previa	23	1.04	0.69-1.58	13	0.90	0.52-1.56
Abruptio placentae	26	1.08	0.73-1.59	14	0.90	0.53-1.53
Antepartum bleeding	32	1.20	0.84-1.20	23	1.43	0.95-2.16
Intrapartum bleeding	46	1.06	0.79-1.43	29	0.99	0.68-1.44
Postpartum bleeding	122	1.05	0.87-1.27	81	1.19	0.95-1.50
Delivery induction	204	0.90	0.78-1.05	127	0.89	0.74-1.07
Caesarean section	349	1.05	0.94-1.18	214	1.02	0.88-1.19

Rates of maternal diagnoses thus do not deviate from expected values.

Outcome after Maternal use of Ophthalmologicals

Infant Sex

After early exposure, 1 063 male and 974 female infants were born, sex ratio 1.09 (95%CI 1.00-1.19). After later exposure, there were 626 male and 589 female infants, sex ratio 1.06 (95% CI 0.95-1.19). The normal sex ratio (1.06) is thus contained in the confidence intervals.

Multiple Births

After early exposure, there were 27 twin deliveries (OR = 0.91, 95% CI 0.62-1.34) and two triplet deliveries. After later exposure, there were 13 twin deliveries (OR = 0.73, 95% CI 0.42-1.26).

Table 61.5. Pregnancy duration and infant birth weight at maternal use of ophthalmologicals

Variable studied	Drug use in early pregnancy			Drug use later in pregnancy		
	Number	OR	95% CI	Number	OR	95% CI
<37 weeks	95	0.98	0.80-1.21	58	1.01	0.77-1.32
<2500g	67	1.11	0.87-1.42	27	0.75	0.51-1.09
≥4500g	79	0.98	0.78-1.23	36	0.73	0.52-1.01
SGA	39	0.90	0.66-1.25	20	0.81	0.52-1.27
LGA	110	0.93	0.80-1.18	67	0.94	0.73-1.21

No deviations are thus seen with respect to pregnancy duration or birth weight.

Table 61.6. Infant mortality after maternal use of ophthalmologicals

Variable studied	Drug use in early pregnancy			Drug use later in pregnancy		
	Number	RR	95% CI	Number	RR	95% CI
Stillbirth	5	0.70	0.23-1.64	4	0.95	0.26-2.44
Early neonatal death	1	-	-	0	-	-

There was no excess perinatal mortality.

Table 61.7. Neonatal diagnoses after maternal use of ophthalmologicals

Diagnosis	Drug use in early pregnancy			Drug use later in pregnancy		
	Number	OR/RR	95% CI	Number	OR/RR	95% CI
Hypoglycaemia	67	0.91	0.71-1.16	32	0.72	0.51-1.02
Respiratory diagnoses	64	1.11	0.86-1.43	64	1.11	0.86-1.43
Low Apgar score	14	0.35	0.21-0.57	14	0.63	0.37-1.06
CNS diagnoses	12	0.96	0.55-1.66	9	1.02	0.47-1.94#
Jaundice	90	1.05	0.85-1.30	54	1.04	0.79-1.37

#observed over expected number with exact Poisson 95% confidence interval.

No signs of abnormalities in neonatal diagnoses are thus present.

Table 61.8. Congenital malformations in infants whose mothers had used ophthalmologicals in early pregnancy

Congenital malformation	Number	OR	95% CI
All malformation	101	1.06	0.87-1.30
Relatively severe malformation	74	1.16	0.92-1.47
Chromosome anomalies	4	1.09	0.44-6.89#
Without chromosome anomalies			
Any CNS malformations	3	1.34	0.28-3.91#
Eye malformations	6	3.28	1.20-7.74#
Ear malformations	5	1.10	0.31-2.58#
Orofacial clefts	3	0.83	0.17-2.42#
Any cardiovascular defect	20	0.93	0.59-1.44
VSD and/or ASD	14	1.20	0.71-2.03
Hypospadias	6	1.01	0.37-2.19
Cystic kidneys	4	5.41	1.47-13.8#
Poly/syndactyly	7	1.69	0.68-3.48#
Hip (sub)luxation, unstable hip	12	0.85	0.48-1.51

#observed over expected number with exact Poisson 95% confidence interval.

There was no excess of orofacial clefts and none of the mothers of the three infants with clefts had used ophthalmologicals containing glucocorticoids.

There are thus two conditions which show risk increases which are formally statistically significant: eye malformations and cystic kidneys. Three of the infants with cystic kidney had been exposed to cromoglicid acid and the fourth for fusidic acid. Two of the infants had infantile polycystic kidneys which are usually genetic, the third a cystic dysplasia and the fourth cystic kidney associated with hydronephrosis. This association is probably random in spite of formal statistical significance.

Table 61.9. Congenital eye malformations observed after maternal use of ophthalmological

Malformation	Ophthalmological	Other drugs
Aniridia + glaucoma	cromoglicid acid	cromoglicid acid, nasal preparation
Cataract	timolol combination	
Cataract + glaucoma	timolol	
Glaucoma	dorsolamide	timolol systemically, ginseng
Anterior segment malformation	dorsolamide+brimonidine+ cromoglicic acid	promethazine with caffeine and ephedrine
Lacrimal duct stenosis	cromoglicic acid	terbutaline and budesonide inhalations

Five of the eye malformations were thus serious. It is doubtful if a causal association exists. No details were known on the maternal eye diseases but four of them had used drugs for glaucoma and a genetic link is possible [2].

SUMMARY

Basically, pregnancy and neonatal outcomes were normal after maternal use of ophthalmologicals. An increased risk for severe eye malformations was noted which needs verification.

REFERENCES

[1] Ballard PD, Hearney EF, Smith MB. Comparative teratogenicity of selected glucocorticoids applied ocularly in mice. *Teratology* 1977; 16: 175-180.

[2] Kwon YH, Fingert JH, Kuehn MH, Alward WLM. Primary open-angle glaucoma. *New Engl J Med* 2009; 360: 1113-1124.

Chapter 62

OTOLOGICALS

There are no indications that treatment with otologicals during pregnancy could affect pregnancy or neonatal outcome. The present material is small but shows no certain deviations in outcomes.

Treatment of external otitis with antiinfective agents and/or corticosteroids will not result in absorption large enough to be able to affect embryonic or foetal development. Little is known on the use of such drugs during pregnancy and in the present material only few such exposures were reported.

Table 62.1. Number of women identified using otologicals

Total	194
Reported use in early pregnancy	128
Got prescription later in pregnancy	83
Both early and later use	17

Type of drug	ATC code	Early use	Later use
Antiinfectives	S02A	6	0
Aluminium acetotartrate	S02AA04	1	0
Acetic acid	S02AA10	1	0
Acediasulfon+dihydroxymethylcarbamide	S02AA30	4	0
Corticosteroids	S02B	100	74
Hydrocortisone	S02BA01	86	61
Betamethasone	S02BA07	15	13
Antiinfectives+corticosteroids	S02C	2	0
Flutmetasone+clioquinol	S02CA02	2	0

CHARACTERISTICS OF WOMEN USING OTOLOGICALS IN EARLY PREGNANCY

Based on women reporting the drug in early pregnancy (n= 128). Each variable is adjusted for all other variables and year of delivery. Comparison with all women who gave birth during the period and with information from the first antenatal care (n=967 742). Due to the low number of women using otologicals in early pregnancy, little clear-cut differences from expected values were seen. Only first parity was significantly increased: OR = 1.60 (95% CI 1.10-2.23).

Table 62.2. Concomitant drug use (early pregnancy)

Drug group	Number	OR/RR	95% CI
Multivitamins	18	1.07	0.65-1.73
Folic acid	15	1.25	0.72-2.16
Systemic corticosteroids	5	13.2	4.27-30.7#
Thyroid drugs	3	1.46	0.30-4.26#
Antibiotics	21	6.56	4.08-10.0#
Naiads	3	1.59	0.33-4.64#
Uploads	3	4.23	0.87-12.3#
Minor analgesics	9	1.12	0.51-2.13#
Drugs for rhinitis	5	2.86	0.93-6.67#
Antiasthma tics	12	3.13	1.62-5.47#
Cough medicine	3	5.08	1.05-14.9#
Antihistamines	15	2.07	1.16-3.41#
For NAP	7	1.24	0.50-2.51#
For allergy	9	5.00	2.29-9.49

#observed over expected number with exact Poisson 95% confidence interval.

There is a strong association with the use of systemic corticosteroids, antibiotics, antiasthmatics and cough medicines, and antihistamines used for allergy. Estimates have wide confidence intervals due to the fact that so few exposures were analysed.

Table 62.3. Some maternal diagnoses associated with the use of otologicals

Diagnosis	Drug use in early pregnancy			Drug use later in pregnancy		
	Number	OR/RR	95% CI	Number	OR/RR	95% CI
Preeclampsia	7	1.11	0.44-2.28#	3	0.80	0.16-2.34#
Ante partum bleeding	3	1.89	0.39-5.51#	1	-	-
Intrapartum bleeding	5	1.63	0.53-3.80#	3	1.60	0.33-4.61#
Postpartum bleeding	9	1.22	0.56-2.323	3	0.62	0.13-1.82#
Delivery induction	17	1.19	0.70-2.00	8	0.87	0.38-1.71#
Caesarean section	32	1.51	1.02-2.24	14	0.92	0.52-1.64

#observed over expected number with exact Poisson 95% confidence interval.

The only significantly increased risk was seen for caesarean sections after early (but not later) exposure.

Outcome after Maternal use of Otologicals

Infant Sex

After early exposure there were 69 male and 61 female infants, sex ratio 1.13 (95% CI 0.80-1.61), after later exposure 42 male and 42 female infants, sex ratio = 1.00 (95% CI 0.61-1.54). The normal sex ratio (1.06) thus lies within both confidence intervals.

Multiple Births

After early exposure there were two twin deliveries, after later exposure one.

Table 62.4. Pregnancy duration and infant birth weight at maternal use of otologicals

Variable studied	Drug use in early pregnancy			Drug use later in pregnancy		
	Number	RR	95% CI	Number	RR	95% CI
<37 weeks	12	1.90	0.98-3.32	4	1.02	0.28-2.60
<2500g	6	1.45	0.53-3.16	2	0.77	0.09-2.77
≥4500g	8	1.73	0.75-3.41	3	0.98	0.20-2.87
SGA	3	0.99	0.20-2.90	1	-	-
LGA	6	0.95	0.35-2.07	2	0.44	0.05-1.58

No deviations reach statistical significance but preterm birth after early exposure is close to it.

None of the infants died perinatally.

Table 62.5. Neonatal diagnoses after maternal use of otologicals

Diagnosis	Drug use in early pregnancy			Drug use later in pregnancy		
	Number	RR	95% CI	Number	RR	95% CI
Hypoglycaemia	7	1.53	0.25-1.61	5	1.74	0.56-4.05
Respiratory diagnoses	6	0.97	0.36-2.12	2	0.53	0.06-1.92
Low Apgar score	1	-	-	0	-	-
CNS diagnoses	0	-	-	1	-	-
Jaundice	7	1.22	0.49-2.50	3	0.82	0.17-2.40

No deviations of neonatal diagnoses were thus seen.

There were only three infants with congenital malformation diagnosis after maternal use of otologicals in early pregnancy: None was severe: one infant had tongue tie, one had nevus and the third had a persistent ductus arteriosus and was born after 38 completed weeks.

Summary

As expected no ill effects could be seen after maternal use of otologicals.

INDEX

A

B

C

D

E

F

G

H

I

J

K

N

O

P

Q

R

S

T

U

V

W

Y

Z